OXFORD MEDICAL PUBLICATIONS

Measurement in Neurological Rehabilitation

Measurement in Neurological Rehabilitation

Derick T. Wade
Rivermead Rehabilitation Centre
Oxford

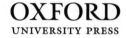
OXFORD
UNIVERSITY PRESS

OXFORD

UNIVERSITY PRESS

Great Clarendon Street, Oxford OX2 6DP

Oxford University Press is a department of the University of Oxford.
It furthers the University's objective of excellence in research, scholarship,
and education by publishing worldwide in

Oxford New York

Athens Auckland Bangkok Bogotá Buenos Aires Calcutta
Cape Town Chennai Dar es Salaam Delhi Florence Hong Kong Istanbul
Karachi Kuala Lumpur Madrid Melbourne Mexico City Mumbai
Nairobi Paris São Paulo Singapore Taipei Tokyo Toronto Warsaw

with associated companies in Berlin Ibadan

Oxford is a registered trade mark of Oxford University Press
in the UK and in certain other countries

Published in the United States
by Oxford University Press Inc., New York

A catalogue record for this book is available from the British Library

Library of Congress Cataloging in Publication Data
Wade, Derick T.
Measurement in neurological rehabilitation / Derick T. Wade.
(Oxford medical publications)
Includes bibliographical references and index.
1. Neuropsychological tests. 2. Brain—Diseases—Patients—
Rehabilitation—Evaluation. 3. Brain damage—Patients
—Rehabilitation—Evaluation. 4. Mentally handicapped—
Rehabilitation—Evaluation. I. Title. II. Series.
[DNLM: 1. Biometry. 2. Disability Evaluation. 3. Nervous System
Diseases—rehabilitation. 4. Neuropsychological Tests. WL 100
W119m]
RC386.6N48W33 1992 91-24268
√ISBN 0 19 261954 3 (Pbk)

Printed in Great Britain
on acid-free paper by
Biddles Ltd., Guildford and King's Lynn

To Liz, Rachel, Rhiannon, and Nathaniel

Preface

Neurological rehabilitation has made little progress over the last few decades, and one reason may be the complete lack of agreed methods of measurement. Improved information is necessary for progress, and usually leads to progress. One way to improve information is to make systematic, detailed observations using well-tested measures. The main aim of this book is to help progress in neurological rehabilitation through aiding anyone looking for a measure relevant to neurological disability, whether for routine clinical use, research, audit, or for any other reason.

The book has several objectives:

(1) to put forward a framework for the management of disabling diseases;

(2) to discuss the principles of selecting and using clinical measures;

(3) to discuss some available assessments;

(4) to act as a reference guide to many commonly used assessments; and

(5) to give specific advice on the choice and use of measures.

A theoretical framework or model of rehabilitation is essential when discussing assessment. Although this is definitely not a textbook of rehabilitation, it is vital that readers have a clear idea of the processes involved when managing neurological disability. The World Health Organization's model of illness is described, emphasizing the importance of the concepts of pathology, impairment, disability, and handicap. Chapter 1 develops this framework in some detail, demonstrating its utility in clinical practice and a classification appropriate for neurological disability is developed in Chapter 3.

The terms measurement and assessment have slightly different meanings. Assessment carries with it an implication that data is interpreted, whereas measurement simply refers to the determination of the extent, quantity, or dimensions of some phenomenon. However, in practice it is difficult to draw any firm distinction between the two, and they will be treated as similar in this book. This is discussed in more detail in Chapter 2.

Measures are vital to everyone involved in the management of patients with neurological disability. Unfortunately most assessments used are particular to the individual department or hospital. Many people still have little idea how to evaluate and choose a measure for their purpose. Therefore the fourth chapter discusses general issues about measurement such as validity, reliability, and, much more importantly, how to choose an appropriate measure.

The second section of the book contains reviews of the practical aspects of assessment in different circumstances and at different levels. In the chapters covering, for example, motor loss, disability, communication, and mobility, some of the available measures are discussed in detail and specific recommendations are given.

The third section only has two chapters. The first considers measurement in relation to some common specific diseases such as stroke and Parkinson's disease. It concludes that disease-specific measures may be useful in terms of prognosis because they concentrate upon impairment. The second chapter gives some final recommendations on the selection and use of measures. This chapter draws particularly upon my own experience in running an in-patient intensive rehabilitation centre and in running a service which aims to support younger severely disabled people in the community. My recommendations should be interpreted with caution.

The fourth and last section contains full details of many measures. One difficulty facing anyone reading research articles is to discover anything about the outcome measure used. Often the original scale was published in some journal or book which is not readily available. Furthermore, there is rarely any review of the scale's characteristics. Hopefully this section of the book will overcome this problem. The measures have been separated into groups in different chapters, but some measures could have been placed in several chapters—it was not possible to devise a perfect way to group the measures.

In order to avoid cluttering the text with too many repeated references and tables, all measures, scales, etc. are only shown once—in the fourth section. Furthermore the reader will need to use the index to locate any measure mentioned in the text; this policy has been chosen to avoid repeated reference to the relevant page.

Throughout the book the emphasis is upon published, clinically relevant measures which can be used by anyone, with the minimum of difficulty. Obviously there is a huge range of measures in use, many unique to one person or place, and many specific to some particular purpose. In general the aim has been to restrict the book to measures which

(1) have been published openly;

(2) have been used in neurological conditions;

(3) are not dependent upon too much (expensive) equipment;

(4) are likely to be useful clinically; and

(5) can be used without too much specialist training.

Another difficulty facing anyone setting out to choose a measure is to discover what measures already exist. Consequently new measures are constantly being devised, often when a very suitable measure is already available. I hope that this compilation of available measures will reduce the proliferation of new measures.

The book is subject to some limitations. Although I intended to include as many measures as possible, it was obviously vital to undertake some selection. Most of the measures included have been used in neurological research or clinical practice. However, a few measures have been included because it seems that they could be useful. A few others are included to demonstrate measures which should be avoided. In addition, measures relating to quality of life and Quality Adjusted Life Years (QALYs) are included because they may influence clinical practice in future.

Selecting the measures to be included was difficult, and many have been excluded. Firstly there are undoubtedly many measures which I am not yet aware of, but I hope to have considered most of the better known ones. Secondly, some measures are only to be used by fully trained professionals, neuropsychological tests being the most obvious example. Next, some assessments are so long that it was not feasible to include them. Other assessments are subject to tight copyright or are only available from the originating organization. This possessive attitude is to be regretted, because it makes it difficult for most readers to evaluate the assessment.

A further limitation is the extent to which each measure is evaluated critically. Ideally any measure should be researched in great detail before use. Unfortunately this takes time and great effort, and it was not practical to undertake such research. Moreover the book would have become enormmous. Therefore an entry to the relevant literature is given wherever possible, but only a few measures are evaluated in any detail.

The book is undoubtedly inconsistent in the amount of attention given to different topics and measures. Throughout, I have tried to steer a course between excessive referencing and academic purity, and simplistic dogmatic statements. I hope that it is clinically useful but sufficiently well referenced to encourage readers to be critical of measures.

Lastly, the reader should be aware that this book has been written by one person, a neurologist whose main specific interests have been in stroke and head injury, in epidemiology, in clinical trials, and in measurement. This may account for some biases and omissions. Any comments, particularly about measures I have missed, will be most welcome so that a second edition might be more useful to you, the reader.

Oxford   D. T. W.
September 1991

Acknowledgements

I have been interested in measurement for many years, and have tended to collect assessment forms wherever I have been. My first acknowledgement must be to the very many people who have helped by telling me about measures they have worked with.

Finding information about some measures requires considerable detective work, and my second acknowledgement is to the many librarians who have, wittingly or unwittingly, helped.

Naming specific institutions is less easy because I do not wish to offend those not mentioned—so I must ask them to accept my apologies. I owe the greatest debt to all my colleagues here in Oxford at Rivermead Rehabilitation Centre and Ritchie Russell House and in Bristol at the Frenchay Stroke Unit; they have provided vital stimulation, encouragement, and information. I must also thank all members of the British Stroke Research Group and the Society for Research in Rehabilitation for their help.

However, my chief thanks must go to one individual: Richard Langton Hewer initiated my interest in research, and nurtured it over the first few difficult years. He continues to provide invaluable advice and criticism, and stimulated me to write this book.

Lastly I acknowledge the hard work undertaken by all those whose measures are discussed here. I hope I have represented your work fairly, and that any criticism is reasonable. I know how hard it is to develop and evaluate a measure.

Contents

xiv Contents

Section 1

Background to the choice and use of measures

Any tool can be used even with limited or no understanding of its development, construction, or working principles. Indeed, many of us use computers and other modern electronic tools in just this way. However, even a slight appreciation of how something works will often enable us to avoid making mistakes in its use and will enhance its value. This is particularly true of the measurement tools described in this book. This section comprises four chapters which give some background information on measures.

The first requirement is to have a framework within which to work. Chapter 1 outlines the World Health Organization's (WHO) system for classifying the consequences of disease, the so-called Pathology, Impairment, Disability, and Handicap model. The chapter explains these terms, and shows how they can be useful in clinical practice, while also outlining their limitations.

The next step is simply to consider why you want to measure at all, as the reason for measuring primarily determines the choice of measure. The second chapter therefore discusses what a measure is, what it can achieve and some general principles of test construction. For detailed instructions on developing new tests, a specialist text should be consulted.

One property of measures is that they isolate one phenomenon and quantify it. A major problem within neurological rehabilitation is the difficulty of defining agreed boundaries between different activities or abilities. For example, is cooking an Activity of Daily Living (ADL) (together with dressing), an Instrumental ADL (together with housework), or should it be considered in isolation? Chapter 3 addresses the issue of classification, and puts forward a solution.

The last chapter of this section looks again at the properties of a given measure, and outlines guidance on the choice of a measure, discussing such features as validity and reliability.

1 Pathology, impairment, disability, handicap: a useful model

Summary

1. The lack of an adequate, comprehensive model of illness has hindered the development of rehabilitation.
2. In the World Health Organization's (WHO) model, any illness can be considered at four levels: pathology, impairment, disability, and handicap.
3. Pathology refers to the damage or abnormal processes occurring within an organ or organ system inside the body.
4. Impairments are the direct neurophysiological consequences of the underlying pathology (symptoms and signs).
5. Disability refers to the functional (behavioural) consequences of any pathology and/or impairments.
6. Handicap is the social and societal consequence of the disease, and refers specifically to the personally relevant consequences.
7. This model leads to many useful insights into the management of any disease with long-lasting effects. For example, the focus of interest changes with time from the pathology to the disability, and from the patient to his environment.
8. Within this model, rehabilitation is an educational, problem-solving process focused on disability but aimed at reducing handicap. The major processes involved are assessment, planning, intervention, and evaluation.
9. There are some limitations to this model, which covers a spectrum without definite boundaries.

Introduction

Traditional medical neurology advanced quickly because a systematic approach was developed early, making it a scientifically-based discipline. The standard neurological examination is now so well established that most hospital departments have printed examination forms which vary little throughout the world.

In stark contrast, when disability is discussed, there is still virtually no common language. Each therapy department and hospital will use its own set of assessments, the only general exception being neuro-psychologists who tend to use the same measures, particularly of IQ.

One problem is the lack of an agreed framework or model. For example, a recent paper (Stein *et al.* 1987) discussing the measurement of severity of illness, put forward the idea that chronic illness could be assessed at four levels: biological, physiological, functional, and burden of illness. Yet the model discussed here was developed precisely for chronic illness many years earlier, a fact that does not seem to be generally known. Even the word 'rehabilitation' has no agreed meaning. Therefore the first task must be to identify a logical and comprehensive system for use in rehabilitation.

The World Health Organization Model

The model to be described has been developed over many years (see Duckworth 1984; Granger 1984). It was published by the World Health Organization (WHO) in 1980 as the basis of a more detailed system for the classification of the consequences of any disease (WHO 1980).

The classification system, known as the International Classification of Impairments, Disabilities, and Handicaps (ICIDH), is too detailed for routine use, and seems biased towards rheumatological disease. However, it forms an extremely good framework for discussing and understanding the management of neurological disability.

The most important concept the model introduces is that any illness can be considered at four levels: pathology, impairment, disability, and handicap. In practice, these levels form a continuum, with many grey areas in between. It is also difficult to define handicap. Although it is easy to get bogged down in sterile semantic arguments, the underlying idea is extremely useful and so the model will be described. Its usefulness will also be illustrated here, which should become increasingly obvious as the book progresses.

The term 'illness' is generally used to refer to all the consequences of any disease and also to a socially recognized behaviour or role. The term 'disease' is usually associated with diagnosis or pathology.

Pathology

This refers to the damage or abnormal processes occurring within an organ or organ system inside the body. Synonymous terms are 'disease' and 'target disorder'. When a diagnosis of stroke or multiple sclerosis is made, the pathology assumed to underlie the clinical syndrome (collection of symptoms and signs) is being referred to.

Pathology is the traditional focus of medical care. Doctors concentrate upon diagnosing the disease, and then upon curing or reducing it if possible. Hospitals are increasingly concerned simply with identifying and treating pathology, and their caring role seems to be diminishing. Pathology is the focus of the International Classification of Diseases (ICD).

Obviously there can be further subdivisions within the level of pathology. For example, one can identify the aetiology, biochemistry, anatomy, or genetics of the disorder. However, the crucial feature is that pathology is restricted to a part of the whole body, usually an organ or organ system.

A pathological diagnosis is vital in rehabilitation for at least two reasons:

- The most effective management of any illness is to stop or reverse pathology, if possible. Therefore, unless there is a firm pathological diagnosis, it is likely that effective and specific treatment will be denied some patients.
- The prognosis and natural history of an illness is determined largely by the underlying pathology. Because the nature and direction of any rehabilitative effort depends critically upon the expected future, management will often be sub-optimal if there is no firm pathological diagnosis.

Measurement at the level of pathology will usually involve invasive testing, such as taking blood or undertaking a biopsy and the use of technological (laboratory) equipment, such as X-rays. Most measurement is for diagnostic reasons but measurement itself is also possible, such as the grading of tumours or of the severity of metabolic disturbance in diabetes.

Impairment

Impairments are the direct neurophysiological consequences of the underlying pathology. They are associated with 'symptoms and signs'. Normal clinical (medical) practice concentrates upon using impairments to deduce the likely underlying pathology. Examples of common neurological impairments are weakness in, or loss of a limb, pain, double vision, ataxia, and reduction in movement at a joint.

The ICIDH definition of impairment is '. . . any loss or abnormality of psychological, physiological, or anatomical structure or function'. And the ICIDH also notes that 'Impairment represents exteriorisation of a pathological state, . . .'. In other words, it is the immediate consequence of pathology as perceived by the individual. Impairments affect actions which in themselves have no meaning.

It is important to remember that not all pathology causes impairment. For example, it is well known that corpses have been found at post-mortem to have widespread plaques of multiple sclerosis with no recorded appropriate history or findings. Similarly, cerebral infarction (stroke) may occur silently (Roberts et al. 1988; Kase et al. 1989).

Equally important, not all impairments arise from demonstrable pathology; but one must realize that patients can present with apparently non-organic impairments (i.e. 'hysterical symptoms') and only months or years later develop evidence of appropriate pathology. There are obviously unknown, intervening influences (level of anxiety, or other psychological mechanisms) which determine the nature of the link between pathology and impairment.

The exact status of some medical diagnoses is difficult to define.

- Is idiopathic epilepsy a pathology or an impairment with no known pathology?
- Is schizophrenia an impairment?
- Is anxiety an impairment or a syndrome at the level of impairment?

As the above conditions are disease diagnoses, and as it is assumed that there are significant underlying pathological processes (probably bio-chemical and so far undetected), it is probably best to classify them as pathologies.

Disability

Most (but not all) impairments will, to some extent, disturb aspects of a patient's behaviour or normal function—otherwise the patient would probably not have consulted a doctor. This functional loss, which manifests itself at the level of the person's interaction with the immediate environment, is termed 'disability'. Examples include slow walking, needing help to dress, and no longer being able to cook a simple meal.

The ICIDH definition of disability is '. . . any restriction or lack (resulting from an impairment) of ability to perform an activity within the range considered normal for a human being.' The ICIDH also notes that 'Disability represents objectification of an impairment, and as such represents disturbances at the level of the person'. In other words, disability is the personal nuisance caused by the pathology: it refers to the effect pathology or impairment has upon actions which have some meaning to the person. It is essentially the external, behavioural consequence of the disease.

As with the link between pathology and impairment, there are many intervening variables which may affect the nature and severity of the disability seen with particular impairments. Two important influences are the local environment and again, psychological influences; there are many more, unidentified influences. A recent study in multiple sclerosis (MS) has illustrated how little relation there is between changes in pathology, as detected on magnetic resonance imaging, and observed changes in disability (Thompson *et al.* 1990).

Handicap

It is often handicap which, from the patient's viewpoint, determines the real severity of any illness. Handicap refers to the social and societal consequence of a pathology, which arises at the level of the patient's own social roles and activities. The most important distinguishing characteristic of handicap is that normality is judged with reference to the patient's own immediate social context, whereas normality for disability, impairment, and pathology is generally judged with reference to the population at large. Examples of handicap include the loss of a job, or marital breakdown, arising as a consequence of the disease.

The ICIDH definition for handicap is '. . . a disadvantage for a given individual, resulting from an impairment or a disability that limits or prevents the fulfilment of a role that is normal (depending on age, sex, and social and cultural factors) for that individual.' The ICIDH also notes that 'Handicap represents socialisation of an impairment or disability, and as such it reflects the consequences for the individual—cultural, social, economic, and environmental—that stem from the presence of impairment and disability'. In other words, handicap is the freedom the patient has lost due to the pathology. (The difficulty in defining handicap is explored further in Chapter 10.)

It is important to realize that handicap can arise directly from an impairment or even from a pathology without impairment, as well as from a disability. For example, a right hemianopia may cause no disability, indeed the patient may not notice it at all, but once detected by a doctor it might lead to disqualification from driving, and thus enormous handicap. Another example is a positive test for HIV. Once known, this pathological finding can severely restrict a person's life-style—loss of job, inability to obtain life insurance, social isolation, etc., can all follow without any intervening impairment or disability.

In the case of handicap, the link with disability can be very slight. Environmental factors such as social expectations and prejudices, the legal framework, family support, the physical environment, and financial support, all have a major effect upon the final handicap.

It is also important to recognize that within the model, handicap and indeed disability and impairment are considered to be a reduction of some pre-existing state that has occurred as a result of the underlying pathology. Particularly in the case of handicap, poor housing or unemployment are not handicaps *per se*; it is the loss of a job, or the deterioration in housing caused by a disease which constitutes the handicap.

Practical consequences arising from this model

Several useful ideas arise from this model:

- As time passes, the focus of attention should pass from pathology to handicap.
- As one progresses from pathology to handicap, the focus of attention should pass from the patient to the environment.
- Treatment should be aimed as close to pathology as possible.
- Assessments (measures) should only contain items relating to a single level.
- As the patient's condition changes from impairment to handicap, the losses become increasingly personal and meaningful.
- The reference frame for judging normality changes.
- Analysis of difficult problems.

Time

When a patient is first seen, whether as an emergency with an acute illness or electively with a longer-standing problem, the doctor concentrates upon pathology. This is obviously necessary and correct, for if pathology can be stopped or reversed, a cure is effected. Even in a chronic illness, new pathology can arise and each new impairment needs to be diagnosed, even though the cause may be obvious in many cases. However, even in the early stages of an illness, and certainly later on, the patient will also be concerned about disability; and later still about handicap.

Therefore, the focus of interest changes with time. Once a pathological diagnosis has been reached, the doctor and the medical system should move on to diagnose and treat the disability in an attempt to reduce handicap. In practice, this means spending more time asking patients in follow-up clinic about their disabilities, not their symptoms, and assessing their abilities, not examining for signs.

Unfortunately most medical institutions, particularly hospitals, are set up to manage acute illnesses which are somehow assumed to be self-limiting, to occur in a social vacuum, and to leave no significant disability. This is rarely true. Yet, for example, in countries where Diagnostic Related Groups (DRGs) are used to determine payment, little or no account is taken of social factors despite the demonstrable importance of such factors when considering hospital use (Wade and Langton Hewer 1985*a*; Epstein *et al.* 1988).

From time to time, attention may need to return to pathology; for example, when a patient with multiple sclerosis develops epilepsy or starts to experience other new symptoms—hence the need for medical neurological input in rehabilitation.

Patient and the environment

As the focus of attention passes with time from pathology and impairment to disability and handicap, so the important intervening variables also change, specifically towards environmental factors. Influences on the links between pathology and impairment, and between impairment and disability, are largely related to the patient. For example, unknown factors determine when a brain tumour first causes symptoms or whether a cerebral infarct manifests as a stroke. Also, personal (for example, psychological) factors, such as anxiety, determine in part how much disability arises from a given impairment.

The environment has a major effect on handicap. For instance, the legal environment determines the degree of handicap arising from the impairments of epilepsy and hemianopia, both of which will prevent driving, yet cause minimal (if any) disability—non-drivers might not suffer any handicap. The pathology of HIV infection may cause severe handicap even if asymptomatic (i.e. not causing any impairment or disability) because the patient might not be able to acquire a job or a mortgage. On the other hand, some patients with severe disability may still lead successful lives—Professor Stephen Hawking FRS is a well-known example. Movements such as the Independent Living movement are attempting to reduce handicap through altering a wide range of physical, social, legal, and financial environmental influences.

Even at the level of disability, environmental factors can be important: the provision of a walking aid, stair rails, or foot-drop splints can all help mobility; the type of clothes worn or the type of food eaten may affect dressing and feeding disabilities; the invention of microwave cookers has alleviated cooking disability.

Level of intervention

It is almost always more effective to intervene as close as possible to the pathology. Removal of a meningioma causing gait problems and foot drop is far more effective than physiotherapy or a splint. In Parkinson's disease L-dopa (given to reduce impairments such as bradykinesia) is the most effective treatment. Rehabilitation services that do not include a neurologist (or other doctor) risk overlooking treatable pathology, so risking possible mismanagement of some patients.

Measurement

As this book demonstrates, there are many assessments available for use in neurological diseases but unfortunately many of these are ill-constructed. The use of the ICIDH model allows one to evaluate measures and to develop better ones.

The first questions to ask when evaluating any measure are:

• what level is it measuring (impairment, disability, handicap)?
• do all component items relate to that level?

The Kurtzke Scale for MS (Kurtzke 1955 and 1983) and the Hoehn and Yahr Scale for Parkinson's disease (Hoehn and Yahr 1967) are examples of widely-used scales which are basically flawed because they include a mixture of impairments and disabilities (Willoughby and Paty 1988; Kurtzke 1989). There are a great many other measures which fall at this first hurdle.

In general, disease-specific measures will concentrate upon impairment because it is the impairments (symptoms and signs) which allow one to deduce the underlying pathology. However, at the level of disability, the specific influence of the underlying pathology has much less effect and it is usually more appropriate to use nonspecific measures. (This is discussed in more detail in Chapter 11.)

Personal meaning

As one moves from impairment to handicap, the losses have increasingly more personal meaning to the patient. For example, when testing strength to determine weakness, the action of flexing an elbow has no intrinsic purpose other than following the instruction given. At the level of disability the underlying constructs have meaning. For example, dressing, walking, and communicating are all actions undertaken to achieve an abstract result: the state of being dressed, going to a different place, expressing an idea to someone else. The subject matter of handicap in such areas as paid employment or social integration is yet more abstract.

Normality

The reference frame for judging normality changes as the patient progresses towards handicap. When considering pathology, impairment, and disability, patients are generally judged with reference to the rest of humanity, with increasing allowance for age, sex, etc. But handicap can only be measured in relation to the individual's own milieu: his or her family role, neighbourhood, friends' expectations, etc.. Indeed, it is this characteristic of handicap which makes actual measurement very difficult. Handicap is probably synonymous with 'quality of life', and the difficulties in measuring it have been acknowledged (for example, Mor and Guadagnoli 1988).

Analysing difficult problems

When faced with a difficult clinical, managerial, research, or political problem, the ICIDH model can be used to clarify matters. For example, at present in the UK people aged 65 or under can apply for a mobility allowance if they are 'unable or virtually unable to walk'. Apart from the imprecision of this phrase (Hunter 1986), there is much scope for disagreement about the eligibility of patients who, though able to walk, might be amnesic, blind and/or deaf, subnormal, etc., and will need someone to supervise or guide them. In the UK, this has led to considerable acrimonious debate, including a legal challenge.

Using the ICIDH model will help to understand why the disagreement arises. The allowance is aimed at people with mobility *disability*, whereas the patients who are blind and/or deaf etc., have mobility *handicap*. The analysis obviously does not resolve the problem, but should allow both sides to discuss their disagreement (or at least help others to understand it).

Rehabilitation: what is it?

There are many definitions of rehabilitation. Here is one based upon the ICIDH model:

Rehabilitation is a problem-solving and educational process aimed at reducing the disability and handicap experienced by someone as a result of a disease, always within the limitations imposed both by available resources and by the underlying disease.

Put another way, it is acting upon pathology, impairment, or disability, or upon the intervening variables in order to reduce handicap. In essence it is the management of change.

The word 'rehabilitation' has, unfortunately, gained many meanings and connotations. Some people restrict its use to patients suffering from conditions where improvement is expected. Others restrict it still further to mean returning to work. For some people rehabilitation is synonymous with 'therapy' (as given by a therapist). It is also used with reference to the reforming of criminals.

The phrase, 'management of (neurological) disability' is perhaps a much better description of rehabilitation. Although the final goal is still to minimize handicap, it is probably easiest and most effective to concentrate upon disability.

In managing a patient with (neurological) disability, the following stages or processes are important:

- assessment: identification and measurement of problems
- planning: analysing the problem(s) and setting goals
- treatment: intervention to reduce disability and handicap
- care: intervention to alleviate consequences of disability
- evaluation: checking on the effectiveness of any intervention

Assessment in rehabilitation refers to the acquisition of information needed to come to some conclusion, whether that is a diagnosis, a prognosis, or a decision on intervention. In other words, assessments are tools and processes to be used, not rituals to be completed. Unfortunately, like rehabilitation, the word 'assessment' has also acquired many meanings. Indeed, some people act as if assessment and rehabilitation were synonymous.

Planning is extremely important, but is often overlooked. Effective planning (goal setting) depends upon:

- an accurate appreciation of all the current problems
- a thorough knowledge of the prognosis (natural history)
- assessing the potential for effecting any change
- knowing how to realize any intervention

Most importantly, however, planning depends upon a full and open agreement between all the parties concerned (especially the patient and his family, but also occasionally lawyers, insurance companies, etc.), as to what the goals are.

Interventions can be active in effecting change by either reducing handicap, or slowing an inevitable deterioration, or they can be inactive by supporting a static situation. The distinction between 'treatment' and 'care' is obviously artificial, but this can sometimes be helpful when facing a difficult problem.

Evaluation is, in essence, a reassessment. The process can be iterative, but it is usually important to consider discharging the patient for various reasons.

- If there is a large risk of fostering an over-dependent attitude, so reinforcing illness behaviour.
- If resources are too limited to allow constant monitoring of a stable situation.
- If the patient has an unalterable disability constant assessment can give them unrealistic and false expectations.

Measures are important at most stages of this cycle. Initial assessment depends upon adequate information both delineating the problems, their severity, and their causes. Planning interventions and evaluating results also depend upon measures.

Community rehabilitation

The purpose of rehabilitation is, or should be, to return a patient to, or maintain a person in, his own chosen environment, usually his own home. Consequently, the ideal is for all rehabilitation interventions to be carried out at home. There are several drawbacks in this. It is difficult to develop and maintain expertise without concentrating patients with professionals. Some patients are too disabled to be at home in the early stages of their treatment. Sometimes specific equipment may be needed. However, the treatments given are often more effective and it is arguably more efficient to give treatment at home. It is important to have measures available which can be used within the community, especially when most patients with disability spend most of their time there, which is, after all, the goal of all rehabilitation.

Difficulties with the ICIDH model

The ICIDH model has its limitations, and these are outlined below.

The four levels are part of a spectrum with no clear-cut boundaries. Even within pathology there is a range from the underlying aetiology, and the biochemical (molecular) abnormalities through microscopic changes and changes in cell behaviour on to gross macroscopic changes.

Distinguishing between impairment and disability can be particularly difficult. For example, in motor neuron disease the following spectrum could be found:

- Death of motor neurons.
- Muscle fibre wasting.
- Weakness and wasting of muscles.
- Reduced movement at joints.
- Loss of use of specific limbs (for example, inability to write).
- Difficulty in dressing and problems with cooking.
- Inability to use public transport, to reach work, or to do such work as assembling cars.
- Loss of job and income.

Where are the boundaries? However, provided one does not waste time in semantic arguments, the problem of defining boundaries does not matter too much. Also, in relation to this problem, it is very difficult to devise an operational definition of handicap to allow its measurement. (This is discussed in Chapter 10.)

In addition, some disease diagnoses do not actually have any known pathology. Most psychiatric diagnoses are labels attached to impairment syndromes. The underlying pathology (if any) is not known. Thus, 'depression' is not really a pathology. There are also few measures of disability in psychiatric illness.

Epilepsy is another illness which is difficult to fit within the ICIDH model. It is presumably an intermittent impairment of awareness. Other intermittent diseases such as recurrent mania are not easily fitted into the system.

Finally, it is necessary to add the dimension of time to any description of a patient's illness. The WHO scheme simply records a static position, so the study of a patient's history is vital when undertaking rehabilitation because it may determine, for example, the patient's expectations.

Despite these difficulties, the WHO scheme is still the best framework available for understanding rehabilitation.

Conclusions

The ICIDH model described in this chapter is powerful, and emphasizes the importance of having a 'holistic' approach to patient care. It also emphasizes the importance of a multidisciplinary approach because each profession brings its own range of expertise. In terms of measurement, it demonstrates that, if at all possible, measures should be restricted to one level. It is important to use the model flexibly, and not to be bound rigidly by it—it is simply another tool.

2 Measurement and assessment: what and why?

Summary

1. Measurement is simply the quantification of an observation against a standard, whereas assessment also includes the process of interpreting measurement.
2. When choosing a measure, the most important consideration is why the measure is being used.
3. The commonest major reasons for undertaking measurement are to establish diagnosis, prognosis, severity, and outcome.
4. Any test has false positives and false negatives, and it is important to know these specifically for the population being tested. Tests cannot necessarily be transferred between different settings.
5. The results of a measure can be simply a categorization, or can give an ordinal, an interval, or a ratio scale and this will determine the statistical tests which can be used.
6. Many measures in rehabilitation are simply an aggregation of individual pass–fail items which sometimes form a hierarchy.

Introduction

To measure is to quantify and to determine the extent of something by comparison with a standard unit. In practice, the word 'measurement' refers both to the process of discovering the extent of the phenomenon and to the result obtained. In the context of neurological rehabilitation, measurement in the pure scientific sense is rarely possible—there are few aspects which can be quantified easily, and standard units are generally absent.

Assessment is the second word in frequent use in neurological rehabilitation. Originally the word 'assessment' referred to the process of calculating the amount of tax owed to the state. However, 'assessment' has now acquired a new usage in rehabilitation. It refers to the process of evaluating a patient's problems, including recognition, and measurement of the problems and determining their cause and their extent. In other words, assessment of disability uses similar processes to those used when determining the medical (pathological) diagnosis of a patient's symptoms and signs (impairments).

The following could form strict definitions and in principle these should be adhered to:

- measurement—the use of a standard to quantify an observation; and
- assessment—the process of determining the meaning of measurement(s).

In practice, assessment and measurement are closely intertwined, and often the words are interchanged (even if they should not be). Some measures are used to determine whether or not a problem (for example, unilateral neglect) is present, and most so-called assessments can be used to determine the extent of a problem. This chapter, and indeed this book, discusses both assessment and measurement.

Many, but not all, measures discussed in this book generate numbers, but often these numbers do not carry the significance of ordinary numbers. Therefore this chapter also discusses briefly the differences between nominal, ordinal, interval, and ratio scales, primarily to illustrate what conclusions can correctly be drawn from any results.

However, the most important consideration when choosing any measure is to know why the information is being sought. For example, a measure suitable for planning the treatment of a walking disability after stroke is unlikely to be useful in auditing the effectiveness of a rehabilitation programme. Chapter 2 therefore starts with a discussion of the reasons for using measures.

Reasons for assessing

Patients may be assessed for many reasons (see Table 2.1), and often measures are used (consciously or unconsciously) for several reasons at the same time. The various reasons are discussed below.

Diagnosis

Tests may be used to determine whether or not some particular feature is present. For example, the Star-cancellation Test may be used to detect unilateral visual neglect (Halligan *et al*. 1989), just as a fasting blood glucose may be used to determine whether a patient has diabetes.

When tests are used diagnostically, it is important to remember that the connection between the finding on the test and the presence (or absence) of the underlying phenomenon is not absolute.

First, most biological phenomena are not dichotomous but form part of a spectrum. For example, after stroke there may be any degree of motor loss, from none to complete paralysis. Memory disturbance may, at one end of the spectrum, simply refer to the patient just forgetting slightly more facts than was originally known, to complete and permanent amnesia at the other end. Yet, in practice, tests are often used to categorize patients into two (or more) groups. Therefore, the results of categorization can exaggerate small differences at the border, and minimize large differences elsewhere.

Table 2.1 Some reasons for using measures

Diagnostic/prognostic
- Is a specific item of interest present or absent?
- Is a specific pathology likely?
- What are the underlying impairments?
- What disabilities are present?
- What change (or outcome) can be expected?
- Is a specific treatment indicated?

Measurement/quantification
- How severe is the problem?
- How much change has occurred?

Process
- What is being done to/with the patient(s)?
- What are therapists/carers doing?

Other
Legal/administrative
- to determine eligibility for/access to allowances
- to determine payment (of therapist, or patient)

Planning and running services
- population screening (e.g. in prevalence survey)
- to set priorities in treatment (between patients)
- audit of a service (perhaps to obtain payment)
- measuring work-load
Research into a specific disability or other problem

Second, when a test is used to detect the presence or absence of a phenomenon, it will inevitably fail to detect the item in some patients who have it (i.e. false negatives) and will classify some patients as being positive who are in fact negative (i.e. false positives). This is shown in Table 2.2.

The ability to classify patients correctly can be measured in several ways —specificity, sensitivity, and predictive value—as shown in Table 2.2. These values can be changed by altering the difficulty of the test, for example by choosing a different cut-off score. Indeed, a score should be chosen that gives the best separation in the population being tested.

Another, often overlooked, factor affecting diagnosis is the prior likelihood of the phenomenon's being present. Chest pain on effort in someone aged 20 years probably reflects anxiety; but at 70 years of age, angina is much more likely. A test with good characteristics when applied to one population, such as patients with stroke, may be poor when applied to another, such as patients with motor neuron disease or the general population. One consequence is illustrated in Table 2.2, where it can be seen that even a 'good' test in one circumstance can be valueless in another. Most patients from the general population who test 'positive' will not have the condition.

Third, the patient's performance on a test is usually only representative of a true overall ability in some wider sphere. The closeness of fit between abnormality on the test and the underlying abnormality being sought is

Table 2.2 Sensitivity and specificity of a test

Assume:
- A test for aphasia giving a score between 0 and 20.
- In the general population 98% of the population score 18–20.
- In 'true' aphasia, 95% of patients score 0–17.
- The 'gold standard' is a speech therapist's diagnosis.

1. Apply test to 100 stroke patients, 40 of whom have aphasia.

Speech therapist: Test score:	TRUE APHASIA	TRUE NORMAL	Total
0–17 ('aphasia')	38	1	39
18–20 ('normal')	2	59	61
Total	40	60	100

2. Apply test to 100 patients with MS, 5 of whom have aphasia but 5 more have generalized cognitive deficits affecting performance and 3 major visual problems affecting performance.

Speech therapist: Test score:	TRUE APHASIA	TRUE NORMAL	Total
0–17 ('aphasia')	5	9	14
18–20 ('normal')	0	86	86
Total	5	95	100

3. Apply test to 1000 of the general population, 1 of whom has aphasia.

Speech therapist: Test score:	TRUE APHASIA	TRUE NORMAL	Total
0–17 ('aphasia')	1	20	21
18–20 ('normal')	0	979	979
Total	1	999	1000

Table 2.2 (*cont.*)

Under these three (hopefully realistic) settings, the characteristics of this test are:

	Stroke	MS	Population
Sensitivity (true-positive)	38/40 (95%)	5/5 (100%)	1/1 (100%)
Specificity (true-negative)	59/60 (98%)	86/95 (91%)	979/999 (98%)
Predictive value, positive	38/39 (97%)	5/14 (36%)	1/21 (5%)
Predictive value, negative	59/61 (97%)	86/86 (100%)	979/979 (100%)
False-positives	1/39 (3%)	9/14 (64%)	20/21 (95%)
False-negatives	2/61 (3%)	0/86 (0%)	0/979 (0%)

referred to as its validity. For example, on the Star-cancellation Test, failing to notice and cross out stars on the left is a formal specific example of unilateral neglect, which is then assumed to occur in other settings when undertaking other activities—the extent to which this assumption is true is the extent of the test's validity. It is important to remember that performance on the test does not usually define the abnormality.

It is therefore important to be aware that:

• all tests can have false-positives;
• all tests can have false-negatives;
• the absolute numbers will depend crucially upon the underlying likelihood of the phenomenon's being present in the population being tested; and therefore
• a good screening test in one high-risk population is likely to give many false positives in a second low-risk population.

Prognosis

Measures may be used to determine who is likely to recover well and thus (possibly) who will need help or not need help. In practice such tests are rarely possible—tests may, however, determine which patient is likely to respond to what treatment. Many of the considerations on sensitivity and specificity discussed here can apply equally to tests for prognosis. However, when considering prognosis one specific additional consideration applies.

Items of prognostic value are not necessarily directly or obviously related to the outcome. A good example concerns the presence of urinary incontinence and the outcome after stroke (Barer 1989a): patients who are incontinent of urine are more likely to die, and those who survive are more likely to be left disabled. There is no obvious connection between continence and being left disabled, but none the less it is a better indicator than loss of consciousness (Wade and Langton Hewer 1985*b*) or severity of paralysis, which is more obviously connected to disability.

Prognostic items are usually derived from studies on large groups of patients. Consequently, rare phenomena, which may be important when present in individuals, will not be identified. In addition, most prognostic items are markers of overall severity, and so only one of several items will be identified. For example, after-stroke patients with the following conditions recover less well: severe paralysis, hemianopia, sensory loss, cognitive deficits, etc. All are interrelated, and so only one is needed. Therefore, if one is concerned with prognosis, it is necessary to review published research to determine which measure is most appropriate. It is not always the most obvious.

Measurement

Most measures will be of a phenomenon which occurs in normal people, with the patients being at one extreme of a continuum. As was discussed above, this enables measures to be used to classify patients as being 'abnormal'—a diagnostic use.

However, because measures quantify the extent of a problem, they can also be used to detect change, to quantify input or outcome, and to evaluate the effectiveness of intervention. In this context the measures are used both repeatedly and often by different people. Consequently an important consideration is their reliability—how much is any difference due to a real change, and how much is random or biased error. Another important consideration is sensitivity: can the measures detect the change expected? (These issues are discussed in Chapter 3.)

Process

There is an increasing interest in the study of what happens in rehabilitation. In countries where services are charged for directly in relation to individual patients, there is an obvious need to measure the input of resources, whether these are physical items or take the form of a professional's time. Even publicly-funded rehabilitation services are increasingly required to provide information on the input provided. In practice, the value of collecting this information could be questioned, especially given the resources needed simply to collect the data. There is little evidence that the frequency and/or duration of patient-contact is necessarily related to patient-benefit (Wade *et al.* 1984), although some evidence does suggest that it is (Smith *et al.* 1981).

The usual method is simply to record each time the patient is treated, for how long, and with what aim. The validity and reliability of these observations have never been tested, but in some countries they form the basis of remuneration. Scientific methods have been devised which can assess the behaviour of both patients and professionals (Kennedy *et al.* 1988; Tinson 1989; Lincoln *et al.* 1989). In general these have found depressingly low rates of direct face-to-face treatment.

Other reasons

Measures may be used for a variety of other reasons. For example, they could, and indeed probably should, be used to determine eligibility for allowances. In practice, legislators seem to be unaware of measures, and often use unsatisfactory criteria for determining eligibility allowances. This has been noted in relation to the Mobility Allowance in Britain (Hunter 1986). This allowance is for the disability of being 'unable or virtually unable to walk'; but some people receiving it are fully mobile, and some with severe problems arising from blindness and deafness are excluded. More recently in the UK, people with 'severe mental impairment' are excused from paying the community charge ('poll-tax'), but no specific guide-lines have been given. One patient of the author's had a long, reasoned, logical argument over the telephone with the responsible council officer, and managed to have himself declared as suffering 'severe mental impairment'!

Any measure used to determine access to resources obviously needs to be as reliable and free from bias as possible. Preferably it should allow separation of patients into various categories of severity, with the resources awarded being similarly graded. Concepts such as '80 per cent disabled', which still forms the basis of some UK allowances, are totally unacceptable given the large number of well-studied measures now available.

Population screening (for example, in prevalence surveys) has stimulated the recent development of well-studied measures of disability, such as the Office of Population Censuses and Surveys (OPCS) scales and the Functional Limitation Profile (FLP). There are now several validated questionnaires (see Section 4). The problems of using measures originally devised for use in high-risk populations have already been illustrated (Table 2.2).

Emphasis upon planning services for the community is growing, especially in the UK. Consequently, there will be an increasing demand for measures which can be used to survey both the extent of disability and, more importantly, the need for services. There are two drawbacks with the survey instruments mentioned above. First, they are not comparable to clinical measures in common use (for example, the Barthel ADL Index), which makes it difficult to interpret the findings. Second, they do not establish need.

Population studies require short simple measures which can be used by non-specialists, including patients and their relatives. The measures will generally be non-specific in their focus. It is unwise to use measures specifically designed for a single disease (such as stroke) because they may give invalid results when applied to other diseases.

Another increasingly important use of measures is to audit a service, perhaps to obtain payment and certainly to determine whether it is being effective. Again, this will require short, simple measures which are applicable to the broad generality of patients going through the service.

Many services have more people seeking treatment than they can fit in, so it is usually necessary to grade patients according to priorities for treatment. Measures might help in this.

Lastly, measures are always needed in research. The choice of measures here depends upon the questions being asked and the resources available to the researchers. In general the measure selected would be specific to the subject under research, but sometimes it may be necessary to devise new measures. If this is done, every effort should be made to demonstrate reliability and validity, and to relate the measure to day-to-day clinical practice.

Levels of measures

The data produced by measures can be classified into one of four distinct levels: nominal, ordinal, interval, and ratio. The meaning of these terms are discussed below, with emphasis upon the practical implications. A summary is shown in Table 2.3. Readers should consult specialist texts if more detail is required, as this discussion is only intended to introduce some of the important points.

Nominal measures

Many measures are not really measures in the true sense of the word. Instead they are simply a way of categorizing items. The most obvious example is gender—patients are either male or female. Another one is medical (pathological) diagnosis, where patients usually have a single disease such as stroke, multiple sclerosis (MS), Parkinson's disease, etc.

The most noteworthy feature of a nominal measure is that there is no particular order which can be superimposed on the two or more categories. It is a neutral classification system. Even though numbers are often used, letters or other symbols would be just as satisfactory. The ICIDH model is an example of a classification where the numbers carry no meaning except as a coding system. Nominal measures, even if numerical, cannot be subjected to any numerical analysis in themselves. They simply allow one to form groups, and to count the numbers of subjects in each group.

Table 2.3 Levels of measurement

Level:	Nominal	Ordinal	Interval	Ratio
Features	Categories For classification	Rank order Non-uniform intervals	Uniform interval No zero	Uniform intervals Has zero
Use/meaning of numbers	Code only, no meaning	Order, but not difference	Order and difference, not absolute	Order, difference, absolute value
Group description	Frequencies Proportions Mode	Median Range	Mean (arithmetic) Variance	Mean (geometric) Coefficient of variation
Group comparison	Chi–square Fisher's exact test Odd's ratio Binomial test	Mann-Witney Wilcoxon Kruskal–Wallis Sign test	t-test Analysis of variance	t-test Analysis of variance
Correlation/ reliability	Phi Cramer	Spearman rho Kendall tau	Pearson r	Pearson r
Inter-rater reliability	Kappa	Kappa Kendall coeff. of concordance	Intra-class R	Intra-class R

Derived from LaRocca (1989)

Ordinal measures

As the name suggests, ordinal data has some order, with one score being in some way better or worse than another. And, if there are three or more levels, they can be put into a logical order. Many, if not most, measures used in rehabilitation are ordinal.

There are two types of ordinal measure in common use. The first relates to one very restricted skill, such as walking, and categorizes patients according to their ability at that skill. For example, the Functional Ambulation Categories are based on the amount of personal help needed. Any scale rating a patient as having severe, moderate, mild, or absent 'X' falls into this category.

The other more common scale is that which comprises many items, each of which is scored usually as pass–fail, and the whole score represents the number of items passed (or failed). The Barthel ADL Index is one of many such scales. The validity of using such scales at all is discussed later, but the results do form an ordinal scale.

In practice the important point to remember is that the different scores cannot be compared in any absolute way. A difference of one point between 5 and 6 is not necessarily the same as the difference between 10 and 11. In the same way a score of 5/20 does not represent being twice as bad (or good) as scoring 10/20. In other words, normal arithmetic manœuvres cannot be practised on ordinal results. Ordinal scales can be analysed using non-parametric statistics (Siegel and Castellan 1988). Unfortunately, it is almost impossible not to consider the results as an interval scale (see below) because numbers are commonly used in that way.

Suggestions on the use of ordinal scales in research have been published (MacKenzie and Charlson 1986), and the main recommendations are:

- states must be clearly defined, mutually exclusive, and hierarchical;
- scales must detect improvement and deterioration; and
- patient scores should not cluster at one extreme.

Interval scales

An interval scale is an ordinal scale with an additional feature—the differences between any two scores are identical. This means that parametric statistics such as averages can be used correctly.

There are few true interval scales in use in rehabilitation, because it is difficult to attach suitable weights to each item. However, there are ways of deriving weights, and the methods have been discussed (Froberg and Kane 1989). If different categories can be given appropriate weights, then an interval scale for disability can be derived. For example, the recently devised British Office of Population Censuses and Surveys (OPCS) scales have weights for items relating to one construct, which also allow comparison of different disabilities (Martin et al. 1988). The Sickness Impact Profile (SIP; also Functional Limitations Profile, FLP) has an interval scale.

The usual way of deriving an interval scale is to ask people to judge the relative value of different disabilities. This can be done in monetary terms, with reference to time, or by use of some arbitrary unit; but the ultimate aim is to be able to compare disabilities. For example, if 'Running' is normally worth 100, 'Running with difficulty' might be worth 95, 'Only walking' worth 80, 'Not walking at all' worth 30, and 'Not being able to transfer from bed to chair' worth 5. This method is often used to derive Quality Adjusted Life Years (QALYs), and the validity of different methods has been reviewed recently (Froberg and Kane 1989).

Ratio scales

There are some ratio measures used in rehabilitation. For example, timing of any activity will give a ratio result—how many metres walked in 10 seconds, how many pegs placed in 60 seconds, etc? Measures of strength using dynamometers also give ratio results. More use of ratio scales is possible— stop-watches are cheap and easy to use—and might improve research and clinical practice. It could also be argued that some QALYs' scales are ratio scales, giving death a score of 0, and (usually) full health a score of 1.

Measure construction

The measures used in clinical practice, and discussed in this book, can be constructed in various ways. The simplest measure is to note the presence or absence of some phenomenon or ability. Such 'measures' include 'Can walk/unable to walk', 'Conscious/unconscious', 'Independent in dressing/ needs help dressing', and 'Has neglect/neglect absent'. Apart from the fact that such simple dichotomy scarcely constitutes measurement, it is rare for any phenomenon to be so absolute. None the less, with adequate definitions measures such as these can be useful at times, particularly when designing individual treatments for patients with unusual problems.

Multi-item indices

The next step taken by many people is to amalgamate a multitude of single items to form an index, and the most common indices amount to a 'more-or-less' detailed description of the patient in one or more areas. A score is given for each item, sometimes with intermediate values to represent partial success, and the scores are added to give a total. The Barthel ADL Index is one of many such indices.

There is always a tendency for these indices to grow, as individuals add items they consider important or try to increase sensitivity (for example, Shah *et al.* 1989). For instance, the simple question 'Does dress, or does not dress' first splits to 'Dresses alone, with help, not at all', then to 'Dresses top half/bottom half alone, with help, not at all', and then to a considera-tion of each garment.

Consequently, it is necessary to restrict items included to those that add information. It is often noted that some items are all passed or failed together, and so only one item needs to be included. For example, patients who can spoon soup to their mouths can almost always spoon cereal to their mouths and even soft food, and so only one of these three items is needed. In this way a measure representative of a patient's abilities can be developed.

Finally, items can be arranged into a hierarchy, such that patients passing items at one intermediate level can be assumed to be passing all easier items, and, conversely, patients failing at a level can be assumed to be failing all more difficult items. Such indices are much quicker to use because one can start at a sensible point, and stop once the patient has failed two or three items. The Rivermead ADL Index and the Action Research Arm Test are two such tests.

Unfortunately, there are not many tests of proven hierarchy. Moreover, it is likely that the particular order is often specific to one pathological condition, and may be different if the scale is used with other patients. Indeed the order may reflect particular local environmental factors. For example, in Rivermead in 1978 early mobilization in a wheelchair was encouraged, and hence independent mobility in a wheelchair appeared early (low) in the hierarchy of the original Rivermead ADL Index; but in an institution discouraging early mobility, it appears later (Lincoln and Edmans 1990).

It is easy to criticize any scale which includes two or more components. First, some people find it difficult to accept that there is any logic in adding items, usually comparing it with adding oranges to lemons. However, provided that the items belong to the same construct (and the construct being measured) such as Activities of Daily Living (or fruit) then this is reasonable. Second, as was discussed earlier, there is a problem in attaching weights to the different components. Analysis of ADL scales suggests that this is not necessarily a major problem in practice (Bebbington 1977).

True ratio measures

The last approach is to use some physical measure such as time, force, or volume, and to measure function with this. Obvious examples include walking speed, force of muscle contraction, and number of words said in one breath. In general, timing of activities is grossly under used, in part because it is felt that 'quality' is more important. This does not apply outside rehabilitation, and it is unclear why it should apply within. Moreover, speed probably often relates closely to quality.

Conclusions

There are many reasons for choosing a measure, and the intended use will (or certainly should) determine which measure is chosen. However, some general considerations are important. If a test is being used to detect a phenomenon, it is important to know its sensitivity and specificity in the population being tested. And if a measure is being subjected to detailed, statistical analysis, its mathematical properties are important.

3   Classification of impairment, disability, and handicap

Summary

1. A logical, consistent system of classification would aid the construction and selection of measures. Such a system has not yet been developed.
2. The standard neurological examination is (to some extent) a systematic categorization of impairments, but it concentrates upon motor and sensory phenomena.
3. Impairment measures will often be specific to a particular pathology.
4. Various standardized systems have grouped disabilities into between 6 and 12 categories.
5. An alternative system for classifying disability is based on two axes—distance from the person and object of interaction (animate/inanimate).
6. The six WHO areas of handicap are physical independence, mobility, orientation, social integration, occupation, and economic self-sufficiency. No better categorization is known.

Introduction

The greatest problem facing anyone devising measures and assessments in rehabilitation is to decide upon a logical, coherent, and inclusive framework for classification. This is particularly difficult in neurology because the nervous system has so many functions, whereas most other organs have a much more limited range of functions. The World Health Organization (WHO) has developed a classification (the ICIDH model), but it is not necessarily always appropriate for neurology. In this chapter the problems are discussed, and the solution used in this book is described.

The ideal method of developing a classification would be to start from the framework or model, and to decide on a logically consistent group of mutually exclusive but comprehensive categories. The measures needed could then be developed. This book does not attempt such an ideal solution. Many people have spent much time attempting to devise such a system, and the WHO ICIDH model represents one such attempt. Any system would require the development of whole new series of measures (the ICIDH model does not include measures).

Also in this chapter a system relevant to neurological rehabilitation will be described. The classification used here is to some extent based on currently available measures, although an attempt has been made to fit them into a systematic categorization. It is not intended that this classification will necessarily be appropriate for use with non-neurological diseases.

Impairments

There are many detailed charts available for recording neurological impairments (signs). These are often designed for specific circumstances, such as a muscle or a sensory chart for peripheral nerve lesions. The classification used is primarily anatomical, and this suits their diagnostic purpose—they are usually used to localize pathological processes. The systems are best for localizing lesions in the brain-stem, spinal cord and peripheral nerves.

It is much more difficult to devise a logical classification based upon cerebral anatomy, probably because cerebral processes are in general much less localized. However, much of neurological rehabilitation relates to central damage, including cerebral damage, and it is difficult to give a comprehensive, logically consistent classification which can be applied generally. Table 3.1 represents a classification attempt which probably needs much further development, and which may eventually prove to be of little use.

A second way to approach the measurement of impairments is to start from the pathology, and to construct measures which concentrate upon those impairments that are specific to the disease. This is perhaps best illustrated by the measures of movement disorders such as Parkinson's disease, but underlies many other measures developed for use in research. The advantage of this approach is that the severity of impairment is usually of prognostic importance, and the measure may also help make the pathological diagnosis.

Disability

There are many potential disabilities, and categorization is difficult as there is no generally agreed system. Table 3.2 outlines four of the more widely used indices which cover all aspects of disability. Two features emerge:

- The range of activities and behaviours included within disability indices vary, with differing emphasis upon work and social behaviour.
- The categories are rarely similar even between these four well-developed indices.

Clearly, it is difficult to devise a coherent uniform classification system.

The classification offered in Table 3.3 considers that the abnormal behaviour which arises as a consequence of neurological pathology and

Table 3.1 A classification of neurological impairments

Function Sub-categories	Impairment	Measures
Arousal/awareness		
Consciousness		Glasgow Coma Scale
Limb motor		
Strength	Weakness	Dynamometry
Control	Ataxia, dysarthria	
Involuntary	Tremor, chorea, etc	AIMS
Tone	Spasticity	Ashworth Scale
Range of movement	Contractures	Goniometry
Limb sensory		
Skin (touch, temp)		Clinical
Joints (position)		Clinical
Cranial motor		
Eyes, range	Gaze palsy	
Eyes, control	Nystagmus	
Face		
Speech (talking)	Dysarthria	Clinical
Swallow	Dysphagia	Swallow water
Cranial sensory		
Eyes	Reduced acuity	Visual acuity charts
Eyes	Field loss	Confrontation, perimetry
Ears	Deafness	Clinical, specialist
Nose	Anosmia	Clinical
Integration (cognition)		
Information processing		PASAT
Sensory perception	Neglect, agnosia	BIT,RPAB
Motor planning	Apraxia	
Language	Aphasia	FAST
Pain		
Psychological		
Mood	Anxiety, depression	GHQ
Motivation		

AIMS   = Abnormal Involuntary Movement Scale
BIT   = Behavioural Inattention Test
FAST   = Frenchay Aphasia Screening Test
GHQ   = General Health Questionnaire
PASAT = Paced Auditory Serial Addition Test
RPAB = Rivermead Perceptual Assessment Battery

Table 3.2 Classifications of disability

OPCS categories $n = 12$
Locomotion; reaching and stretching; dexterity; continence; seeing; hearing; communication; behaviour; intellectual functioning; consciousness; eating, drinking, and digestion; and disfigurement.

WHO categories $n = 7$
Behaviour; communication; personal care; locomotion; 'body disposition' (domestic activities and body movements); dexterity; and 'specific situations'.

FLP and SIP categories $n = 12$
Sleep and rest; eating; work; home management; recreation and pastimes; ambulation; mobility; body care and movement; social interaction; alertness behaviour; emotional behaviour; communication.

FIM categories $n = 6$
Self-care; sphincter control; mobility; locomotion; communication; social cognition.

OPCS = Office of Population Censuses and Surveys (Martin *et al.* 1988)
WHO = World Health Organization (WHO 1980)
FLP = Functional Limitation Profile (Patrick and Peach 1989)
SIP = The Sickness Impact Profile (Bergner *et al.* 1981)
FIM = Functional Independence Measure (Granger *et al.* 1986)

impairments can be viewed as occurring in one dimension along two parallel axes. The first axis relates to interactions between the person and the physical, inanimate, environment. The second axis refer to psychological interactions (information transfer) within and outside the patient; in other words to internal mental states and external communication with others. The other dimension, which applies to both axes, is the physical distance from the individual, starting internally or peripersonally. The categories span a wide range of behaviours, some of which could be construed as being within handicap.

The first major area is personal physical disability, which combines mobility (ICIDH 40–47) and personal care (ICIDH 30–39). This combination is necessary to reflect normal clinical practice, because most Activity of Daily Living (ADL) indices (see below) include items on both mobility and personal care. Specific assessment of mobility and manual dexterity (ICIDH 52–54, 62–64) is also useful in practice, because these abilities underlie so many others.

Next come behaviours that are sometimes referred to as Instrumental Activities of Daily Living (IADL), but which the author prefers to term 'Extended ADL' (see Chapter 9). These activities are subdivided into

Table 3.3 Neurological disability—a classification and some measures

A. Physical interactions		Distance
Category	Measures (or comment)	Location
Personal physical behaviour		*Peripersonal*
Overall	Barthel ADL Index	
• personal care		
• mobility	Gait speed, Functional Ambulation Categories	
• dexterity	Nine-hole Peg Test, Frenchay Arm Test	
Domestic behaviour		*Inside home*
• kitchen	Rivermead ADL Test	
• housework	Rivermead ADL Test	
• money affairs		
Outside home behaviour		*Outside home*
Overall	Frenchay Activities Index	
• work	i.e. specific skills	
• home maintenance	e.g. shopping, gardening	
• leisure	i.e. specific activities	
• mobility	e.g. car driving, transport use	

Table 3.3 (*cont.*)

B. Information transfer		
		Distance
Category	Measures (or comment)	Location
Self-awareness		*Intra-personal*
• monitoring behaviour/safety		
• insight/planning/foresight		
• orientation	Hodkinson Mental Test or Short OMC test	
Analysis		*Intra-personal*
• memory/learning	Rivermead Behavioural Memory Test	
• problem solving	Any IQ test	
Communication		*Specific people*
Overall	None available?	
• speaking (dysarthria)		
• expression	Frenchay Aphasia Screening Test	
• comprehension	Frenchay Aphasia Screening Test	
• reading		
• writing		
Social interaction		*Inter-personal*
Overall	frequency	
	content	
• specific	measures poorly developed	

ADL = Activities of Daily Living
OMC = Orientation-memory-concentration

domestic disabilities (ICIDH 50–51) and out-of-house activities. Environmental factors might restrict mobility outside the house, and thus be the main cause of disabilities in this area, whereas difficulties with domestic abilities arise more directly from impairments (both motor and cognitive) and also often determine the need for help.

Definition and classification of cognitive disabilities is difficult. The ICIDH model only recognizes cognitive impairments (ICIDH 10–19, 23, 24), and not disabilities. However, it does recognize language impairment (ICIDH 30–34), speech impairment (ICIDH 35–39) and communicative disability (ICIDH 20–23, 27–29). It would seem easiest to have an overall group of disabilities centred in information handling and transfer, with the 'disabilities' shown in the table. This may represent a non-standard use of terminology, and is itself not entirely consistent. Nevertheless, the author does not know, nor could he devise, a better simple system.

The definition and classification of 'psychiatric' states such as depression, anxiety and motivation is also difficult. The WHO system suggests that these are impairments (ICIDH 25–29), and here they have also been categorized as impairments. However, one could categorize 'psychiatric states' as behavioural disabilities with two major subtypes: intra-personal (subjective; for example, depression, motivation, anxiety, insight) and interpersonal (objective; for example, aggression, disinhibition). The WHO classification also recognizes behavioural disabilities (ICIDH 10–19), but these are not easily used and only personal safety (ICIDH 13; for example, loss of consciousness, altered self-awareness) has been retained.

Sensory and visual disabilities can be important in neurological diseases, for example due to the impairment of nystagmus or optic atrophy in multiple sclerosis or hemianopia after stroke. However, most of these will be included within the classification already outlined.

Handicap

The World Health Organization recognized six areas of handicap:

- orientation
- mobility
- physical dependence
- economic self-sufficiency
- occupation
- social integration

The ICIDH model also gave a scaling system for each, ranging from 0 (least handicap) to 8 (most severe handicap). No other detailed classification of handicap has been proposed.

Conclusions

Classification of impairment, disability and handicap is difficult for various reasons.

1. There is only a general, not specific, relationship between disturbances at each level. Indeed, if there were more direct relationships there would be no need to develop this model with different levels. Furthermore, the interactions between different impairments (or disabilities) leads to different patterns of disability (or handicap).

2. A systematic approach to the consequences of disease has only been developed in the last decade, but measures have been around for much longer. Consequently, classification is constrained, in practice if not in principle, by the measures already used and their implicit classification system.

3. A complicating factor is the need to develop a system relevant to clinical practice. This concentrates on personal abilities and independence. Moreover, it focuses on areas that are amenable to intervention at a personal level (in contrast to political or societal actions).

4. Most classification systems have been developed by non-neurologists, usually either rheumatologists, or sociologists interested in community surveys. Neurological diseases cause particular impairments and (though less so), particular disabilities, and so require a particular classification system.

   This chapter has proposed a system which might be of general use, and certainly is of use with neurological diseases. The system is based on the premise that two fundamental areas of behaviour exist—that with the physical environment, and that involving information handling and transfer both within the individual and also with others. (This system could benefit from further development.)

4 Choosing a measure

Summary

1. The first important factor dictating the choice of measure is that it should be relevant and sensible—it should provide the information wanted, no more and no less.
2. The second step is to consider the measures already developed to determine if any of them suit the purpose—there will usually be a suitable measure.
3. Next, one must decide whether the measure being considered actually measures the phenomenon it is intended to measure, and if it will achieve the purpose required; is it valid?
4. Reliability refers to the extent to which two observations agree; unreliability may arise from patient variability, observer variability, and variability in measuring instruments. Bias, a systematic variation between results obtained in different ways, should particularly be guarded against.
5. Any measure used should be of sufficient sensitivity to detect the differences expected or required.
6. A good test should be simple, which encourages reliability but often reduces sensitivity.
7. Finally, the results obtained should be capable of being communicated to others without difficulty.

Introduction

This chapter discusses how to assess a measure. There are many measures mentioned in this book, and many cover similar areas. Therefore it is necessary to have a system for choosing which measure to use.

Most articles considering the choice of measures will concentrate upon the characteristics of the measure itself. Indeed, there are whole books devoted to the construction and characterization of measures. However the most important consideration is often neglected, perhaps because it is felt to be self-evident. Unfortunately, the author's own experience in advising others would suggest that this consideration is often completely overlooked. Therefore this chapter starts with a discussion emphasizing the central importance of knowing what information is wanted and why. In other words, the 'sensibility' of the chosen measure should be considered (Feinstein *et al.* 1986).

The other necessary characteristics of a measure are then discussed: validity, reliability, sensitivity, simplicity, and communicability. This discussion is necessarily brief, simply highlighting the major issues. (For a more detailed analysis, reference is made to other texts.) Finally a series of questions are given that were found useful by the Medical Research Council for judging questionnaires.

Identify necessary information and data

The most important step when choosing any measure is to decide precisely what information is required, and why. This has been discussed in some detail in Chapter 2, but a few particular points will be made here.

Measures may be needed for three reasons:

- To define the type of patient being studied (input), particularly with regard to prognosis. The prognosis will certainly relate to the natural (untreated) outcome, and it may include features which identify patients likely to respond to the treatment.

- To measure various parts of the process of treatment, such as the amount and timing of treatment given and effects on presumed intervening variables (usually impairments).

- To measure the outcome, and this outcome should always be at the level of disability, and might include handicap if at all possible.

Sometimes only process is measured (for example, time given to the patient, or procedures carried out), forgetting that process is separate from outcome (and may bear little relationship to it). Health service managements and politicians often confuse process (for example, waiting lists, throughput) with outcome.

It is vital to determine the specific data appropriate to your needs. This requires a reasonable background knowledge about the patient's specific illness. For example, if it is necessary to establish a patient's prognosis, then the measure chosen must be able to establish the best prognostic information, and not be a second-best measure. For patients with stroke the presence of urinary incontinence is a good prognostic indicator (Barer 1989a). If mobility is the outcome of interest, then specific measures of mobility should be chosen, not global measures which include (among other items) mobility.

It is also important to decide upon *the least information necessary* to achieve the purpose. Many people collect too much information, and forget that it is expensive in time and effort to collect data. In addition, collecting excessive information will probably reduce the accuracy and completeness of the data collected.

Therefore, before considering specific measures, it is necessary to determine the minimum information needed on *prognosis*, *process*, and *outcome*. It is then necessary to start identifying the data which are relevant, and it is important to resist the temptation to collect other, irrelevant data. Only then can the actual measures be chosen.

Choosing a specific measure

The first step is to discover what measures already exist. If possible, it is always best to use an existing measure, provided it is valid (for the use you require), reliable (under the circumstances proposed), and is appropriate to your needs and resources. This way, much effort will be saved in establishing validity and reliability. Moreover, at least a few other people (i.e. those familiar with the measure) will then better understand the results.

When choosing an existing measure (or developing a new one), the following questions should be asked:

- Is it actually relevant (see last section)?
- Is it a valid measure of what I wish to assess?
- What is its reliability?
- Is it sensitive enough to detect the change/difference expected?
- Is it simple enough to be used?
- Can the results be communicated to others?
- Is there a better measure available?

Validity

Validity is a concept which is probably over-stressed in the context of measures used within neurological rehabilitation. In essence a valid measure is one which can measure whatever it is supposed to, and can achieve the purpose wanted. For example, a measure of strength might include grip strength but should not contain items concerned with visual acuity. In other words, for any measure there should be a construct (idea) which is generally accepted, and the measure should quantify some aspect of that construct. Three main types of validity are generally recognized: construct, criterion-related, and content validity.

1. *Construct validity* refers to the extent to which results obtain using a measure concur with the results predicted from the underlying theoretical model. If it is accepted that manual dexterity is affected by ataxia, then the results of a measure of ataxia should correlate with an independent measure of dexterity. Of course, if the correlation is perfect, the measure

becomes redundant but this is rarely the case. If there were no correlation at all, then one of these two measures would probably be invalid.

2. *Criterion-related validity* refers to the testing of a measure against some outside criterion or 'gold standard'. The criterion can take many forms: another measure of accepted validity ('concurrent validity'); the opinion of experts; or the ability to predict the expected future (so-called 'predictive validity'). This type of validity is most important in screening measures and in prognostic measures.

3. *Content validity* refers to the items included within a multi-item measure. The component items should not only relate to the construct being measured, but also cover all aspects of that construct. One way of checking this is to ensure that all the component items come from the same level of impairment, disability or handicap. For example, the widely-used Rankin Scale has poor content validity, mixing, as it does, impairment, disability, and handicap in one scale.

There are two more terms used occasionally:

1. *Face validity* refers to the apparent sensibility of the measure and its components. For example, the severity of paralysis has more face validity than urinary incontinence as a predictor of outcome after stroke (but it has a less good predictive validity).

2. *Ecological validity* refers to the suitability of the measure in the environment it is to be used in. For instance, measures of mobility derived in a specialist gait laboratory might have low ecological validity if it is only possible to assess a small minority of patients.

It can be seen that the term 'validity' encompasses many different ideas, and that it cannot simply be classified as a measure that is valid or invalid. Instead, it is a question of asking whether the measure chosen will achieve the intended purpose. This reinforces the importance of deciding first what is to be measured, and why. In other words, validity is not an absolute property of any measure, but only a relative one. A measure may be valid for one purpose, but invalid for some other purpose. For example, the Star-cancellation Test is probably a valid screening test for visual neglect (Halligan *et al.* 1989), but it is not a valid measure of prognosis after stroke, nor of visual acuity.

Reliability

There are three main sources of uncertainty when comparing two results obtained using one measure:

- there may be variation in the patient's state;

- different observers may differ when measuring; and
- if there is a mechanical tool being used, it too may vary over time.

In addition, it is important to remember that variation may be random or non-random (i.e. biased). Therefore any data can be considered as having two components: a 'true' reading and an 'error' reading; the error being either biased or unbiased.

Measures of reliability may refer to how closely two obtained results relate to each other, and should also refer to how much bias affects the error component. For example, two observers may have high correlation, but one may consistently mark the patient 10 per cent lower than the other. A straight correlation coefficient would show high 'reliability' and would not reveal the major bias (see Sheikh 1986). Although reliability is now often assessed, there is little agreement on how to express reliability. Further, the methods used should depend upon the type of measure being studied: nominal (categorical); ordinal; interval; or ratio.

The types of statistical measures used include kappa statistics (of increasing sophistication) (Fleiss 1971; Landis and Koch 1977), correlation coefficients, coefficients of concordance, Cronbach's Alpha, intra-class coefficients (Shrout and Fleiss 1979), and coefficients of variation. These statistical measures are used to summarize much data, and to determine whether two or more observations agree more than would be expected by chance alone. (For more details, readers should consult statistics textbooks or (preferably) statisticians; see also: Bland and Altman 1986; Sheikh 1986; Siegel and Castellan 1988; Streiner and Norman 1989.)

Agreement between observations with high statistical significance does not necessarily mean that the individual readings are all that close. For example, it was found that the timing of walking over 10 m was 'reliable' on test–retest ($r = 0.98$) with no bias, but none the less results in individual patients varied by as much as 20 per cent (Collen *et al.* 1990). Equally important, statistically significant correlations can easily arise in the presence of bias; for example, with one observer consistently rating patients either better or worse.

In practice, clinicians want to know what difference in the results is the one likely to reflect the real difference, and this is rarely disclosed by the traditional statistical tests. For example, when studying the use of the Barthel ADL Index in a rehabilitation setting, a Kendall's Coefficient of concordance of 0.93 was found ($p < 0.001$). However, this does not identify that differences of 4 points (out of 20) might have arisen from observer variability, and that differences of 5 points or more will almost always reflect real change (Collin *et al.* 1988).

Consequently, statistical analysis should be used to establish that the agreement seen is better than by chance alone, and also to establish that there is no bias present. Other analysis should be used to determine the actual limits of reliability, and these limits should be stated.

Sensitivity

Much less attention has been paid to the measurement of sensitivity, yet it is obviously necessary to choose a measure which can detect the change expected. For example, if mortality is the only outcome measure, then reductions in morbidity can not be detected! Recently, there have been attempts to assess sensitivity, being based upon the statistical variance found in groups of patients (Guyatt *et al*. 1987). For example, Wood-Dauphinee *et al*. (1990) used the coefficient of variation (Standard Deviation/Mean) to show that the Barthel ADL Index was the most sensitive measure for assessing morbidity after stroke.

The likelihood of detecting change can be increased in several ways. For example, an intrinsically, very sensitive single measure can be used such as grip strength after stroke (Heller *et al*. 1987; Sunderland *et al*. 1989) and walking speed (Wade *et al*. 1987*a*). Unfortunately such tests are rare, and those proposed are often very complex and unreliable.

One alternative is to use several complementary outcome measures. For example, in a study evaluating the reduction of neglect, measurement could be made of Activities of Daily Living (ADL), speed and accuracy of reading, ability to negotiate doorways, and speed and ability in completing a simple jigsaw. The price paid is the time involved in measuring, and the increased risk of obtaining a false-positive result. In a recent controlled trial of treatment after stroke, measures of arm impairment and disability were used; the reasons were to detect both process (was weakness reduced?) and outcome (was function improved?) (Sunderland *et al*. 1991).

Lastly, if the change of interest can be specified precisely, then that skill can be measured directly. For example, if the purpose of a rehabilitation programme was to achieve independence in a wheelchair about the home, then simply observing the person in their home would be the way to do this. It is best to avoid the temptation to use a more complex scale to assess, perhaps, many aspects of mobility, and also the temptation to assess mobility about a special course (in hospital).

Simplicity

Wherever possible, the measures that are used should be simple, particularly if more than one person is going to use the measure. Simplicity will improve the patient (and user) compliance, and will increase reliability. Simple measures are usually quick and therefore more readily used.

Unfortunately there is usually a trade-off between the three requirements of simplicity, reliability, and sensitivity. Sensitivity often requires more complex measures, but unless great care is taken these are often less reliable.

Communicability

Measures should give results which are easily understood by others. Colleagues (or readers of the study) cannot be expected to have the interest, experience, and the innate understanding. (In his ward rounds the author finds it difficult to attend to and remember any report on a patient's assessment which lasts over two to four minutes, and which does not contain simple numerical or categorical data.)

Results which are presented numerically with zero representing the worst level and 10 or 100 the best level are most easily understood. It is unwise to design a measure where 57 is the worst level and 17 the best (Sheikh *et al.* 1979)—readers will simply not get used to the meaning of the numbers.

There are several measures which use visual display to improve communicability. Most are not used widely. Visual displays depend upon having the correct forms available at the time, and they need a separate piece of paper. Medical notes are already overburdened with paper, which often gets lost. For these and other reasons (for example, the need to buy copies of the display), visual displays do not appear to have achieved their potential.

Alternative measures

It is always worth considering whether there are other, better measures. Time spent asking colleagues about measures, and reading around the subject is time well spent. If two or more similar measures are used, the results of any comparison of the two measures should be published so that others may know which is better. There are now some studies being published which do compare different measures and, interestingly, simple measures of disability do seem to be more sensitive than measures of impairment (Goodkin *et al.* 1988).

Assessing a measure

The British Medical Research Council have an informal but standardized method for assessing any questionnaire measure proposed. In practice it is difficult to carry this out completely, because it takes time to acquire all the relevant data—the author has not attempted such a detailed analysis for any measure in this book. The headings and questions are given below, and these are similar in content to the heading used above.

Context of use

- Is the measure appropriate to the aim of the study?
- Who can use the measure?

- Who is the questionnaire to be completed by?
- Can a proxy respondent complete it?
- What is the method of administration?
- How long does it take to complete?
- Is the measure acceptable to patients?

Development

- How were the included items selected?
- What populations have been sampled?
- What is the format of the questionnaire?
- Is the format suitable for your study patient(s)?
- How is the questionnaire scored?
- Are the scores skewed (ceiling or floor effects)?
- Are item scores weighted and if so how were weights derived?
- Are normal values from a control population available?
- Are there separate subscales?

Validity

- Has construct validity been established?
- Has concurrent validity been established?
- Has predictive validity been established?

Reliability

- Test–retest reliability?
- Inter-observer?
- Different modes of administration?
- Is there any bias?
- What are the limits?

Sensitivity

- Used in placebo-controlled trials?
- Used in a trial of treatment of known efficacy?
- Compared with other measures?

Conclusions

The criteria for selecting measures are well-established, but one thing is often overlooked—will the measure provide the information needed? This depends upon formulating a clear-cut question at the outset. Data collection simply 'for the record' is rarely, if ever, worthwhile, however good the measures used. Time spent considering exactly what it is that the user wishes to discover is time well-spent.

The other attributes measures should have, such as validity and reliability, are not absolute but relative. It is important to know the limits of these attributes, and then to decide if the measure will achieve the aim.

Section 2
Measurement at different levels

This section looks at measurement from the viewpoint of the four levels previously identified—pathology, impairment, disability, and handicap. It reviews the specific implications of choosing and using measures at each level. Some recommendations are given.

Chapter 5 reviews briefly the use of measures at the level of pathology. Measures can either establish the likelihood that a specific disease is present or can, sometimes, establish its severity (prognosis). Clinical measures at the level of pathology are uncommon, and are only occasionally relevant to neurological rehabilitation.

Chapters 6 and 7 review measures of impairment. The major part of Chapter 6 is devoted to measures of motor loss, recommending greater use of measures of strength (power). It also covers arousal and sensation. Chapter 7 concentrates upon the measurement of more complex cognitive impairments, and moods.

Chapter 8 is devoted to the measurement of physical disability which necessarily is the major focus of much rehabilitation. It strongly recommends three particular measures:

- The Barthel Activities of Daily Living (ADL) Index as an overall measure of physical dependence.
- Gait speed as a measure of mobility.
- The use of the Nine-hole Peg Test to measure manual dexterity.

Measurement of most other aspects of disability is covered in Chapter 9. The topics covered range from the use of very specific measures when studying individual patients through to the use of comprehensive measures covering the whole range. Included within this chapter is some discussion of disability questionnaires and of the measurement of extended ADL activities.

The last chapter in this section (Chapter 10) covers the measurement of handicap. Included within the chapter is a discussion of the assessment of quality-of-life. It is recommended that quality-of-life measures are abandoned in favour of more specific and restricted measures.

5 Measures of pathology

Summary

1. Pathology is the damage or disruption which occurs within an organ or organ system within the body.
2. Measures at the level of pathology are useful in establishing the likelihood of the pathology being present.
3. Measures at the level of pathology can also establish disease severity, specifically in the patient with a tumour or a life-threatening acute illness. However, impairments are usually better at measuring severity.

Introduction

Many neurological diseases have microscopic abnormalities within the central or peripheral nervous system, or muscle which can be demonstrated at post-mortem, if not before. This is the pathology. Others have functional abnormalities shown only during life; for example, the characteristic electrical discharges seen (and heard) on electromyography (EMG) in patients with myotonia.

In some diseases the pathological functional abnormalities at the organ level can occur in the absence of any demonstrable structural changes. In other diseases, such as epilepsy and depression, there is rarely any demonstrable pathological function or structure. In these cases, it is assumed that there must be an underlying pathology (perhaps of the cell membrane), but it is presumably possible that there are illnesses which only arise at the level of impairment.

This brief chapter simply outlines that there are measures applicable at the level of pathology. A few of these are included in the book, particularly in relation to stroke.

Disease diagnosis

Many neurological diagnoses cannot be confirmed with a definite, specific test. Sometimes it is impractical to conduct the theoretically possible test. For example, multiple sclerosis could be confirmed by biopsy of the brain, optic nerves, or spinal cord but it is obviously not sensible to undertake such a procedure—the increase in diagnostic certainty would not lead to any specific change in management; the cost (in terms of increased impairment) does not lead to enough benefit. For other neurological conditions, there is at present no definite pathology identified. For example, no specific lesion has been found in spasmodic torticollis. The cause of most cases of epilepsy is unknown. Headache rarely has an identified pathology. Transient ischaemic attacks may leave no trace.

Therefore the great majority of neurological diagnoses (of pathology) are clinical, and depend upon the doctor recognizing the syndrome, and excluding realistic alternative diagnoses. This leaves considerable scope for error and disagreement. For example, Tomasello *et al.* (1982) and Garraway *et al.* (1976) have shown problems in the diagnosis of stroke, although physicians do usually agree (Gross *et al.* 1986). In practice, most neurological diagnoses are probably correct.

Nevertheless attempts have been made to formalize the criteria which need to be fulfilled when making some diagnoses. These criteria are effectively a measure of diagnostic certainty. The most well-known are probably the diagnostic criteria for multiple sclerosis (MS) published by Poser *et al.* (1983). Others include criteria for diagnosing Alzheimer's Disease and dementia (for example, see Molsa *et al.* 1985), criteria for separating cerebral haemorrhage from cerebral infarction (Allen 1983), and criteria for localizing the area of infarction after stroke (Bamford 1988).

The measures of certainty of pathological diagnosis will not be discussed further in this book. However, it is important to realize that they do exist, and that exactly the same considerations apply to them as to all other measures. In particular, issues of sensitivity and specificity are important. Most of these measures are based on impairments which are more or less specific for the disease.

Disease severity

Measurement of the severity of the disease can also occur at the level of pathology. The best example is that of grading tumours. Gliomas are usually graded on a four-point scale, based on microscopic features such as number of mitoses (dividing cells) seen, degree of necrosis, and capillary abnormalities.

One example of a pathologically-based measure of disease (or rather illness) severity is the APACHE II system (Knaus *et al.* 1985). This measure is based upon a variety of pathological measures such as arterial oxygen and pH, and it is a measure of disturbance of basic cardio-respiratory physiology.

Its importance is twofold. First, it gives an idea of prognosis in almost any life-threatening acute illness, and is thus useful in research into new treatments, and provides a method for judging likely outcome and ensuring comparable groups. Second, it may be used (in future?) to decide who should or should not be admitted to intensive care units, though at present it is probably not sufficiently sensitive to allow such decisions; indeed, one study found clinical assessment to be as accurate (Kruse *et al.* 1988), and its utility must still be in doubt.

A further example of pathological measurement is the use of CT scans to measure the extent (volume) of brain loss after stroke or head injury. Although possible, this information is not of clinical value in rehabilitation: there is less connection between extent of brain loss and disability than there is between easily measured impairments and disability or prognosis. In other words, the connection between pathology and impairment is too weak to allow measures of pathological severity to be of much use in neurological rehabilitation.

For example, it is not uncommon to see a patient with a large cerebral infarct on CT scan who has relatively minor disability, or, conversely, a severely disabled person with minimal infarction visible on CT scan. Instead, in most diseases, measurement of disease severity and prognosis will occur at the level of impairment. The important point is that the pathological diagnosis gives vital information on the expected natural history of the illness.

Conclusions

Measurement at the level of pathology can and does occur. There are relatively few such measures at present, and they have only a peripheral influence upon most neurological rehabilitation. However, it is important to remember that:

• there is uncertainty attached to any diagnosis;
• the severity of pathological loss is poorly related to disability; but
• the pathology has a major influence upon prognosis.

6 Motor and sensory impairments

Summary

1. Impairments are symptoms or signs, the subjective and objective immediate manifestations of any pathology. They are often disease specific.
2. The level of arousal (consciousness) is best measured using the Glasgow Coma Scale. Formal measures of orientation (for example, post-traumatic amnesia), include the Galveston Orientation and Awareness Test, and a test of learning.
3. Measurement of muscle strength is valid, reliable, and sensitive, but is not widely undertaken.
4. Muscle tone can be measured using the Ashworth Scale, but the clinical relevance of tone needs investigation.
5. There are many measures of abnormal movement, most relating to Parkinson's disease.
6. There are few useful, reliable measures of sensation.
7. Specialist measures of some cranial nerves exist, such as visual field perimetry, or orthoptic assessment of eye movements.

Introduction

Impairments are the external or conscious manifestations of a disease. They are abnormalities in the functions of the whole body, with these functions usually having no personal meaning to the individual. This contrasts with disabilities, where it is goal directed behaviour that is altered.

There are (in principle) two types of impairment:

- subjective (i.e. symptoms), which cannot always be observed directly, and
- objective (i.e. signs).

Usually attempts are made to detect signs which corroborate the patient's symptoms. For example, a symptom of altered sensation may coincide with a reduction in the ability to detect vibration.

Impairments are often specific to a disease (or to a relatively small group of diseases). Consequently, many specific measures of disease severity are, in fact, measures of impairment. Disease-specific measures are considered in Chapter 11. In this chapter the emphasis is on the general impairments identified first in Chapter 3, Table 3.1, and shown again here (Table 6.1). The next chapter considers detailed measures of cognitive impairment and

Table 6.1 A classification of neurological impairments

Function Sub-categories	Impairment	Measures
Arousal/awareness		
Consciousness		Glasgow Coma Scale
Limb motor		
Strength	Weakness	Dynanometry
Control	Ataxia, dysarthria	
Involuntary	Tremor, chorea, etc.	AIMS
Tone	Spasticity	Ashworth Scale
Range of movement	Contractures	Goniometry
Limb sensory		
Skin (touch, temp)		Clinical
Joints (position)		Clinical
Cranial motor		
Eyes, range	Gaze palsy	
Eyes, control	Nystagmus	
Face		
Speech (talking)	Dysarthria	Clinical
Swallow	Dysphagia	Swallow water
Cranial sensory		
Eyes	Reduced acuity	Visual acuity charts
Eyes	Field loss	Confrontation, perimetry
Ears	Deafness	Clinical, specialist
Nose	Anosmia	Clinical
Integration (cognition)		
Information processing		PASAT
Sensory perception	Neglect, agnosia	BIT, RPAB
Motor planning	Apraxia	
Language	Aphasia	FAST
Pain		
Psychological		
Mood	Anxiety, depression	GHQ
Motivation		

AIMS   = Abnormal Involuntary Movement Scale
BIT   = Behavioural Inattention Test
FAST   = Frenchay Aphasia Screening Test
GHQ   = General Health Questionnaire
PASAT = Paced Auditory Serial Addition Test
RPAB   = Rivermead Perceptual Assessment Battery

mood because these form a particular group of impairments, which are difficult to measure.

Level of arousal

A patient's level of consciousness is obviously of great importance to the doctor or surgeon who is managing any acute neurological illness, especially head injury. However, it is also of great importance in the later management of many patients because the extent and duration of coma is of considerable prognostic importance in many conditions, both surgical and medical (Levy *et al*. 1981). It is therefore vital to use a reliable measure of consciousness.

The Glasgow Coma Scale (Teasdale *et al*. 1979) has all the characteristics of a good measure. It is clinically very useful, has proven validity, good reliability, and is simple yet sensitive enough for clinical purposes. In addition, the results are easily communicated and widely understood. The scale can also be used in children, although alternatives designed for children do exist (Raimondi and Hirschauer 1984). There are one or two other scales, such as the Edinburgh-2 Coma Scale (championed in Japan), but they have not been shown to have any great advantage. Therefore, the Glasgow Coma Scale (GCS) should always be used, and the results of each section recorded separately.

In general a GCS score of 9–15/15 is taken as indicating some awareness, whereas lower scores are referred to as indicating coma. However, the scale simply measures the level of arousal, and any divisions are arbitrary.

Post-traumatic amnesia (PTA)

A second, related disturbance of arousal is level of orientation (awareness). This is particularly disturbed in the state of post-traumatic amnesia (PTA) which occurs after head injury, but similar disturbance is found after any general cerebral insult, such as cerebral anoxia. Precise definition of PTA is difficult, but in essence a patient who does not have continuous day-to-day memory is in PTA. The measurement of duration of PTA (time from injury to return of continuous memory) is often retrospective, but attempts have been made to determine the end of PTA prospectively.

One method is to use the Galveston Orientation and Amnesia Test (GOAT), which essentially rates a person's awareness clinically at regular intervals. Using the GOAT, the end of PTA is defined as achieving a score better than 78/100 on three successive days. This method is only practical in a well-staffed unit, because administration of the GOAT takes time. It is also probably less useful in patients who have prolonged PTA, for example extending for three weeks or more, because PTA ends gradually. It could be administered less frequently.

Another method is to test repeatedly the ability to learn, using three pictures (Artiola i Fortuna *et al.* 1980). The patient is shown three pictures during one day, and 24 hours later is asked what was shown the day before. The end of PTA is defined when the patient is successful at recalling the pictures shown on three successive days.

The difficulties and uncertainties in assessing PTA, especially in patients with mild head injury, have been discussed (Gronwall and Wrightson 1980). Despite the limitations in accuracy, it is still important to assess PTA after head injury because it is probably the best single measure of severity.

Motor impairments

The motor impairments usually assessed are muscle bulk, muscle power, muscle tone, control of movement (for example, ataxia), and the presence of involuntary movements (for example, tremor, dystonia). In addition, the range of movement at a joint can be measured, either as an indication of muscle strength or, more usually, to measure abnormalities in joint mobility (i.e. contractures) which may restrict function.

Muscle bulk is very difficult to measure reliably. Moreover, it rarely forms an important measurement within neurological rehabilitation. Therefore muscle bulk measurement will not be discussed further, except to stress that it is probably an unreliable and insensitive measure. Measurement of strength is much more useful.

Muscle strength

The Medical Research Council (MRC) grades are widely used as an ordinal measure of power (they are very similar to the so-called Oxford scale). Power is graded as follows:

0 = no movement
1 = palpable contraction, but no visible movement
2 = movement but only with gravity eliminated
3 = movement against gravity
4 = movement against resistance, but weaker than other side
5 = normal power

These scales were initially devised for use in patients with peripheral nerve injuries usually occurring after war wounds. In these circumstances the need is to detect signs of any innervation, because usually innervation is either present or absent and, if present, will recover well. The scales therefore concentrate upon the lowest 3 per cent of the range of strength (Van der

Ploeg *et al*. 1984). They were not designed to be used with upper motor neuron problems.

One solution has been to derive new weights for the original MRC grades (0–5), these weights being more appropriate for use in patients with upper motor neuron lesions. This has been undertaken (Demeurisse *et al*. 1980) and a Motricity Index devised which has been shown to have good validity and reliability at least with stroke patients (Collin and Wade, 1990; Collen *et al*. 1990). This index derives summed scores for each limb, and for each side. A similar process has been used for measuring motor loss after spinal cord injury (Lucas and Ducker 1979).

An alternative is to measure the force generated directly, using dynamometers. Although controversial (Bohannon 1989*a*), this has several advantages. It gives a ratio measure; the measurable range can extend from minimal force to full force, giving high sensitivity; reliability is reasonable provided standard techniques are used (Andres *et al*. 1986; Bohannon and Andrews 1987*a*); it is a valid measure, in that force is related to performance on other tasks (Bohannon 1989*b*); it is simple and easily communicated.

The major disadvantage of measuring strength is the intuitive resistance of many therapists to the measurement of strength in patients with upper motor neuron disease (Bohannon 1989*a*). However, there is good evidence to support its use in many neuromuscular diseases such as stroke (Bohannon 1989*b*), motor neuron disease (Andres *et al*. 1986) and myopathies (Wiles and Karni 1983).

In conclusion, much more use should be made of measurement of strength either clinically or, preferably, using dynamometers. As an alternative, the MRC grades can be used utilizing the weighted scores given in the Motricity Index.

Tone

Assessment of tone is central to almost all physiotherapeutic assessment, and it is therefore disappointing how little effort has been given to the development of reliable measures or establishing reliability of current clinical practice. Assessment of tone within the Motor Assessment Scale is unreliable (Poole and Whitney 1988), and this is probably the method used clinically. The Ashworth Scale is the only clinical measure which has been evaluated to any extent (Bohannon and Smith 1987); it is reliable.

The validity of assessing and treating tone must also be questioned, because there is no good evidence that the disturbance of tone is the primary problem. Recent research suggests that disability is more closely related to weakness than it is to spasticity (Bohannon and Andrews 1990). Spasticity seems quite likely to be an epiphenomenon (McLellan 1977).

Electromechanical devices for measuring spasticity have been developed. They are not in widespread use and cannot be used easily on a day-to-day basis, and so will not be reviewed here.

Movement control: ataxia, tremor, etc.

Clinical measurement of ataxia and abnormal movements is not easy. Ataxia, like any other phenomenon, can be graded as absent, mild, moderate, or severe, but this is often done with reference to the consequent disability (Klockgether *et al*. 1990). The best approach is probably to note the presence of ataxia, and to measure the disability using tests of mobility and manual dexterity.

Many clinical measures of abnormal movements have been devised in relation to movement disorders. Parkinson's disease has been a specific focus for the development of measurement, presumably because treatments exist which reduce impairment. Unfortunately, most of the scales which have been developed tend to mix the impairments with their resultant disabilities, using the disability to rate the severity of the impairment. Many are included in this book, and discussed in Chapter 11, as well as being shown in Section 4.

Involuntary abnormal movements, especially tremor, are particularly amenable to measurement using equipment, and so this will not be pursued further here.

Movement range

Measurement of the range of movement at joints has been well developed for orthopaedic and rheumatological diseases. Most measures use mechanical or, increasingly, electronic goniometers. These can be used in two circumstances in neurological diseases. First, patients may have associated orthopaedic pathologies, such as contractures or fractures reducing the range of joint movement. Second, the range of active joint movement can be used as a measure of motor power particularly at the early stages of recovery after stroke (Bard and Hirschberg 1965).

Sensation

Measurement of sensation is difficult, and not very satisfactory for clinical purposes. There are special electronic devices which can measure sensory thresholds (see Lindblom and Tegner 1989; Dyck and O'Brien 1989). These will not be discussed further as they are not practical in routine clinical service.

Clinical assessment of sensation using standard tests (for example, pin-prick, light touch) has not been evaluated for reliability in any detail but has been included in test batteries for use after stroke. In most of these, sensation is tested using a pin and is rated simply as 'normal', 'impaired', and 'absent'. In general, global assessments of sensory disturbance seem reliable, though less reliable than motor measures (Duncan *et al.* 1983; Shinar *et al.* 1985; Brott *et al.* 1989; Goldstein *et al.* 1989). However, Tomasello *et al.* (1982) found a low rate of agreement about sensory loss after stroke, and Sisk *et al.* (1970) demonstrated poor agreement when simply relying on the history.

The thumb-finding test (the patient has his eyes closed, and one arm is passively moved and the patient is then asked to 'find his thumb' using the other arm) has been found of prognostic value after stroke (Prescott *et al.* 1982; Smith *et al.* 1983). Reliability has not been assessed, and it is unclear as to what the test is measuring.

Depth-sense aesthesiometry (Smaje and McLellan 1981) has been developed as a simple but sensitive test of sensation and used in patients after stroke (Parker *et al.* 1986). Unfortunately, it is not widely known or used, perhaps because the simple piece of equipment needed is not readily available.

In patients with MS, clinical tests of joint position sense, vibration sensitivity and superficial sensation were found to be reliable on test–retest over a week (Kuzma *et al.* 1969).

In conclusion, it is probably reliable to use gross measures of sensory loss, with three categories not specifying particular modalities. The reliability of more detailed clinical assessments must be open to some doubt at present. Fortunately it may not often be all that important.

Cranial, motor and sensory

Most studies on the assessment of cranial nerve impairments have been as part of a larger test battery for use after stroke, and most concentrate simply upon separating normal from abnormal. Simple clinical measures of the severity of motor or somatic sensory loss in cranial nerves are rare. This probably arises for two reasons:

- Measurement of severity will rarely be relevant.
- Reliable measurement is difficult.

However, there are specialist measures available for several specific cranial nerves, such as vision and hearing, and other aspects such as bulbar control and eye movement.

The reliability of testing the sense of smell (using perfumes) and taste has not, to the best of the author's knowledge, been tested. In the context of neurological rehabilitation, measurement of these is not particularly important. (This is not to deny the distress associated with loss or alteration of these senses; there is simply no remedy available.) However, it is vital to remember that patients left with anosmia after head injury should be advised to install a smoke alarm at home.

Simple clinical assessment of eye movements is limited, though may be reliable at detecting major abnormalities. An orthoptic examination can give much very useful detail but takes much time. Visual acuity is easily tested, both for near and far vision, using standard ophthalmological measures. Visual fields can be assessed by simple confrontation techniques, using moving fingers or coloured objects, and this is probably reliable at detecting major field losses from hemisphere damage (Goldstein *et al.* 1989; Brott *et al.* 1989). However, this technique is not very reliable at detecting abnormalities arising from compression of the optic chiasm (Trobe *et al.* 1981). A more detailed measurement using perimetry is available, but it takes much time to do.

Weakness of facial movement is probably not assessed very reliably (Goldstein *et al.* 1989) although some studies show better agreement (Cote *et al.* 1989; Brott *et al.* 1989). Assessment of fifth nerve weakness has not been evaluated.

Bulbar abnormalities are best measured in detail by using measures of disability, and the author is not aware of formal studies of the reliability of assessing bulbar motor loss. Clinically, swallowing can be observed and rated on a three-point scale (normal, impaired, unable) (Shinar *et al.* 1985); and it can also be noted whether the patient chokes (Gordon *et al.* 1987; Barer 1989*b*). More detail can be obtained from timing the swallow of a fixed volume of water. Dysarthria can be rated clinically, and reliability is fair (Shinar *et al.* 1985; Goldstein *et al.* 1989; Brott *et al.* 1989). Auditory acuity can be assessed using specialist equipment.

Simple clinical assessment and rating of cranial motor loss (present/absent) is reasonably reliable, but more detailed nonspecialist measurement is probably unreliable. It is also rarely needed. Clinical assessment of special senses (visual field loss, visual acuity, colour blindness, smell, hearing) is possible.

In practice, it is important to accept the limitations of routine clinical measures and to obtain more specialist detailed measurements when this is needed. Current experience suggests that routine orthoptic evaluation reveals major unsuspected and clinically important abnormalities in many patients (S. Fowler, personal communication), but this has not yet been published.

Integration and mood

The more complex level of cognitive function relating to sensory input and motor output are difficult to classify. Many measures have been devised, but most are very specialist. These will be discussed in the next chapter, as will mood disturbance which is also difficult to classify.

Conclusions

The clinical measurement of impairments is still relatively weak and few have been subjected to much critical evaluation. In part, this is because impairments are primarily used to deduce pathology, and it is the overall pattern of a patient's history, symptoms and signs which is useful rather than the isolated severity of a specific impairment. However, there are many disease-specific measures that are primarily based upon impairments; these are discussed later.

Level of consciousness should be measured using the Glasgow Coma Scale (GCS). Motor impairment is best assessed by measuring power, directly or through the Motricity Index. Measurement of tone is probably unreliable and irrelevant. Gross clinical assessment of sensation is probably acceptably reliable, but for detailed measures it is necessary to use expensive and specialist equipment which takes too long to be used routinely.

Detailed specialist assessment of eye movements, visual field loss, other visual impairments and auditory function should be sought if problems are suspected, because clinical assessment is probably not sufficiently reliable or sensitive. Orthoptic evaluation may be particularly useful.

7 Cognitive and emotional impairments

Summary

1. There is no simple coherent model of cognitive function, which makes it difficult to describe the measures in a logical way.
2. Memory includes three components: attention, orientation (past memory), and learning (new memory).
3. There are several simple, short tests of orientation, and they are all similar. Measuring attention is less easy, though the Paced Auditory Serial Addition Test (PASAT) and digit-symbol test might be useful. Tests of learning necessarily take time, and paragraph recall may be the best single simple test.
4. Aphasia is best detected and measured using the Frenchay Aphasia Screening Test (FAST). Speech therapists then have many well developed tests for performing more detailed measurements.
5. Perceptual problems can be very complex, and though test batteries exist their utility is in doubt. However, there are simple tests for neglect, such as the Star-cancellation Test and clinical testing for inattention using double simultaneous stimulation (visual and tactile).
6. Apraxia is a difficulty in planning complex motor activities, but until clear and rigorously defined diagnostic criteria become available, it will not be possible to measure apraxia. At present it cannot even be diagnosed reliably.
7. Intelligence is the ability to solve problems. There are short non-specialist tests of both verbal and non-verbal IQ. Estimation of pre-morbid IQ can be undertaken through measuring vocabulary, though the validity of this approach may not have been checked.
8. There are many measures of mood, but none has been well validated for use in patients with chronic neurological disability, either as diagnostic instruments or to assess severity of disturbance.

Introduction

Detailed definition and measurement of cognitive impairments is the responsibility of neuropsychologists and speech therapists (speech pathologists), and several major textbooks exist on the topic (for example, Lezak 1983). This chapter is restricted to measures which can be used by relative non-specialists such as doctors or occupational therapists. Detailed assessment of mood is in theory the province of psychiatrists but in practice no one seems to have much expertise in assessing patients with brain damage or disability.

The main difficulty is to devise a suitable coherent, logical classification of cognitive functions. This arises because, in practice, the brain acts as a whole, and localization of specific functions is rarely precise or consistent. Even damage to the left temporo-parietal areas has an inconsistent effect upon language, the most localized of functions. Furthermore, in most neurological diseases damage is rarely localized to one small area.

In addition, it is difficult to draw definite distinctions between impairment and disability in the cognitive or emotional spheres. For example, is poor memory a disability? The behavioural consequence is usually *not* undertaking some task which should be performed, but this is difficult to measure or conceive as a disability. For instance, what are the behavioural consequences of depression?

This chapter will therefore be structured around the measures available, rather than around a coherent theoretical model. It will discuss measures which focus on cognitive problems, including language disorder. Only a few tests will be discussed, though very many exist (see Lezak 1983). Assessment of mood and motivation will also be discussed; more information can be obtained from Thompson (1989).

Concentration and memory

Disturbances of concentration and learning are almost universal impairments in any chronic disease of the central nervous system. This has been well-known for many years for patients after head injury, but it is now becoming increasingly well recognized in such common diseases as stroke (Wade *et al.* 1986*a*), multiple sclerosis (Peyser *et al.* 1990) and Parkinson's Disease (Mayeux *et al.* 1988) and may also be seen in such diseases as motor neuron disease (Iwasaki *et al.* 1990). It is therefore vital to have and use tests when assessing any neurologically-disabled patient. Failure to detect or recognize poor memory is quite common and may lead to problems in management. In particular, the results may well determine the practicality of undertaking treatments because most require learning of new techniques.

There are three functions which are closely related and probably interdependent: attention (concentration); memory for previously learned material; and ability to learn new material (Skilbeck and Woods 1980). Unfortunately, the word 'memory' often includes both the last two functions, despite their obvious differences. In addition, other terms relating to memory such as 'short-term memory' and 'amnesia' often have different meanings to different people. It is best to be as specific as possible when discussing memory and its measurement. The original Information–memory–concentration Test of Blessed *et al.* (1968) recognized these distinctions.

Attention and information processing

The concept of attention can itself be subdivided, for example, into focused attention, divided attention, sustained attention, and supervisory attention (Van Zomeron and Brouwer 1987). Measures of attention also, necessarily, assess the ability to process complex information. It is obviously difficult to delineate exactly what is being measured by any test.

Clinically, the simplest and most widely used test of attention is the digit span, both forwards and backwards. Further information can be obtained by comparing performance in the two directions. This test, part of both the Weschler Memory Scale and the Weschler Adult Intelligence Scale, is easy to administer and score but probably bears little relationship to any memory disability.

The Paced Auditory Serial Addition Test (PASAT) is designed to measure attention and information processing (Gronwall 1977). The test requires the subject to add consecutive pairs of random numbers presented regularly. For example 3, 5 (3 + 5 = response 8), 6 (5 + 6 = response 11), 1 (6 + 1 = response 7), etc. The numbers are presented using a tape recorder at a fixed rate, and the measure is of the number of correct responses.

The PASAT has been found useful after mild head injury (Gronwall and Wrightson 1974, 1975), but it is not in widespread clinical use, in the UK at least.

More complex tests exist. For example, the digit-symbol test is part of the Weschler Adult Intelligence Scale, but it is also available in isolation. This timed test takes 90 sec to complete and is easily scored. It probably assesses speed of information processing. It is a paper and pencil test, which makes it difficult in the presence of major motor impairments. On the other hand, the test is simple yet sensitive.

At present there is no well tested, valid and reliable test of attention and information processing that can be used by anyone on a wide range of patients. It should be possible to develop one, and it could be very useful, for example, in screening the many patients who have suffered a mild to moderate head injury. It would be important that the test be simple, short, and be able to be used by any profession.

Orientation

Assessment of orientation is sometimes considered synonymous with assessment of memory, but it is only a measure of how good memory is for well-learned information from the past. Most simple orientation measures scarcely measure the ability to learn or memorize new information in any detail.

There are many measures of basic orientation, most having been developed for use by geriatricians in the detection and management of dementia. However, some measures also include items that test other functions, such as new learning or concentration. Only recently have the component items of these measures been studied in detail.

The most well-established test, validated against neuro-pathological evidence, is that of Blessed *et al.* (1968). Various tests have been derived from the original Information–Memory–Concentration section, such as the Hodkinson Mental Test and the short Orientation–Memory–Concentration Test. The former has probably been more widely used, but the latter is probably the better test.

A second widely-used test is the Mini-Mental State Examination (MMSE). This has been analysed in Alzheimer's disease, where it was found that the orientation and recall sections were the most important (Galasko *et al.* 1990). The major problem with the MMSE is that it attempts to compress assessment of too many functions into one test, making interpretation of an isolated score difficult. Clinically, it can be very useful, provided the patient's performance on each item is noted, rather than the total score.

The third test shown in this book is the Clifton Assessment Procedure for the Elderly (CAPE) subtest, concentrating on orientation. The similarity of all three tests is obvious.

In conclusion, there is little evidence to help chose between the various measures of orientation, but one of the tests derived from the original Blessed measure is probably best.

New memory (learning)

Traditionally, memory has been measured using the Weschler Memory Scale (WMS), but this is a long test which requires a trained neuro-psychologist. There is evidence that the logical memory (paragraph recall) sub-test correlates well with the patient's day-to-day behaviour (Sunderland *et al.* 1983), and some typical paragraphs are shown in Section 4.

The Rivermead Behavioural Memory Test (RBMT) was developed as a more ecologically valid, clinically-useful test and it has achieved its aims. It is more specific than the WMS in distinguishing between patients living independently. It takes only 20 to 25 minutes to complete, and can be used by anyone.

The behavioural consequences of memory failure (i.e. memory disability) can be measured using such scales as the Subjective Memory Questionnaire or the Cognitive Failures Questionnaire. Such scales necessarily depend upon obtaining information from relatives or other witnesses.

The Blessed Dementia Rating Scale also records the behavioural consequences of dementia. Recent analysis of its component items has identified a distinct cognitive factor, as well as items relating more to personality change, apathy and basic self-care (Stern *et al.* 1990). The Clifton Assessment Procedure for the Elderly (CAPE) also includes a behavioural measure, derived from the Stockton Geriatric Rating Scale (see Section 4).

Separation of true dementia from depressive pseudodementia is difficult. The Anomalous Sentences Repetition Test (ASRT) is supposed to achieve this in the elderly (Weeks 1988), but a recent report disputes this (Rai *et al.* 1990). This test requires the subject to repeat sentences which are meaningless (for example, 'The stream burns the hair seriously now.'). It is the accuracy of repetition which is measured.

In conclusion, there are many tests of memory (ability to learn new material) ranging from the relatively short to the long and complex. The Rivermead Behavioural Memory Test (RBMT) has several advantages: it is relatively short (25 min), simple, able to be used by anyone, widely used, and its validity in various settings has been assessed. It is, despite its title, essentially a measure of impairment and disability can only be measured using such tests as the Blessed *et al.* (1968) dementia rating scale, or the cognitive failures questionnaire. If a single test is required, paragraph recall (for example, from the RBMT) is probably best.

Language

Assessment and measurement of language disruption (aphasia) is bedevilled by too many long and complex measures, coupled with too many theoretical distinctions between different types of aphasia. One consequence is that most non-experts have become very poor at recognizing and understanding aphasia. For example, most people overrate the comprehension ability of a patient with aphasia (McLenahan *et al.* 1990). Doctors can become obsessed with trying to distinguish different aphasic syndromes, despite the fact that such distinctions do not help make a pathological diagnosis, nor do they help in improving the patient's communication. In practice, many patients do not have any specific type of aphasia.

The Mini-Mental State Examination (MMSE) contains a section which tests language specifically, and for some clinical purposes this may be sufficient.

The Frenchay Aphasia Screening Test (FAST) is a brief test specifically developed to screen for aphasia among stroke patients (Enderby *et al.* 1986). Although an interested clinician may be as good at detecting aphasia (O'Neill *et al.* 1990) it is the author's experience that many doctors fail to recognize even the presence of, let alone the severity of, aphasia. As with all tests, abnormal results need to be interpreted in the light of all available information: a low score can arise from visual neglect, confusion, low intelligence, etc. Also, a high score does not exclude aphasia, but does suggest that communication is at least reasonable. The FAST score is closely related to the Functional Communication Profile score, suggesting it may measure both impairment and disability.

There are many specialized tests such as the Porch Index or Communicative Ability (PICA), the Boston Diagnostic Aphasia Test and the Whurr. Unfortunately all are long tests, and give results which are difficult to interpret. Speech therapists need to agree on a way of communicating with their linguistically normal colleagues.

Perception and neglect

Psychologists and occupational therapists have developed many tests of perception, the interpretation of sensory input. These vary from simple tests like double simultaneous stimulation (tactile or visual) through tests such as object recognition on to figure-ground tests. The Rivermead Perceptual Assessment Battery (RPAB) contains 16 tests which are generally representative of most other tests (Whiting *et al.* 1985).

The measurement of perceptual ability poses great difficulty. There is no agreement on what exactly should be included within the construct of 'perception'. Almost all tests are visual. In addition, other traits such as intelligence and concentration also influence performance on any test.

Considering the RPAB, some of the tests are testing intelligence at least as much as perception: for example, the cube-copying test is identical to the block-design test of the Weschler Adult Intelligence Scale (WAIS). Others are concentrating upon visual neglect, and others assess the ability to sequence correctly. The whole test takes at least two hours to complete; this in itself being a good test of sustained concentration!

The solution is probably for everyone involved in neurological rehabilitation to be aware of, and sensitive to, the existence of complex perceptual disorders. Therefore, when a patient appears to have some disorder (for example, when he has disability which is not easily explained), more specific testing may be undertaken to investigate the specific impairment underlying the disability. The approach should be logical and diagnostic, and not simply to test everything. Help will often be needed from an expert psychologist.

Neglect

The phenomenon of neglect has been shown to be very complex, and it is difficult to be certain what any particular test is assessing. Indeed, neglect might be better referred to as selective inattention, and many patients are aggrieved at being told they are 'neglecting' their left side; arguing (reasonably) that they cannot neglect something they are not aware of.

Many single tests have been developed, such as copying drawings, drawing figures, line bisection, letter cancellation, and line cancellation (Albert's Test) (Albert 1973; Fullerton *et al.* 1986). It is apparent that, although these tests do seem to be measuring a single underlying construct, they vary in sensitivity (Halligan *et al.* 1989). There is now a test battery which includes tests of both impairment and disability. This is the Behavioural Inattention Test (BIT), which can be used by anyone.

Clinically, the Star-cancellation sub-test of the BIT is probably the most sensitive single test (Halligan *et al.* 1989). It is easy to perform, and only takes a few minutes. Alternatively, clinical testing for visual or tactile inattention (using double simultaneous stimulation) may be as useful. Although neglect is not synonymous with visual field defects (hemianopia or inattention), in practice most patients exhibiting neglect and other perceptual problems after stroke will have had visual and/or tactile inattention to double simultaneous stimulation at an earlier stage (Barer *et al.* 1990).

In conclusion, it is important to be aware that impairment of perception can occur, particularly when the right cerebral hemisphere is damaged, and that tests do exist to help detect and measure perceptual problems. However, these tests should be used selectively, and great care taken in interpreting any results. For screening purposes it may be best to use the Star-cancellation task, to test for hemianopia, and to test for visual and tactile inattention to double simultaneous stimuli.

Apraxia

Apraxia refers to an inability to undertake voluntarily complex movements in the presence of normal motor and sensory functioning. It is assumed that the brain cannot plan the correct sequence of movements. Like perceptual impairment, apraxia is very difficult to define operationally, and so is very difficult to measure (and to diagnose). Moreover, it is more often seen with left hemisphere lesions, and so is often associated with aphasia which makes assessment even more difficult.

There are many tests, but these usually consist of tasks intended to demonstrate apraxia and not to measure it. Indeed, one book devoted to the topic basically concluded that often diagnosis (and measurement?) depended upon an expert seeing the patient, the expert being someone who could recognize apraxia (Miller 1986).

Until more definite diagnostic criteria are available, it is going to be difficult to measure this possibly illusory phenomenon. Even the reliability of clinical recognition (diagnosis) of the phenomenon has yet to be established.

Problem-solving: intelligence

Measurement of IQ (Intelligence Quotient) is almost always undertaken by neuro-psychologists using the Weschler Adult Intelligence Scale (WAIS), a series of eleven tests divided into two groups measuring performance and verbal IQ. This test will not be discussed further, but the component items are shown in Section 4.

There are two tests available for more general use: Raven's Progressive Matrices, and Raven's Coloured Progressive Matrices (Raven 1960, 1965). These are tests for non-verbal problem-solving ability, which can be used by anyone, and the tables allow the results to be transformed into an approximate IQ. The tests take about 20 min to complete, and are simple to score.

In many patients with brain damage it is useful to have an estimate of their intelligence before injury. In the absence of any formal tests, there are two ways to deduce previous intelligence.

• take an educational history, noting what examinations were passed or failed;

• use a measure of vocabulary such as the New Adult Reading Test (NART) (Nelson and O'Connell 1978), and assesses the patient's knowledge of the pronunciation of increasingly unusual words.

The test is based on two assumptions: vocabulary is closely related to IQ; and vocabulary (past memory) is preserved after brain damage. To the best of the author's knowledge there have been no detailed studies to validate the use of the NART as a measure of pre-morbid IQ in younger patients with recent acquired brain damage.

Mood

Clinically there is a general acceptance (as yet unproven) that features, or adjectival descriptions, of the patient such as 'low motivation', 'depressed' and 'apathetic', probably have a major influence upon outcome. Consequently, it would seem of vital importance to be able to measure these phenomena. Unfortunately there are few measures available, partly because it is very difficult to define precisely what is to be measured.

The first difficulty arises in drawing a distinction between disabilities (observed maladaptive behaviours), and impairments and underlying presumed pathologies. The typical patient might, for example, not interact with others, may cry, and frequently make statements of hopelessness (for example, 'I'll never be able to work again'). These are behaviours at the level of disability. When asked, the patient may admit to feeling miserable, unhappy, etc. These are presumably the impairments underlying the disabilities. The whole syndrome might (or might not) warrant the label 'depression'. Three questions arise:

1. *Are these feelings in fact a realistic response to the situation, and hence not 'abnormal' at all?* This clinical decision is, in practice, very difficult, and no useful measures have been developed to help. Although increased 'misery' is associated with increased disability, the relationship is weak and does not 'explain' (or account for) most 'depression' (Wade *et al.* 1987*b*).

2. *Is there a single underlying change or phenomenon such as 'depression' or 'lack of motivation'?* If so, is it an impairment or a pathology? Alternatively, are many of the symptoms just isolated phenomena without any underlying cause? There are no easy or certain answers to these questions.

3. *Are the various problems seen a direct consequence of brain damage?* It is thought that euphoria seen in MS may be (Minden and Schiffer 1990) and emotionalism seen after stroke may also be (House *et al.* 1989*a*). However, it is unlikely that the majority of emotional disturbance can be attributed directly to specific, focal brain damage (see House 1987 and Minden and Schiffer 1990 for further reviews).

In practice, it is easiest to assume that there are unitary phenomena such as depression and anxiety, and that 'low motivation' and irritability are probably specific sub-types of these phenomena. Moreover, they are probably syndromes at the level of impairment and certainly sometimes arise as secondary, realistic reactions to the disability being experienced.

Most available measures have been developed in the field of psychiatry and many have recently been reviewed (Thompson 1989). Very few have been developed specifically for use with physically ill or disabled people. Almost all consist of a series of items relating to specific impairments that, taken together, comprise the underlying 'diagnosis'. For example, most depression inventories include questions on feeling unhappy, crying, difficulty in sleeping, and considering suicide. Further, most are designed primarily to assess the severity of the problem, rather than to detect the phenomenon.

One scale has been developed for use with medically ill, hospitalized patients: the Hospital Anxiety and Depression scale (HADs). It is designed to detect depression and anxiety. However, there are some who dispute its validity, and certainly there is insufficient evidence to support its uncritical use. None the less, using this questionnaire at least reminds the clinician (and the patient) that depression and other emotional problems need to be considered and discussed.

The General Health Questionnaire (GHQ) is a second measure which has been used to screen neurologically ill patients. It is a well-studied, widely-used measure and in its 28-question version is relatively short, easily administered (and commercially produced). Although often used with disabled patients, it has not had its validity assessed for such use. It has also been used to assess stress in carers (Carnwath and Johnson 1987; Wade *et al.* 1986*b*).

There are several other measures shown in this book which have been used in neurologically-disabled patients: the Beck inventory, the Wakefield self-assessment depression inventory, and the Hamilton inventory. Although all are valid measures of depression in a psychiatrically ill population, their use as diagnostic measures and as severity measures has not been fully established for a disabled population.

A different approach is to use a visual analogue scale, a line of fixed length (often 100 mm) with two extremes marked (for example, 'As depressed as I can imagine' and 'Not at all depressed'); the patient is asked to mark their present state on the line. This has been evaluated (Folstein and Luria 1973) only once, and doubts must remain concerning its validity. House *et al.* (1989*b*) found that many patients simply could not understand the scale, despite its apparent simplicity.

Specific measures of motivation do not exist. There are two indirect ways of assessing motivation:

1. Measure depression on the assumption that low motivation is simply one aspect of depression.
2. Use a so-called 'locus of control' measure which assesses the extent to which someone feels in control of their destiny. One such measure has been used recently (Partridge and Johnstone 1989).

Measures of other phenomena also exist. Probably the most common emotional disturbance experienced is, in fact, anxiety, not depression and self-assessment scales have been developed (Snaith *et al.* 1978, 1982). The author is unaware of any studies on neurologically disabled patients that have used these or similar scales.

Conclusions

Measurement of cognitive impairments is not easy. It is difficult to isolate, define, and measure agreed specific functions. Instead, most measures will be affected by impairments in several domains. At the same time, it is impossible to draw up a logically consistent, mutually exclusive system of categories of cognitive abilities.

There are some measures of orientation and learning, and of problem solving that are widely used, valid, and reliable. There are too many detailed tests of language, but only one clinically useful, valid reliable screening test (i.e. the Frenchay Aphasia Screening Test). Perceptual and motor planning deficits (for example, neglect and apraxia) probably cannot be assessed easily, using standard tests. Instead, it is important that they are considered and, if necessary, a detailed logical analysis of the problem should be undertaken by an expert.

Measurement of mood disturbance can be undertaken, using one of a range of scales, but interpretation of the result is difficult and may not be reliable. Separation of normal adjustment from abnormal mood states is difficult, and usually a matter of opinion. The physical disabilities also complicate interpretation of many questionnaires. At present evaluation of mood disturbance remains a subjective (clinical) process.

8 Personal physical disability

Summary

1. Activities of Daily Living (ADL) refer to the basic, physical functions which underlie normal living, such as continence, going to the toilet, dressing, and walking. Although developed empirically, there is evidence that ADL do represent a valid single construct.
2. Measures of ADL should record a person's actual performance, not their presumed potential ability.
3. Information should be collected in the most economic way possible, usually by questioning the patient and/or the carers.
4. ADL indices measure need for help, and can act as a check-list and as a measure of general progress. They cannot give specific details, for example, on the cause of dependence.
5. The Barthel ADL Index is recommended as the best one to use.
6. Mobility is of vital importance, and can be recorded simply by noting whether the patient can walk, or by counting the number of falls experienced.
7. There are several itemized scales or classification systems for measuring mobility, such as the Hauser categories and the Rivermead Mobility Index.
8. Measures of walking speed over 10 m or 6 min (for endurance) are extremely good measures, and grossly under-used.
9. Measures of arm function usually assess impairment of motor control, manual dexterity or a series of tasks involving both proximal and distal abilities. The Nine-hole Peg Test is the best single measure of manual dexterity.

Introduction

While it is true that achieving independence in basic activities of daily living, such as dressing and mobility, is not equivalent to complete success in rehabilitation, without this independence further progress is difficult. Consequently, many rehabilitation measures focus on activities of daily living (ADL). Indeed, some so-called 'quality of life' measures are also primarily concerned with ADL. This chapter reviews both measures of overall function, and measures of the major sub-components; mobility and arm function.

The first part of this chapter is centred on the Barthel ADL Index, shown on pp. 175–6, because this is recommended as the best measure available. (This choice is defended within this chapter.)

What are 'activities of daily living'?

The meaning of the phrase 'activities of daily living' (ADL) is perhaps one matter in rehabilitation where there is general agreement. There have been many reviews of ADL and its measures (for example, Donaldson *et al.* 1975; Deyo 1984; Law and Letts 1989; Eakin 1989; Barer and Nouri 1989). The core of ADL is usually established by looking at published measures and there is general agreement that the items shown in Table 8.1 constitute the activities of daily living; activities that everyone will need to accomplish every day (or at least every week with some items).

The activities shown in Table 8.1 are the ten activities covered in the Barthel ADL Index, and this is now probably the most widely used and best standard measure of ADL (Wade and Collin 1988). However there are variations in the activities included in different scales. Some ADL scales exclude continence (for example, the Nottingham Ten-point Scale) while others include simple domestic activities such as making a cold drink or snack (for example, the Rivermead ADL Scale).

The question 'Are activities of daily living a single construct, or are they an artificial, if convenient grouping?' arises because the concept of ADL

Table 8.1 Activities of Daily Living (ADL)

Impairments affecting ADL	Self-awareness	Arms	Legs
Disabilities			
Excretion			
Bowels	+		
Bladder	+		
Toiletting	+	+	+
Mobility			
Transfers		+	+
Wheelchair	(+)	+	
Walking			+
Stairs			+
Cleanliness			
Grooming	+	+	
Bathing	+	+	+
Feeding		+	
Dressing	+	+	+

has followed from the general development of scales, rather than being developed from any consistent theory or framework. It seems likely that ADL is in fact a valid unitary phenomenon. Studies which have analysed the component items of a scale do find that a single ADL factor emerges on factor analysis (Minderhout *et al.* 1984; Wade and Hewer 1987*a*; Norstrom and Thorslun 1991); ADL indices are not mixing chalk and cheese, as has been suggested. In addition, the scales have been developed in response to perceived clinical needs, and this greatly enhances their validity.

However, ADL scales often include items which could be considered impairments; in particular, continence. Moreover, to some extent, the items included depend upon each other. For example, independence in toiletting will generally require at least some independence in dressing. At the same time, different impairments can affect different activities, as illustrated in Table 8.1.

Therefore ADL scales are probably measuring a valid and important sphere, that of dependence upon others in fundamental (necessary) daily activities. They are certainly so well established (and also so useful) that it is now difficult to return to a theoretical framework to develop a more logical system.

Nevertheless, it is important to recognize the limitations of any ADL index; in other words, the things an ADL index does not measure:

- It does not measure, or identify, the reasons why patients fail to achieve tasks—there is no attempt to measure the underlying impairments and other measures should be used if this is wanted.

- It does not measure the other aspects of disability, such as communication, orientation, or domestic abilities. Other measures do this, and should therefore be used.

- It does not assess how someone achieves independence, but again this is not intended.

While these comments may seem obvious the author has included them because many people suggest that ADL measures are of no use for these reasons, and many other people attempt to devise 'better' measures that do achieve these ends. The author hopes that it is clear that simple measures of ADL independence have their uses but that they are not attempting to measure everything in one measure.

'Can or does' measurements

One issue frequently discussed is whether ADL scales should measure what someone does achieve, or what they can do (for example, Andrews and Stewart 1979). This should not be an issue. Disability measures should concentrate upon actual, observed behaviour and not potential abilities.

Just as when choosing a sports team, the sensible captain looks for people who have done well, not those who could or should do well. The same principle applies when assessing disability; emphasis should be placed upon what the patient does do, for this will determine the stress upon the carer, and not what they could, or should do.

Therefore, ADL indices should record actual performance in the relevant setting. The most appropriate setting is the patient's own home environment; but in a hospital or rehabilitation centre, the ward would seem the most appropriate area for assessing ADL. If there is a discrepancy between observed performance and expected ability, then it constitutes an opportunity for rehabilitation; it is not a failure of the index.

Sources of information

Information may be gathered by direct observation or indirectly, for example, through questioning relatives. Most research which has compared various ways of collecting information has found the results comparable whatever method is used (Sheikh *et al.* 1979; McGinnis *et al.* 1986; Collin *et al.* 1988), although patients with poor memory or insight may over-rate their abilities (Lincoln 1981). Therefore, in clinical practice, information can always be obtained by direct questioning, rather than observation. Moreover, questioning can be done by telephone or letter (Ebrahim *et al.* 1985), and can be directed to the patient, or relatives, or others.

The best clinical approach is to use the best source(s) of information available, including simple observation and common sense. Major discrepancies between stated behaviour and expected behaviour should be explored in more detail.

Use of ADL indices

All ADL indices in this book, and indeed almost all published ADL indices, are limited in the detail they give about a patient's actual abilities and problems. Consequently, many occupational therapists (OTs) and others consider ADL indices of little use, forgetting that different purposes require different measures.

Most ADL indices are in effect measuring the need for help, rather than a patient's positive abilities. To this end they are very pragmatic and can be useful in judging such matters as suitability for discharge, the ability to live alone, or the need for additional support. From the point of view of the carers, the main consideration is whether or not the patient needs any help; the precise nature of that help is often of secondary importance. Of course, some disabilities are especially stressing, particularly urinary incontinence (Sandford 1975), but identifying the exact level of stress is a clinical matter. The ADL index is a tool to help; it does not give absolute truth.

Therapists, on the other hand, are usually concerned with two other questions: why is the disability present and what can be done to remedy the matter? ADL indices cannot answer these questions, nor should they; they can detect (diagnose) the presence of a problem and crudely measure its severity, but no more. In addition, therapists are often concerned (correctly) that items within ADL indices are not sufficiently sensitive to monitor response to specific therapy directed at a particular disability, such as dressing. In such instances, a therapist should either find a specific measure (rarely available), or measure the activity directly.

There are many other possible uses for an ADL index, such as studying the performance of a service or identifying population need (Hanley and McAndrew 1987).

One last, vital, often contentious matter, needs discussion: how is the data collected to be used? The problem of misuse of data is present with every measure, but seems to generate most concern when discussing ADL indices. For example, some people feel that collection of data will encourage doctors to discharge patients who do not show progress, or who have reached some threshold; or that managers will judge a service on the rate of change seen over time.

Interpretation of data is always the responsibility of the individual using the data, but it is the responsibility of professionals to draw attention to factors which must be considered when making an interpretation:

- Almost all ADL indices provide ordinal data. Consequently changes in score cannot be compared, for example, between different centres.
- Changes can only be interpreted in the light of the patients being studied; information on prognostic factors is vital.

The response to potential misinterpretation is not to refuse to collect data, but to collect all relevant data and to offer an explanation of any results.

In summary, *ADL indices can*:

- monitor progress within a rehabilitation programme
- measure overall dependency, for example, for discharge or admission
- act as a simple check-list, for example, in surveys or follow-up

but *ADL indices can not*:

- determine the cause of dependence
- measure detailed changes in specific items
- guide specific treatment approaches

Interpretation of data provided by ADL indices requires:

- an appreciation of the ordinal properties of the scale

- knowledge on the way data was collected
- an understanding of all relevant circumstances

Choice of ADL index

There are certainly hundreds, if not thousands of ADL indices in use around the world, and there are certainly tens, if not hundreds of researched, published ADL indices; Feinstein *et al.* (1986) identified 43. Choice is therefore difficult. There have been very few studies which have compared two (or more) ADL indices, and there are no standard measures available to form a useful basis for making the choice.

The author would strongly recommend the use of the standard Barthel ADL Index as shown in this book and published with guide-lines (Collin *et al.* 1988). The reasons have been argued in detail (Wade and Collin 1988), and so only a summary will be given here.

The Barthel ADL Index includes ten most common areas included within ADL scales, and specifically covers continence of bowels and bladder, which some indices omit. Therefore, it is at least as useful as any other index, and more useful than those which exclude continence (for example, the Rivermead ADL Index) given the stress incontinence can cause to carers.

Its validity has been well-established. The score correlates with clinical impression; with motor loss after stroke; and with scores on other ADL indices. As expected, a low score predicts a low likelihood of discharge home; a less good outcome after stroke; and a lower level of social, domestic and leisure activities.

Although not perfectly reliable, its reliability has been studied in several ways and settings, including within a rehabilitation setting. It is reliable on test–retest, between observers, whether asked or observed, on telephone use, and in different settings. In practice, a difference of 4/20 points or more will usually reflect a real difference; smaller differences might arise from errors.

It is extremely simple to use and, for most patients it takes no more than two or three minutes to complete. The scoring is simple, and it can be presented in a way easy to score repeatedly.

Its sensitivity is limited in two ways:

- It has definite floor and more importantly, ceiling effects (however, this is inherent to any ADL index, and simply requires the use of other measures when appropriate).

- It is insensitive to small differences and some efforts have been made to improve sensitivity (for example, Granger *et al.* 1979; Shah *et al.* 1990).

However, such modified indices are likely to be less reliable (thus losing the apparent sensitivity) and they are more complex.

The score is easily communicated, and as the Barthel index is now the most widely-used ADL index, the score is likely to be understood. The original scoring was 0–100, in five point increments. This gives an impression of great sensitivity, and it seems more honest to use a 0–20 score which can always be multiplied up if percentage scores seem better.

There is one specific problem: there has been a proliferation of 'Barthel' indices such that the word has almost become synonymous with ADL. It is important to identify which Barthel ADL index is being used, and the author hopes (naturally) that the simple one shown in this book is used. The guide-lines given here have been tested, although they differ a little from the original guide-lines (which had not been tested).

Included within this book are two types of competing indices. The first group are the straight competitors such as the Katz ADL Index, the Northwick Park ADL Index, and the Nottingham Ten-point Index. One study comparing the Kenny, Katz, and Barthel indices concluded that the Barthel was probably the 'best buy' (Gresham *et al.* 1980). Second, there are also more comprehensive measures which include ADL items among a very wide range of items. Two such scales are the Sickness Impact Profile, and the Functional Independence Measure.

It is the author's hope that in future the Barthel index will be tested against other measures, so that the relative merits of different indices can be established, and also that improved versions of the Barthel index may be developed, but within the following constraints.

• Specific guide-lines that are used in any new version are published.
• Comparison is made between the basic Barthel and the new version, so that such matters as reliability, simplicity, and sensitivity, are compared.

Moreover, a way of converting and comparing scores should be given. Eventually it may become necessary to refer to the specific version of the Barthel ADL index being used.

Mobility

Loss of normal mobility is of crucial importance. To most individual patients, it is perhaps the one ability on which they place the most stress (Chiou and Burnett 1985). This is perhaps quite understandable given the minimal allowance made in most public areas for people who have restricted mobility. Also, poor mobility is the most common single disability seen in the community (Martin *et al.* 1988).

One problem exists with most measures of mobility; they concentrate upon 'normal' mobility, in other words they measure the use of legs. There are, to the best of the author's knowledge, no well standardized measures of mobility which include the use of other means of getting about, notably wheelchairs. On the other hand, more general measures of functioning, such as the Nottingham Extended ADL Index or the Frenchay Activities Index do not specify how activities are carried out. Therefore they do indirectly measure mobility achieved in alternative ways.

Some specific measures are discussed below, but there are other obvious ways of measuring mobility that should not be overlooked. Medical notes, for example, rarely record even the simple observation of whether the patient can walk. A record of the number of falls experienced in a set time-interval is another important way of measuring mobility.

Finally, one should note what aids and equipment are used (including nearby furniture and people), and recognize that mobility items do feature in all ADL indices.

Categories and itemized scales

There are various systematic classifications, usually based upon the amount of personal help required. The Functional Ambulation Categories (FAC) form one useful system, designed for use in therapeutic environments, which records the amount of personal assistance needed. The Hauser index was developed for use in a trial of treatment for MS, and measures mobility away from the therapeutic environment. These measures are simple, but of limited sensitivity. Subsections of many global disability measures concentrate upon mobility, for example the OPCS scales and the Functional Limitations Profile.

More recently, a specific index aiming to measure mobility has been developed—the Rivermead Mobility Index. This concentrates upon those aspects of mobility that are 'fundamental', in other words it concentrates upon activities that most people will undertake if they possibly can. Walking, or going up stairs, are two such examples.

A second index was originally devised that concentrated upon other aspects of mobility which are more elective or personal (i.e. some people do not undertake an activity, even though they could if they wished). Shopping and gardening are two such examples. The development study showed that only the index of fundamental mobility was reliable.

Another recently developed scale is the Gait Abnormality Rating Scale. This concentrates upon describing underlying impairments and the visual appearance of walking (Wolfson et al. 1990). This scale seems to offer no advantages, and is therefore not reproduced in this book.

Timed walking tests

Mobility implies moving from place to place. Consequently the time taken
to move a certain distance can be measured, and it is surprising how rarely
people time their patients walking over a set distance. There are two types of
timed measure:

- that over a short distance (2–20 m); and
- that over a longer time (2–12 min), which measures endurance and
  cardiorespiratory fitness.

The 10-m timed walk is remarkably simple, reliable, valid, sensitive,
communicable, useful, and relevant—almost the perfect measure! It in-
volves asking the patient to walk over a set distance (5 m and return, or
10 m) at their own preferred speed, using their own preferred aid (including
personal support if wished); the help used should be recorded. A brief
review will be given.

Validity has been established in many studies, albeit often unintentionally.
Gait speed relates strongly to other measures such as cadence and stride
length (Goldfarb and Simon 1984; Bohannon, 1989c), balance (Bohannon
1989b), Functional Ambulation Categories (Holden et al. 1984), clinical
assessment of gait pattern (Wade et al. 1987a; Wolfson et al. 1990), use of
walking aids (Holden et al. 1986; Wade et al. 1987a), falls (Wolfson et al.
1990), and extent of personal mobility (May et al. 1985). It is related to
strength in the leg (Goldfarb and Simon 1984; Bohannon and Andrews 1990).

Reliability has also been established in many studies, both for test–retest
and between observers (Holden et al. 1984; Wade et al. 1987a: Bohannon
and Andrews 1990). However, it is worth noting that the high correlation
coefficient ($r = >0.95$) hides considerable individual patient variability, of
the order of 20 per cent (Collen et al. 1990). Moreover, it is important to
give consistent directions to the patient, because overt encouragement can
increase speed (Guyatt et al. 1984).

Simplicity is obvious. All that is needed is a stop-watch and a 10-m space.
Indeed, a 5-metre space within a house can suffice (5 m and return), meaning that walking speed can be a useful outcome measure in domiciliary
settings (Collen et al. 1990).

Sensitivity is reasonable. There is an obvious ceiling effect once the
patient has reached normal walking speed, but it is possible then to consider
measuring running speed or endurance. Measurement of gait speed has
detected the beneficial effects of Ankle Foot Orthoses (Corcoran et al.
1970), and operations to correct abnormal foot posture in cerebral palsy
(Shapiro et al. 1990). Results can be presented as speed, but in practice the
time taken to cover 10 m is more easily understood.

The main criticism levelled against speed is that it is more important to
assess the 'quality' of the gait. Unfortunately, quality cannot be measured

reliably (Goodkin and Diller 1972). Moreover, it is likely that good quality is associated with greater speed (Wade *et al.* 1987*a*). Lastly, the patient is probably more concerned to get from A to B than in the quality of his or her gait (although in the long-term a grossly abnormal gait pattern may increase the risk of falls or the development of arthritis).

There are minor variations on the 10-m timed walk; for example, using a 5-m walk with return, or, as often used with patients with Parkinson's disease, a 20-m walk (10 m, turn, 10 m). A third variation is to use much shorter walks with electronic timing. However, shorter walks are probably unreliable if timed using a stop-watch.

Endurance is also important, and is best measured by asking the patient to walk for a set time, and then recording the distance covered in that time (and when the patient stopped, if before completion). Three different times have been compared: 2, 6, and 12 min, and all give similar information (Butland *et al.* 1982; Lipkin *et al.* 1986). The best compromise is probably to use the 6-min walk test, giving standard instructions to ensure reliability (Guyatt *et al.* 1984). The 6-min test has been used to evaluate the British mobility allowance (Hunter 1986).

There are many papers reporting studies of gait speed in the normal population (Cunningham *et al.* 1982; Wade *et al.* 1987*a*; Bendall *et al.* 1989).

Other measures of gait

Clinically feasible ways of measuring cadence and stride length have been described (Robinson and Smidt 1981), and there are many, much more sophisticated ways, of assessing gait. Indeed there are gait analysis laboratories. The clinical utility of any of the information provided must be seriously questioned. The money spent is probably wasted, except in the context of well-designed research projects.

The 'step–second' test has been used in research on Parkinson's disease. The patient is asked to rise from a chair, walk 5 m, turn, and return to the chair and sit down again. The observer times the patient from rising to sitting, while counting the number of steps taken. The two figures are multiplied to obtain 'step–seconds' (Webster 1968) and normal people are said to score between 50–100, with scores in Parkinson's disease extending from 100–500 or more. Although this seems, potentially, a simple, sensitive test for use in Parkinson's disease, the author is not aware that reliability has been evaluated, or that it has been simply compared with measuring speed.

Arm disability

The measurement of 'arm function' initially seems difficult because the arm and hand have so many uses from gesture through balance, gross strength-related functions and on to fine manual dexterity. Many of these functions have not been measured in any detail. However, there are good measures available. The topic of measuring arm function has recently been reviewed (Wade 1989), and this section reiterates the main points.

The available measures can be divided into three main groups:

- voluntary motor control (i.e. focal impairment);
- those of specific arm abilities (i.e. focal disability); and
- those of general abilities which usually depend upon well-preserved use of the arm.

Measures of impairment

Many of the tests used to assess arm function are measures of impairment. None the less they are useful in two ways. First, some such as motor control, relate quite closely to disability, and second, measures of impairment can also give useful prognostic information.

Measures of voluntary motor control are often useful as measures of arm disability. The arm section of the Motricity Index relates closely to most other measures of disability in the arm (Parker *et al.* 1987), and is almost as sensitive in detecting change after stroke (Sunderland *et al.* 1989). The sections of other motor assessments which relate to the arm can also be used; for example, the Motor Club Assessment, or the Brunnstrom–Fugl-Meyer assessment (Fugl-Meyer *et al.* 1975; DeWeerdt and Harrison 1985). Indeed, one study of recovery after stroke has simply recorded the range of voluntary movement (Bard and Hirschberg 1965). However, this study probably only recorded the early stages of recovery of voluntary power.

Other measures of motor control include dynamometry to study strength at various joints (Bohannon and Andrews 1987*a,b*), and grip strength (Kellor *et al.* 1971; Mathiowitz *et al.* 1975). Grip strength is useful prognostically, after stroke (Heller *et al.* 1987; Sunderland *et al.* 1989), and is probably a sensitive measure of recovery able to span the whole range of recovery (Sunderland *et al.* 1989). Incidentally, grip strength also predicts mortality in the elderly (Philips 1986).

Measures of focal disability

One approach to testing arm disability is to measure (in detail) the patient's performance on one single skill. Three tests are discussed: peg tests, tapping tests, and the 'box and block' test.

The various peg tests (see Section 4) all involve timing the patient's performance at placing (and/or removing) a set number of pegs into holes. Their advantages are their simplicity, coupled with their potential to be sensitive measures, particularly at the upper range of ability and in the later stages of recovery (Sunderland *et al.* 1989). They are also useful for measuring the disabling effects of sensory loss and ataxia, two impairments which are difficult to measure in isolation.

Peg tests have limitations. They concentrate upon manual dexterity, and thus cannot detect loss of proximal strength. They may be affected by major cognitive problems, such as neglect. They cannot measure gradations of moderate to severe disability, having a relatively high floor level of performance.

The Nine-hole Peg Test (NHPT) is described in Section 4, and is probably as good as any other test, and has the advantage of simplicity. The Ten-hole Peg Test (Annett and Kilshaw 1983) is an alternative, and forms part of a test battery (Turton and Fraser 1986).

A second approach, which is sometimes considered, is to measure tapping speed, usually using the index finger. This is simple, but it seems to be unreliable (Heller *et al.* 1987), probably because it is affected greatly by motivation. Tapping tests cannot be recommended.

The 'box and block test' is a timed test of transferring blocks from one part of a box to another (Mathiowitz *et al.* 1985). It has been used in studying deterioration in multiple sclerosis (Goodkin *et al.* 1988).

Test batteries

There are many test batteries which contain a greater or lesser number of individual items. The Action Research Armtest (ARA), an abbreviated form of a test battery first devised in 1965 (Carrol 1965) assesses proximal and distal strength and dexterity. The Frenchay Arm Test (FAT) assesses proximal control and dexterity. The Cambridge test battery (Turton and Fraser 1986) assesses impairment and manual dexterity. The Jebsen test battery, originally devised for use with patients suffering arthritis, primarily assesses hand function (Jebsen *et al.* 1969). It has been used after stroke (Spaulding *et al.* 1988).

There have been a few studies comparing the utility of the different measures in different circumstances. DeWeerdt and Harrison (1985) compared the ARA with a test of impairment (the Brunnstrom–Fugl-Meyer (BFM) assessment): the results were closely correlated, but the ARA usually took less time to administer. Sunderland *et al.* (1989) compared the Motricity Index, Motor Club Assessment, Frenchay Arm Test, NHPT, and grip strength; all gave similar results, but grip strength was best. Another study compared the original Frenchay Arm Test (De Souza *et al.* 1980) with the BFM (Berglund and Fugl-Meyer 1986), and found a very close correlation between results.

Conclusion

Activities of Daily Living are a single construct, and in practice form the focus of much rehabilitation. The best single measure for general use is the Barthel ADL Index. More detailed information on mobility is best obtained through timing walking over 10 metres, and using the Rivermead Mobility Index.

Manual dexterity, the other important component of ADL, is easily measured using the Nine-hole Peg Test. Measurement of grip strength is a second good measure that is able to detect the early stages of recovery, for example after stroke.

9 Global disability measures, extended ADL, and social interaction

Summary

1. There are several well-developed comprehensive measures of disability, including the Sickness Impact Profile, the OPCS disability scales, and the Functional Independence Measure.
2. There are few well-developed extended ADL measures, sometimes known as Instrumental ADL measures. Three indices which have been well studied are the Nottingham Extended ADL Index, the Rivermead ADL Index and the Frenchay Activities Index.
3. Disturbances of (disabilities in) social interaction are often referred to as behavioural problems, and the few measures available are largely derived from studies on head injury.
4. In studying clinical interventions it is necessary to use measures specific to the patient's problem(s), which often means developing measures for use with that patient.

Introduction

Rehabilitation is not simply concerned with achieving independence in personal activities of daily living. Ideally, it should also consider all other aspects of disability, such as communication, social interaction, domestic activities, work, leisure, etc. Assessment of communication is discussed in Chapter 7.

The phrase 'instrumental ADL' (IADL) has been coined to cover such activities as cooking, shopping, housework, and work. The author is not sure of the derivation of this phrase, nor does he know whether it has been defined in terms of activities included or excluded. For these reasons he feels the phrase 'Extended ADL' (EADL) is better, because it uses the word 'extended', which is clear in its meaning.

This chapter discusses a few measures which attempt to cover all aspects of disability. It also discusses the measurement of extended activities of daily living, and some other aspects of disability not already covered. It also discusses the use of questionnaires to ascertain disability, and the problem of measuring very specific areas of function in single-case studies (whether for research or in clinical practice).

Global measures of disability

There are many more or less comprehensive measures of disability which cover most activities. One has already been mentioned—the WHO ICIDH. Although this is primarily a classification system, an optional method of measuring severity is included. Only one study has investigated the reliability of its severity ratings, finding them reasonably reliable (Van den Berg and Lankhorst 1990). Until further studies evaluate this measure, it is probably best to use other measures.

A good example of a well-evaluated global measure is the Sickness Impact Profile, or Functional Limitations Profile. This profile not only covers 12 different areas of function, using 138 questions, but it also gives a weighted score to each item. Though the profile must take an hour or so to complete, it can be used to give a good measure of the level of disability. It has been used in a community study (Charlton 1989).

Another well-developed measure designed to cover all aspects of disability is that used by the British Office of Population Censuses and Surveys (OPCS) in their survey of the levels of disability in the community (Martin *et al*. 1988). Their measures have several advantages. They have been given weighted scores, which allows different disabilities to be compared. Further, an overall severity score can be calculated. It has been used in one large national survey, and so any findings can be interpreted in the context of a national prevalence survey. Lastly, the scales have been adapted for use with children (not reproduced in this book).

The main limitation of the OPCS scales is that they cover activities that are definitely at the disability end of the spectrum (disability–extended disability–handicap). This follows on from the requirements of its original use, which was to aid the development of governmental policies towards the disabled. Governments naturally want measures which minimize environmental influences (because these are expensive to remedy, and often politically sensitive).

A third measure, which is not used much in the UK, but which is possibly widely used in the US, is the Functional Independence Measure. This is intended to be used as a standard assessment within rehabilitation centres, so that comparisons can be made. Its reliability has been established for use with four level responses, but not for the seven level responses.

A fourth measure is the PULSES profile. This has been used in a rehabilitation network (Granger and McNamara 1984). It is a simple classification system, but it mixes disability with impairment.

Other measures exist, but the first three mentioned above are probably as good as (if not better than) most others. However, most people will probably want measures of more limited areas, such as domestic abilities, or work. Measures of extended ADL abilities will be discussed next.

Measuring extended ADL

As one moves away from personal ADL, it becomes increasingly difficult to classify or categorize activities undertaken. In addition, an increasingly large range of impairments can influence these more complex activities and personal choice and circumstances play a much larger role. Indeed, it is, in practice, difficult to decide whether problems with some aspects of extended ADL constitute disabilities or handicaps, or whether activities such as cooking are ADL or EADL.

Recent research suggests that there is a separation between ADL and EADL, and that bathing is probably part of EADL (Norstrom and Thorslund 1991). This finding is not too surprising, because there is a much greater influence of choice (one can live without regular baths) and because the environment has a considerable influence (for example, use of showers, provision of bath aids). In addition, it is the most complex (difficult) activity within Barthel ADL Index (Wade and Hewer 1987*a*). Despite the evidence that bathing may be more appropriately placed within EADL, it should remain within ADL indices if only because it is too late to alter tradition.

The items to be included within EADL are less well agreed. In a recent review, Barer and Nouri (1989) identified the activities shown in Table 9.1 as being usually included in EADL indices. (The author has moved 'making a hot drink' into EADL.) They identified five EADL measures, two of which are discussed below: they classified the Rivermead ADL Index as an ADL index.

Three relatively short measures of EADL are:

- the Nottingham Extended ADL Index, which has four subsections (mobility, domestic, kitchen, leisure);
- the second part of the Rivermead ADL Index; and
- the Frenchay Activities Index (FAI).

Table 9.1 Items included within Extended ADL (Barer and Nouri 1989)

Getting about	Household activities	Other activities
Carrying a hot drink	Washing up	Gardening
Walking outside	Washing clothes	Managing money
Crossing roads	Housework	Going out socially
Getting in/out of the car	Shopping	Employment/work
Using public transport	Making hot drinks/snack	Hobbies/leisure
Driving a car		Reading
		Using the telephone
		Writing

The first two were developed as hierarchical scales with many pass–fail items covering such domestic activities as cooking and shopping. They are sufficiently short, simple, and reliable enough to encourage use of all items. The Frenchay Activities Index is a 15-item questionnaire covering mainly domestic, leisure, and social activities, but including work. It can easily be used in clinical practice.

An alternative approach to the assessment of EADL is to use the appropriate sections from the comprehensive measures already reviewed.

Social interaction

In practice it is often patients' personalities which determine their success in living outside institutional care: family or other carers will do almost anything for someone who is 'nice', but will only give minimal assistance to someone who is 'difficult' or in other ways unrewarding to help. Oddly, although this is widely known, it is rarely admitted openly and there are few useful measures. This is reminiscent of the status of motivation, another important unmeasurable factor.

Patients with poor social interaction are often referred to as having 'behaviour problems'. These problems are difficult to characterize and within the model described earlier they are really inappropriately named 'behavioural difficulties'. In practice, the problems relate largely to social interaction, and the difficulties may be positive (for example, aggression), or negative (for example, withdrawal).

Social interaction is most commonly disturbed after closed head injury, and it is specialists in this field who have developed the most measures. However, similar difficulties must be faced in the fields of mental illness and mental handicap but the author has not yet found any useful, well-developed measures from those fields.

Aggression is perhaps the most disturbing abnormality in social interaction. A clinically usable scale (the Agitated Behaviour Scale) has recently been published, with some evidence as to its validity, reliability, and sensitivity to change after head injury. It was developed for use with patients still confused and in post-traumatic amnesia.

Two other measures have been used to study patients after head injury: the Behavioural Rating Scale, which covers 28 different social behaviours; and the Katz Adjustment Scale which measures changes in behaviour noted by relatives, and samples 127 different personality characteristics. The Social Functioning Exam has been used after stroke (Starr *et al.* 1983) and the original study investigated reliability and validity. The author is unaware of any further use of this scale.

An alternative method of measuring social interaction and changed behaviour is to use visual analogue scales, with the items being different aspects of behaviour. The end points can be whatever characteristics are of interest. There have not been any good studies investigating the validity or reliability of this technique, but it has the great virtues of being simple and direct as well as being tailored to the area of interest (to the investigator).

Communication is an important component of social interaction. Some measures focusing on the impairment of aphasia have already been discussed. There are no well-developed measures of the ability to communicate *per se*, but the Speech Questionnaire is probably the nearest measure available.

Specific disabilities—single-case studies

In clinical practice, and also in much rehabilitation research, the main emphasis is upon ameliorating specific problems faced by an individual patient. Naturally the treatment is also individual. It is important to determine whether or not the treatment is helping.

The design of single-case investigations is still in its infancy, but good textbooks are available outlining the possibilities (Barlow and Hersen 1984). In essence, the investigator or therapist needs to establish an initial steady state in at least the item being studied (and usually in some 'control' items). The steady state can include a regular improvement or decline. Only then is the intervention carried out.

Sunderland (1990) suggests the following steps be taken when undertaking single-case studies:

- select and investigate methods of serial assessment
- select an experimental design
- decide what will determine the boundaries between (for example) treatment and no treatment
- complete a written protocol
- perform the experiment, recording any uncontrolled external events
- perform a graphical analysis
- only undertake numerical analysis if graphs fail; and
- repeat the study

Notice that the first step is to 'select and investigate methods of serial assessment'. In other words, all designs depend crucially upon measurement, but in fact it will often not be appropriate to use one of the measures described in this book. The essence of any study on an individual is that a very specific impairment or disability is being investigated, and most measures are not sufficiently specific to apply to the individual. Therefore, therapists often need to develop their own measure. For example, if the intervention is supposed to teach someone how to put on an item of clothing, then the measure must record the ability to put on that item.

None the less, the therapist should remember the following principles:

- Consider the available measures, for example, recording gait speed might be appropriate in many treatments of walking disability.
- Always consider timing an activity, as this gives much greater sensitivity.
- At least one outcome measure should be at the level of disability; patients and their carers most appreciate a reduction in disability.
- It is important to consider reliability and bias in measurement, and it may be best for one unbiased investigator to undertake all assessments.

Conclusions

There are several reasonable measures which succeed to a greater or lesser extent in sampling all aspects of disability. Extended ADL probably includes mobility outside the home, household activities, and miscellaneous other activities. There are some measures of extended ADL. There are few well-developed measures of social interaction, and it would be worth developing some simple measures for use, for example, in head injury rehabilitation. Specific measures for use in studying the single patient will often need to be developed for use with the particular patient.

10 Handicap and quality of life

Summary

1. Defining handicap is difficult, but one way is to consider it similar to 'quality of life'.
2. The International Classification of Impairments, Disabilities, and Handicaps (ICIDH) suggests six areas of handicap, but the validity of this categorization and the reliability of the grading of severity have not been tested.
3. Measuring handicap using other measures means comparing expected with observed results, but it can be difficult to establish an expected level.
4. Measures which could be used include the Nottingham Health Profile, and the Rankin Score.
5. The environment has a major impact upon handicap, but there are no well developed measures of environmental support or obstacles.
6. Quality of life measures have been developed, but in the absence of a good theoretical framework, they are probably faulty. In practice, most record disability.
7. Quality of life probably refers to the patient's reaction to the discrepancy between actual and expected achievements arising as a consequence of illness.
8. Quality Adjusted Life Years (QALYs) are, at best, Disability Adjusted Life Years (DALYs) and are probably both invalid and unreliable.

Introduction

The ICIDH defines handicap as 'a disadvantage for a given individual, resulting from impairment or disability, that limits or prevents the fulfilment of a role that is normal (depending upon age, sex, and social and cultural factors) for that individual'.

There are two major differences between disability and handicap. The first relates to the metric (standard) used to measure severity. For disability, the frame is usually the abilities of all other comparable humans with some allowance for age, gender, and other demographic features. Handicap, on the other hand, is judged with reference to the expectations of the specific individual patient with some reference to the expectations of the limited group of people occupying the same cultural, social, economic, and physical environment as the subject. Consequently there is no absolute against which to judge handicap, and this leads to great difficulties when trying to measure it.

The second difference is in the level of abstraction. Disabilities refer to skills, actions, and behaviours which can be observed directly, such as working as a doctor, cooking food, shopping, taking part in games of tennis, etc.

Handicaps relate to the social roles which are restricted, such as no longer able to work, the ability to run the home and enjoyment of leisure being reduced, no longer being the main breadwinner, etc.

Another way of considering handicap is to consider it as referring to the change in a patient's quality of life. Quality of life is an ill-defined, nebulous concept with many meanings, but in essence it probably refers to the emotional or personal response of a patient to the perceived difference between their actual and desired activities. Yet another way is to equate handicap with loss of autonomy or freedom of action.

This chapter reviews the problems of measuring handicap and quality of life. Given the difficulty in defining these concepts, it was difficult to know what to include. However, this chapter does discuss measures of social activity and measures of adjustment, as well as measures of handicap.

Handicap: the ICIDH measures

The ICIDH identifies six 'survival roles', and gives a nine-point scale of severity for each:

- orientation
- physical independence
- mobility
- occupation of time
- social integration
- economic self-sufficiency

This classification warrants further study and development but unfortunately it is not really developed well enough for research use at present. There are no studies to support its validity as a systematic categorization, nor to support the reliability of the grades proposed. However, clinical experience suggests that it is easy to use once one knows a patient reasonably well (for example, after a one-hour interview).

Other handicap measures

A few other measures do, to a greater or lesser extent, assess handicap. However, as stressed in Chapter 9, it is often difficult to separate the extreme end of the spectrum of disability from handicap.

Whatever measure is used to 'measure' actual handicap, it should be necessary to compare 'expected' performance with actual performance. The expected performance could be the results on the measure which held before the onset of the illness. This has been done for stroke (Ahlsio *et al*. 1984; Wade *et al*. 1985; Viitanen *et al*. 1988), and could apply to many illnesses starting in adult life. However, it is particularly difficult to establish the extent of handicap in a condition which arises at birth or during development, or indeed in any illness which spans any period of significant change in life-style (for example, at the time of retirement).

Available measures include two which are discussed in Chapter 9 (the Frenchay Activities Index (FAI) and the Nottingham extended ADL index), and three others: the Life Satisfaction Index (LSI), the Nottingham Health Profile (NHP), and the Rankin Scale. Each has been tested for reliability to an extent, and each is simple. They were developed independently of the WHO ICIDH framework, and include items from different areas of handicap, and items more usually termed 'disabilities'.

The LSI started with 20 items, but has been reduced to 13. Many studies have investigated or used the LSI, but its validity is not proven. The NHP has 38 questions covering sleep, pain, emotion, energy, social isolation, and mobility. Using weighted scores to give a 0–100 scale, the NHP is similar to the more traditional quality of life scale with all the problems already discussed. However, it has been used as a measure of quality of life after stroke (Ebrahim *et al*. 1986). The Rankin is the simplest index, having only six categories, but it is also the worst:

- it is inherently insensitive;
- it mixes objective and subjective items;
- it spans impairment, disability and handicap.

However, it does have the two great virtues of simplicity and reliability, making it ideal for large multicentre trials.

Another measure, not yet used in neurological rehabilitation, is the Edinburgh Rehabilitation Status Scale (ERSS) (Affleck *et al*. 1988). This covers four dimensions:

- independence (and need for support);
- activity (and inactivity);
- social integration (and isolation); and
- the effects of current symptoms on life-style.

At present its utility has not been proved.

Finally, stress on the carer is an important aspect of the quality of life and can be measured using the GHQ, or other measure of emotional upset. There is one specific measure, the Caregiver Strain Index. Changes in family income could also be used as a measure.

Environmental measurement

When measuring handicap, it is likely to be necessary to assess the environment because any handicap arises from the interaction between the patient's disability and the environment. This will include not only obvious physical influences, such as the structure of the house or the accessibility of public buildings to people in wheelchairs, but many other influences such as public attitudes, financial allowances, the law, the economic climate, etc.

Clinically, it is important to consider these influences because they might be amenable to change. For example, someone who cannot walk might obtain a mobility allowance in order to buy a car. For clinical purposes, a simple screening system reminding the clinician of major areas will be needed.

In research, or other evaluations involving large groups of patients, the need is for some method of making allowance for the wide variation of environments patients come from. For example, after stroke one hospital might return 90 per cent of survivors to their own homes, whereas another might only achieve 75 per cent. One influence, easily accounted for, will be stroke severity (i.e. disability). More importantly, the social background will have a major influence—one hospital might only take private patients who will usually be wealthy, whereas the other might be in a deprived, inner city area.

The author is unaware of any well-researched measures which have been used in either context, beyond simply recording single items (such as number living alone). Some suggested clinical measures are given in Section 4.

Quality of life

We all think we know what we mean by the quality of life, but no-one can define it. And without a definition, it is impossible to measure it. Many articles have been written about measuring the quality of life, and useful entries to the field include two issues of the *Journal of Chronic Diseases* (1987, **40** No. 6, and 1987, **40**, Suppl. 1) and two recent reviews (Mor and Guadagnoli 1988; Van Knippenberg and De Haes 1988). Many research studies involving quality of life assessments have been reported, most considering patients with cancer or other progressive diseases with a poor prognosis. There are relatively few in the field of neurological disability.

Assessments of quality of life have been used in two main ways:

- to judge the clinical value of treatments which involve significant risk and side effects, such as treatments for cancer; and
- to evaluate different health interventions from an economic point of view.

In the latter role, the measures are used to define Quality Adjusted Life Years (QALYs) which are proposed as one way of allocating health resources, though not without disagreement (Smith 1987).

Measuring quality of life

Most assessments of the quality of life are based on the assumption that there is a unidimensional construct, a 'state of health' (or 'quality of life') which can be measured. Two problems arise:

- how are different states of health compared?; and
- is there a single underlying construct at all?

One approach to valuing different health states is as follows:

The investigator posits a range of states of illness, usually about 10 states, and usually based upon a single progressive disease. These are then presented to individuals who are asked to rank them in order, and in relation to two anchor points— usually death and perfect health. Sometimes subjects are asked to trade between different components of quality of life, such as a shorter life but one free of pain (Torrance 1987).

The method allows states worse than death, such as prolonged coma or severe pain. The 'value' of each state is then calculated as a score between 0 (death) and 1 (perfect health), sometimes with negative values (worse than death).

This method was used by Rosser and Kind (1978), and is similar to the method used by the OPCS to give weights to different types of disability (Martin *et al.* 1988). The patient is then categorized into one of the states and a weight given. In practice, most such scales are strongly based on physical disability.

A second approach is to construct a multi-item index including component items that are thought to contribute to or affect the quality of life. Within any scale, each component needs to be given a weight reflecting its contribution, also often achieved using a utility or trade-off approach. However, many factors must influence the quality of life. There is often great variation in the nature and importance of the contributing variables between individual subjects. Consequently it is unlikely that any composite scale will be reliable and valid.

A third approach is to ask the patient directly. This has been undertaken for stroke, although only in a study of natural history (Viitanen *et al.* 1988).

Problems measuring quality of life

All attempts to measure quality of life suffer several fundamental flaws. First, although the individual members of the judging panels needed to attribute weights to different health (or disability) states do sometimes achieve good agreement, the members have often been very selected people, typically of higher social class and familiar with health care or illness.

Second, most scales focus on physical disability, and there is certainly no obvious similarity between different measures purportedly measuring the same phenomenon. Many measures have been used to assess quality of life, some developed specifically for the purpose and others simply being interpreted as measuring quality of life. Examples include the Karnofsky Index, the QL-index, the Nottingham Health Profile and the Life Satisfaction Index. Simple inspection of these four indices will reveal the wide differences between different measures all of which are supposedly measuring the same phenomenon, therefore it seems unlikely that there is a unified underlying construct. This was also noted in a recent paper which compared three measures and again noted they had very different component items (Read *et al.* 1987). In practice, many studies are in fact measuring simple disability.

This is particularly important given the increasing use of Quality Adjusted Life Years (QALYs) as a means of allocating resources and evaluating treatments. The term QALY implies a scientific assessment of quality. In practice they are no more than Disability Adjusted Life Years (DALYs). Indeed, if this ugly acronym—DALY—had been proposed and used (rather than the euphonious QALY), the whole concept might never have gained the popularity it now has.

Third, it is sometimes assumed that judgements relating to one illness can be transferred to other illnesses which may have a completely different prognosis. However, the evidence suggests that judgements are influenced by disease labels, prognosis, and having the disease (Sackett and Torrance 1978; Slevin *et al.* 1988).

Fourth, many scales are unreliable and the results differ according as to who undertakes the measurement, the doctor or the patient (Slevin *et al.* 1988). In their study, Slevin *et al.* (1988) found the Karnofsky Scale, the QL-index, and linear analogue self-assessment scales to be unreliable between different observers (doctors).

Therefore there is little evidence to support the assumption that the quality of life does form a unidimensional scale. The first step towards measuring quality of life should be to develop a model which would then allow a more detailed definition of the quality of life. Unfortunately, there is no generally accepted model, nor an agreed definition and both are desperately needed.

What is quality of life?

There are probably three factors contributing to quality of life:

1. The patient's own wishes and expectations (and possibly those of family members). These can only be measured through direct questioning and

might be difficult to establish reliably. Furthermore, each patient will attribute different degrees of importance to different expectations and there may be differences of opinion between different members of one family.

2. The limitations there are on a patient's ability to achieve his or her wishes; these limitations arising either naturally (for example, being too short to enter the police force), or from the environment (for example, widespread unemployment or economic decline), or from a disease. In the context of rehabilitation, it is only the consequences of disease which are of interest and so it may be important to control for pre-morbid limitations.

3. The patient's reaction to the limitations. Some might define this as being the quality of life itself. This presumably includes both emotional reactions (for example, despair) and also other reactions, such as taking up a different career.

A 40-year-old male journalist had a head injury and consequently lost his job. He and his wife took up interior decorating and design, renovating old houses. Their income was considerably increased and in all other aspects (for example, hobbies, holidays) they continued to lead a similar life to that before the injury. The new work was less stressful. Yet he returned to ask for further 'rehabilitation', wishing to return to journalism. This was not possible. *What is his quality of life?*

Therefore the basic problem, probably insoluble, is to find a (unidimensional) scale which can take one particular loss, such as the loss of a single finger, and distinguish its effects upon different people, such as a pianist and a labourer. The scale must also equate different losses in different people; for example, hemianopia in a professional driver and aphasia in a journalist. Furthermore, any attempt to define and measure quality of life needs to take into account the subject's culture, expectations, beliefs, and desires, as well as the many limitations to achieving his or her wishes and state of mind (reaction to limitations). Quality of life is, in other words, extraordinarily individual.

Therefore, accepting that any assessment of the quality of life must attempt to summarize the interactions of a patient's expectations, limitations and reactions, it might be best also to accept that quality of life cannot be measured, certainly in the context of clinical practice or research.

Measuring quality of life, a solution

The difficulties in assessing quality of life have arisen from the lack of any coherent underlying theory or conceptual framework. However, a framework is now available—the model of pathology, impairment, disability, and handicap used in this book.

It is notable that quality of life itself does not feature within this model, although some people might wish to refer to handicap as being quality of life itself. Instead, the model suggests that one has to focus on the component items which may contribute to quality of life—disabilities (physical, emotional, etc.) and handicaps.

The researcher looking for an overall measure of the quality of life should be specific about his aims.

- What difference in outcome does he expect to find?
- What aspect of disability or handicap is he interested in?
- Is he really referring to anxiety and depression, physical disability, the need for support at home, the stress upon the carer, or what?

The researcher should then use the appropriate measure(s) and *not* call the phenomenon measured the 'quality of life'. Instead, the researcher should make explicit what it is he is measuring.

In conclusion, it is necessary to resist the natural constant desire to summarize and quantify quality of life as a single number or result. Instead, one should use the WHO ICIDH model of pathology, impairment, disability, and handicap, to analyse the nature of any information being collected. Then one needs to decide exactly what specific information is required in relation to the hypothesis being tested. Decide what aspects of life are of interest—social adaptation, income, physical functioning, emotional stress—and measure them individually.

Conclusions

Measuring handicap is very difficult. It is dependent upon an individual's psychological coping mechanisms, and the extent to which the patient adapts his or her life-style. Much further research is needed to develop clinically useful, valid measures of handicap.

Measuring quality of life using a single unidimensional scale is impossible. The term 'quality of life' is probably referring to an illusion that cannot be defined or measured. Quality Adjusted Life Years (QALYs) should be renamed Disability Adjusted Life Years (DALYs) to recognize reality, and should be abandoned as a way of allocating resources because they are of unproven validity and most measures used are also not very reliable. At present it is usually going to be most appropriate and efficient to focus on measuring specific areas of disability.

Section 3
Measurement in practice

This section approaches the use of measures from a third angle: that of the practising clinician. The first chapter discusses the choice of measures in different diseases, and suggests that as far as possible one should use the same measures for all patients. However, disease-specific measures may be necessary in order to measure disease severity (and prognosis). Even then, it is often possible to use non-specific measures of impairment.

Chapter 12 discusses the author's own choice of measures for use in different circumstances: running a specialist rehabilitation centre; running a young disabled unit (long-term support facility); seeing out-patients. Again, it is possible to use a relatively small number of measures successfully in these different circumstances. The author would like to point out that Chapter 12 is based almost entirely upon personal experience, with all the limitations that imposes.

11 Measurement in some specific diseases

Summary

1. Diseases often determine the impairments that will be experienced, but have less influence upon disability.

2. Disease-specific measures are usually based at the level of impairment, and may be useful in determining disease severity, prognosis, and the effectiveness of some interventions.

3. Stroke impairments are best measured separately using such measures as the Motricity Index (for motor loss) and urinary incontinence (for overall prognosis).

4. There are several measures specifically designed for use with Parkinson's disease, including a Unified Scale, but this is probably flawed and a better approach is to use McDowell's Impairment Index and general measures of disability.

5. Multiple sclerosis is an unpredictable disease with poor correlation between pathology and impairment as well as a wide range of impairments. The Kurtzke Scale has little to recommend it, and clinical assessment of individual impairments should be combined with general measures of disability.

6. There is only one published measure of the impairment associated with epilepsy, and its major effects, which are at the level of handicap, cannot yet be measured.

7. Head injury causes an extremely variable and wide range of impairments. Overall severity is best measured through measuring level of consciousness using the Glasgow Coma Scale (GCS), and by determining the duration of post-traumatic amnesia.

8. Diseases affecting muscles or motor units cause more or less pure weakness, and so dynanometry should be used.

9. There are many measures developed for other less common diseases.

Introduction

Specialist clinicians or researchers whose main interest is in one particular condition will, naturally (and correctly), wish to tailor their use of measures as precisely as possible to the patients they see. Most clinicians see patients with a wide range of pathologies and disabilities, and do not have the luxury of choosing precisely the most specialist measure for every situation. Instead, they require measures which they can use with as many patients as possible.

This chapter discusses the nature of the conflict between specific and general measures, and then discusses the choice of measures for a range of common conditions. The chapter cannot cover the topic of measurement for every single neuromuscular disease.

Disease-specific measures

The underlying disease (pathology) determines two major aspects of rehabilitation:

- the natural history of the illness, and
- the impairments seen.

In terms of measurement, it is at the level of impairment that disease-specific measures are most likely to be appropriate.

Different diseases will tend to cause different individual impairments and different groups of impairments. Consequently, disease-specific measures will usually contain items covering the usual impairments seen with that pathology. For example, most measures developed for use in Parkinson's disease contain items relating to tremor, bradykinesia, rigidity, and sometimes seborrhea. These items never appear in measures relating to stroke.

On the other hand, the disability measures developed specifically for use with one disease are usually remarkably similar to the disability measures developed specifically for use with other diseases. For example, the disability sections of comprehensive assessments of Parkinson's disease are similar to most other disability indices. Of course, there will be some differences in the patterns of disability seen in different diseases, but these are relatively minor. For example, urinary incontinence is relatively uncommon in Parkinson's disease or motor neuron disease, but is common in multiple sclerosis. None the less, the areas of interest are similar.

In rehabilitation, measurement of impairments may be needed for two main reasons:

- to determine disease severity and prognosis, and
- to investigate whether impairment specific treatment is having the desired (or expected) effect.

In other words, it may be necessary to measure impairments to determine the input to a rehabilitation programme (or load on a rehabilitation service), and it may be necessary to monitor some aspects of rehabilitation process using measures of impairment. However, the measurement of rehabilitation outcome should always be at the level of disability and, in general, disability is not closely related to the nature or severity of the pathology.

The major differences between different diseases at the level of disability will be in the specific areas of disability that need to be assessed. For example, after head injury, measures of social interaction and extended ADL will often be most needed, whereas after stroke it will usually be necessary to assess personal ADL or communication. None the less, if measurement is needed in one particular sphere then the same measure should be used with all patients regardless of pathology. For example, if a stroke patient exhibits anti-social behaviour then it would be appropriate to use a measure originally developed for use after head injury.

In conclusion, it is important to be aware of, and familiar with, a range of simple impairment-based measures for most common diseases as a way of establishing disease severity. However, it is also important to use standard measures of disability for patients whatever the disease. Exceptions are inevitable; for example, in spinal cord injury where disability is arguably very tied to pathology (i.e. the level of complete injury is of over-riding importance).

The rest of this chapter considers some diseases, giving an outline sketch of the important features of the disease as a prelude to recommendations on measures which might be useful. Standard textbooks should be consulted for medical (pathological) details about any particular disease.

Stroke

Stroke is a vascular disease in which a localized volume of brain is suddenly damaged, leading to the sudden onset of focal neurological impairments. Because it is an anatomically defined volume, determined by the blood supply, that is damaged, there are characteristic associations between different impairments. The most obvious is between right hemiparesis and aphasia.

There are many well-developed measures of stroke severity, and some are shown in Section 4 of this book. Most mix a variety of impairments without considering their interactions, and this makes it difficult to interpret any global score. For example, depression of consciousness will preclude most other testing and aphasia makes some other assessments difficult. Moreover, stroke has been studied sufficiently well for the determinants of prognosis to be well established. Consequently global measures of disease severity are probably redundant because simpler more specific measures exist.

Instead of using global ratings, it is probably best to choose measures appropriate to your needs from a basket of recommended measures. Table 11.1 is derived from the measures recommended by the British Stroke Research Group in 1987 (no prizes for guessing who proposed these measures!).

Table 11.1   Standard data in stroke research: adapted from British Stroke Research Group recommendations (1987)

Section
    Essential—should *always* be recorded
        Desirable—something from the group that should be recorded
            Only for special purposes

Demography

Age	I
Gender	I
Source of patient (community, general hospital, etc.)	I
Pre-morbid disability	I

History

Loss of consciousness (worst Glasgow Coma Scale)	I
Urinary incontinence (at 3 days)	I
History of arterial disease (e.g. angina, claudication)	I
History of hypertension	I
Previous stroke or TIA	I

Pathology

First, or recurrent stroke	I
Side of weakness (*not* 'side of stroke', it's ambiguous)	I
Haemorrhage/non-haemorrhage (Guy's Score)	I
Clinical type (Bamford classification)	I
CT scan	I
Glucose	I
Haemoglobin and haematocrit	I
Evidence of arterial disease (clinical, investigation)	I
Other diseases	I
Specialized neuroradiology, etc.	I

Impairment

Death	O
Level of consciousness (Glasgow Coma Scale)	I
Motor loss (Motricity Index, Motor Club, RMA)	I
Visual field loss (confrontation)	I
Swallowing difficulty (drink glass of water)	I
Neglect (Albert's Test, Star-cancellation)	I
Memory—paragraph recall (RBMT or WMS)	I,O
Sensation—thumb-finding test	I
Perceptual problems (RPAB)	I

Disability

Physical ADL (Barthel, Nottingham ten-point)	I,O
Aphasia (FAST)	I,O

Table 11.1 (*cont.*)

Confusion (Hodkinson, short OMC test)	I,O
Mobility (FAC, RMI)	I,O
Walking (10-metre walk)	I,O
Arm dexterity (Nine- or Ten-hole Peg Test)	I,O
Mood (HAD, Wakefield, GHQ)	O
Mobility (6-min walk test)	O
Arm (Frenchay Arm Test, ARA)	O
Memory (RBMT)	O

Handicap

Housing/accommodation/placement	O
Frenchay Activities Index *or* Nottingham EADL	O
Carer—identity	O
Carer—stress (GHQ, Caregiver Strain Index)	O

Timing—in relation to stroke onset
Time of admission to study
Time of intervention
Time of assessments

I = initial assessment   O = outcome assessment
Recommended minimum timing: Initial, 3–4 weeks, 6 months

Abbreviations

ARA	= Action Research Arm Test	OMC	= Orientation–Memory–Concentration (test)
BIT	= Behavioural Inattention Test		
EADL	= Extended Activities of Daily Living (ADL)	RBMT	= Rivermead Behavioural Memory Test
FAC	= Functional Ambulation Categories	RMA	= Rivermead Motor Assessment
		RMI	= Rivermead Mobility Index
FAST	= Frenchay Aphasia Screening Test	RPAB	= Rivermead Perceptual Assessment Battery
GHG	= General Health Questionnaire	TIA	= Transient Ischaemic Attack
HAD	= Hospital Anxiety and Depression Scale	WMS	= Wechsler Memory Scale

A clinical system of making an accurate anatomical (pathological) diagnosis has been devised (Bamford 1988) and it is shown in this book. The clinical anatomical diagnosis relates strongly to prognosis. A clinical system for making a pathological distinction between haemorrhage and infarction has been devised (Guy's Score) (Allen 1983), but it is not sufficiently accurate for practical use with individual patients (Sandercock *et al.* 1985).

Prognosis after stroke in general is related directly to the severity of the initial impairments (and disabilities). This applies both generally (for example, for survival) and specifically (for example, to aphasia). However, specific markers have been identified:

- urinary incontinence (probably the best single marker (Wade and Hewer 1985b));
- loss of consciousness; severity of paralysis, etc., and
- a global prognostic scoring system which gives the likelihood of survival free of severe disability has been devised (Allen 1984).

In general it is better to measure the individual impairments than to use a global mixed index. There are short simple assessments available. There is good evidence that motor loss is of great importance, and this can be measured using the Motricity Index. Other impairments can be measured using the Frenchay Aphasia Screening Test (FAST), the Star-cancellation Test (for neglect), Hodkinson Mental Test (for confusion) etc.

Parkinson's disease

Parkinson's disease is a gradually progressive disease in which one specific part of the motor control system (the substancia nigra) gradually degenerates. Later there may be more general neurological degeneration. Consequently, the major impairments are motor, with cognitive impairments developing later. The drug treatments often also exacerbate cognitive impairments.

The development of specific drug treatment for Parkinson's disease has stimulated the development of many measures for use with this disease, some of which are shown in this book. A unified Parkinson's disease rating scale has been devised, and it is probably now the only scale used in large-scale research projects. However, it does have problems and could be improved and simplified.

The first section of the Unified Scale (mentation, behaviour, mood) relates to secondary features of the disease, and these could best be measured using short specific scales; for example those used to detect dementia. The second section, entitled Activities of Daily Living, includes some impairments (for example, tremor) which also occur in the third section. Conversely the third section, which concentrates upon motor impairments, also includes some disabilities (for example, gait) covered in Section 2. The Hoehn and Yahr Index should not be used—it is a logically inconsistent scheme for clinical categorization, of historical interest only. The Schwab and England ADL Scale has no justification either.

The author's recommendation would be to use the McDowell Impairment Index to assess disease severity, and the Barthel ADL Index, the Nine-hole Peg Test, and walking speed as measures of disability (see Table 11.2).

Table 11.2 Recommended measures in Parkinson's disease

Section
  Essential (clinical *and* research)
    Research only

Impairments
  Hodkinson's Mental Test—*or*
  Short Orientation–Memory–Concentration Test
  McDowell's Impairment Index
    Mechanical/electronic/video recording of motor impairments

Disability
  Barthel ADL Index (best and worst)
  Ten-metre walk
  Nine-hole Peg Test
    Rivermead Mobility Index
    Self-report disability scale
    Step-second test
      Timing of any specific activity

Handicap
  Housing (describe)
  Personal support (describe)

Research
  Considering using unified Parkinson's disease rating scale

Unfortunately, the Unified Scale is probably too well established and supported by too many people to be dropped, despite the problems outlined.

One further major problem occurs in measuring problems in Parkinson's disease: fluctuations in clinical state become increasingly prominent, leading to variation in any measure. There are two complementary solutions.

- The disability can be recorded both for the worst and the best state.
- The patient or carer can record the amount of time spent in the two states—bad and good.

Multiple sclerosis

In multiple sclerosis (MS) there are widespread small lesions within the white matter of the central nervous system. These occur acutely, but are (clinically) unpredictable, scattered both in time and anatomically, throughout the CNS. Consequently, a very wide range of impairments can occur—motor, sensory, emotional, cognitive, etc. Although certain patterns of disease are recognized, they are not sufficiently consistent to be useful clinically.

Multiple sclerosis is one of the most common severe disabling conditions, particularly in the young. There have been many attempts to devise useful treatments. Surprisingly, there are only a few specific scales, and only one is particularly well-known or widely used—the Kurtzke Expanded Disability Status Scale (EDSS) derived from the Kurtzke Functional Systems (FS) Scale.

The EDSS has been correctly criticized as a measure of disability on theoretical grounds (Willoughby and Paty 1988). It mixes impairments (of dubious significance and reliability) with disability, predominantly walking disability. In addition, one study has shown that the EDSS is insensitive to change when compared with simple measures of manual dexterity (for example, the Nine-hole Peg Test) (Goodkin et al. 1988).

Measures of disease severity are poorly developed. There is little connection between activity of the underlying pathology and the appearance of impairments (Thompson et al. 1990). Prognosis is still unpredictable. Therefore it is best to measure specific impairments using such measures as the Motricity Index, the Hodkinson Mental Test and the Ashworth Scale for spasticity. Other impairments, such as double vision, nystagmus and ataxia are probably best recorded clinically. Disability should be measured using standard measures.

Epilepsy

Epilepsy is a condition in which the patient experiences sudden unpredictable stereotyped periods of alteration in level of consciousness, often (but not always) with associated involuntary motor phenomena. As such, it is presumably a medical diagnosis at the level of impairment rather than pathology. Certainly in some patients the epilepsy is secondary to some structural damage (pathology), but in many there is no identified pathology.

Despite its frequency in the population, its importance as a cause of misery and distress, and the existence of effective drug treatments, there are remarkably few measures available for use in epilepsy. Indeed, the only simple published scale the author is aware of is that used by the OPCS in their survey of disability in Britain. This is based on frequency of fits, timing of fits, and predictability of fits.

A complex standard measure has been devised that takes into account such important influences as frequency of fits, timing, and predictability, side-effects of drugs, and types of fit (Cramer et al. 1983). Although well thought out, giving weights to almost all factors, it is far too long for routine use.

However, epilepsy does have the advantage of being countable. Various options exist:

- number of seizure-free days;
- number of seizures in a unit of time (month, year);
- interval (in days) between attacks;
- severity of attack (time not functioning normally).

The major complicating factor is that attacks are probably random, and so clustering can occur easily. This means that sophisticated statistical techniques are needed to evaluate changes or differences. More importantly, most measures do not take into account the personal significance of an attack—some people would be happy with a seizure once every two months but others would be devastated by one every year, especially if they wished to drive.

Consequently, the major effects of epilepsy are probably at the level of handicap, particularly because epilepsy has major legal implications in terms of denying access to many occupations, driving licences, etc. There are no good measures available for use at this level with epilepsy.

Head injury

In non-penetrating head injury patients sustain four major types of pathological damage:

- diffuse axonal tearing;
- frontal lobe contusion;
- temporal lobe contusion; and
- shearing of white matter at the level of the mid-brain and pons.

Focal damage is rare, but may follow penetrating injury or haemorrhage. Additional diffuse anoxic damage is probably common (but should be preventable). Consequently, most problems arise from generalized damage and specific isolated pure impairments are rare.

The most serious initial impairment is loss of consciousness, and this must be measured routinely using the Glasgow Coma Scale (GCS). Once the patient has recovered consciousness, he or she may have a wide range of impairments arising from the different areas of damage. The types and severities of impairment will vary widely between patients, and also with time. Consequently, it is unrealistic to expect one multi-item index to reflect accurately the severity of the injury. Instead, it is necessary to measure the specific impairments found in each patient.

Overall severity is best assessed in two complementary ways:

- time to recovery of ability to respond consistently and appropriately to external stimuli (or time to regain consciousness); and
- time to regain continuous day-to-day memory (i.e. duration of post-traumatic amnesia).

Neither of these measures is sufficiently reliable to make definitive statements about individual patients, but they are probably the best prognostic guides available at present.

Measurement of disability in patients who have sustained head injury is not easy, but it should be done using the standard measures as far as possible. The major long-term impairments after head injury (and also after anoxic brain damage) are not physical. They are cognitive and behavioural (i.e. affect social interaction). Patients have difficulties in solving problems (coping with the unexpected), planning, and executing long-term activities, maintaining social relationships, remembering etc.

Consequently, some patients' disability is very dependent upon their environment—within a protective, structured (family) setting a patient may function well, but may fail if expected to cope independently. This is difficult to measure easily, and one is often forced into measuring the impairments (such as reduced IQ). In practice, measures such as the behavioural rating scale probably have much to commend them. In patients with severe injuries it may be necessary and appropriate to use standard ADL and EADL indices, and measures of mobility and dexterity.

Disease of motor units

Diseases affecting muscle directly (for example, myopathies) or affecting motor units (for example, neuropathies, myaesthenia gravis) will inevitably lead to weakness as their predominant impairment. Motor neuron disease (amyotrophic lateral sclerosis) is a progressive degenerative disorder affecting (clinically) only the pyramidal motor system (upper and lower motor neurons). In practice there may also be cognitive impairment. Neuropathies may be acute, relapsing, or chronic and progressive, and myaesthenia gravis usually fluctuates.

In all these conditions the impairments relate predominantly to motor strength. Quantitative measures of severity based on strength have been developed for motor neuron disease (MND) where the severity of disability is also related to loss of strength (Andres *et al.* 1986). Undue muscle fatigue is a common associated impairment in many of these conditions, and reduction of ventilatory capacity may occur in some diseases.

Therefore the predominant measure of severity will be through use of muscle dynanometry (sometimes with repeated testing to detect fatigue). Other measures useful at times may include tests of respiratory function such as peak flow, vital capacity, the number counted in one breath and even blood gases, and tests of bulbar function such as ability to swallow, or say difficult sounds.

Disability measures are likely to concentrate upon mobility and manual dexterity because, in many of these diseases, progress is so slow that the patient adapts his environment to his needs so that disability is minimized.

Table 11.3   Recommended measures in multiple sclerosis

Section
  Routine clinical practice *and* research
  Research only

Impairments
  Motor loss—Motricity Index
  Mental state—short Orientation–Memory–Concentration Test
    Spasticity—Ashworth Scale
    IQ—WAIS if possible
    Memory—Rivermead Behavioural Memory Test
    Any individual impairments; for example, ataxia

Disability
  Barthel ADL Index (note individual items, especially bladder)
  Rivermead Mobility Index
  Ten-metre walking time
  Nine-hole Peg Test
    Nottingham EADL (or Frenchay Activities Index)
    Timing of any activity

Handicap
  Housing (describe)
  Personal support (describe)
  Employment

Research
  Consider using Kurtzke scales, but *only* to maintain comparability with other studies

---

Conclusions

It is impractical to use different measures for each disease. Few clinicians will be able to remember the measures needed for each condition, and they certainly will not be familiar with them all. A busy clinician may see many patients with many different diseases each day. It is also impractical to store ready for immediate use the large number of forms which disease-specific measures would require. Lastly, there are many diseases for which there are no specialist measures.

Fortunately, in rehabilitation, it is usually possible to use the same disability measures, whatever the underlying disease. However, measures of severity and prognosis are sometimes specific to the disease but even then, some measures of impairment can be used in many diseases. Motor loss is common to most diseases causing disability and the Motricity Index and measurement of strength using dynanometry are useful in almost all.

12   Measurement in some specific circumstances

Summary

1. For in-patient rehabilitation it is possible to use a sheet summarizing each patient's state, using some simple measures and abbreviations. It helps to maintain a critical attitude towards each patient's progress.
2. The routine use of simple measures also allows the development of an audit of a service, recording input and outcome.
3. Similar measures can also be used when devising a brief summary sheet appropriate for patients entering a long-term care programme.
4. The author's own recommended measures for these circumstances are given. They are measures which have proved their worth by being used regularly for months and years after they were first tried.

Introduction

So far in this book an attempt has been made to outline the choices available and to present relatively unbiased comments. In this chapter the author intends to outline the use he makes of measures and other formal documentation at Rivermead Rehabilitation Centre and Ritchie Russell House, the two units he is closely involved in, and in other circumstances. The views expressed reflect the author's experiences at the time of writing. He is influenced particularly by the need to be economic: there are not sufficient resources available to allow us to waste time on measures and assessments that are not useful.

In-patient rehabilitation

Rivermead Rehabilitation Centre specializes in the assessment and treatment of patients with severe, usually complex neurological disabilities. It serves a population of 2.5 million people. It has approximately (in whole-time equivalents) 21 nurses, 10 occupational therapists, 8 physiotherapists, 2.5 social workers, 2.5 doctors, and one each of speech therapist and psychologist. Its in-patient load is 24–28 at any one time, with a turnover of two to three patients each week, and patients may remain as in-patients from 1 to 60 weeks. About one-third of patients have sustained head injury, with the majority of the remainder suffering stroke, but many other pathologies are seen.

In this setting it is vital to maintain good communications both within the centre and with others involved in the community. It is also vital to be certain that all problems are identified and that progress is monitored so that the expensive resource (Rivermead) is used effectively. However, it is equally important not to devote disproportionate effort to measurement for its own sake.

Over the last four years (1986–90) a system has evolved that suits Rivermead and its needs, though it is still changing. Each week there is a meeting ('ward round'), at which all patients are discussed. In order to facilitate communication, and to aid fallible and failing memories a weekly sheet is used giving details on every patient. This is brought up to date each week. A sample sheet (with false names) is shown (Table 12.1), indicating the type of information given. Note that only a limited space is given to each patient and that abbreviations are used extensively. The abbreviations are explained on Table 12.2 which shows the measures most commonly used.

Rivermead has also started recording, in a limited way, details of the work undertaken. (American colleagues may be shocked to realize how little we have to record.) Table 12.3 shows the standard format. All the information is collected by the admitting doctor, including all measures of impairment and disability (but obviously in collaboration with and having help from other staff).

Codes are used for categorical data, and standard codes are used when data cannot be obtained or is not relevant. For example, for the 10-m time, patients who cannot walk are scored '0' if not independently able to wheel their chair, and '1' if wheelchair-independent; aphasic patients are scored '20' on Hodkinson Mental Test; stroke patients are scored '0' on PTA.

Chronic care

Ritchie Russell House is a 15-bed, young disabled unit (YDU) sited (at present) on the Churchill Hospital site in Oxford. It serves a population of 500 000 and its aim is to assess and support all people in Oxfordshire aged 16–64 years with severe disability; over 95 per cent of its patients have neurological disability. It offers assessment, advice, and also both in-patient relief care and out-patient day care. At any one time there are 100–120 patients actively involved with Ritchie Russell House and turnover is approximately 30–40/year.

The main problem to contend with is to keep a reasonably up-to-date summary of all relevant facts on each patient. Change is slow or non-existent

Table 12.1 Routine in-patient information for ward round

IN-PATIENT WARD ROUND   Date: 18 Sept. 90

DAVIES, James. 65 yrs, Banbury   CVA 15.7.90 Ad 21.8.90 CC/dis
  Pathology: Stroke, BP↑, diabetes, osteo-arthritis
  Impairment: Rt hemi arm 11% leg 32% TCT 51%, aphasia, hemianopia
  Disability: Barthel A 5 L 8, FAC 1 10m 215s, FAST C4 E2, WCh indep
  Handicap: Married, retired builder, house, no children
  Goals: %home # walk indoors # toilet indep # ask for help
  Notes *B*:   *Rx aspirin, insulin, anti-BP *Splint arm *Wife ill *AFO

HERBERT, Jane. 22 yrs, Reading   HI 2.3.90 Ad 28.5.90 CC 5.10.90
  Pathology: RTA/HI, # Rt tibia & fibula, epilepsy
  Impairment: PTA 4/12, ataxia, dysarthria, diplopia
  Disability: Barthel A 3 L 13, FAC 0, WCh indep, RBMT 3/12, stand 5s
  Handicap: Student (law), lived in flat, parents, boy friend
  Goals: %to parents # dress indep # leisure
  Notes *R*:   *Rx nil *disinhibited *Electric WCh *many friends

---

WARD, Charles. 30 yrs, Witney   HI 31.7.89 Ad 17.9.90 CC 28.9.90
  Pathology: Fall/HI, # skull, extradural, coeliac disease (1980)
  Impairment: PTA 5/52, conc reduced, Lt arm spastic, anxiety
  Disability: Barthel A 20, FAC 5, 10m 8s, NHPT Lt 32s
  Handicap: Married, 2 Ch, wife works, ex-carpenter (self-employed)
  Goals: %Advice on work # assess cognition # assess carpentry
  Notes *G*:   *Rx gluten-free diet *marital stress *insurance claim

---

in many. Some have very large, poorly organized hospital files. A lot of
them are seen by several doctors in addition to their general practitioners
(family doctors). Many different members of staff are likely to see the
patient.

The solution has been to devise a summary sheet, confined to one page
for each patient. An anonymous, fictitious example is shown in Table 12.4.
The observant reader will note that the disability classification is not that
shown earlier in this book. The form was devised at the start of this book,
and the author's ideas have altered since then.

Other circumstances — measures used by the author

Each individual is going to develop his or her own preferred measures; and
the author's are as follows. These are used not only in his work at Rivermead

Table 12.2   Rivermead in-patient notes: explanation

Uses WHO ICIDH headings, but note:

Line 1   Gives main diagnosis, and dates of onset, admission and any planned
              case conference or discharge

Pathology   Gives relevant medical diagnoses, starting with main diagnosis (cause
              of disability)

Impairment   Gives main symptoms and signs on admission
              All head injuries start with PTA (main prognostic factor)
              All strokes start with side of weakness

Disability   Starts with Barthel ADL index (A = on admission; L = last)
              Updated regularly (weekly initially, then every 4 weeks)

Handicap   Records social factors likely to affect handicap
              Not a measure of handicap

Goals   Sets out our goals
              % = primary goal, usually discharge destination
              # = secondary goals (weeks)

Notes   Anything of interest, including drugs (Rx)
              B = Primary Nurse Team (Red, Blue, Green, Yellow)

Abbreviations

Ad   Date admitted
AFO   Ankle Foot Orthosis
Barthel ADL index score (as patient is on ward)
       A = score on admission
       L = last score (checked weekly initially, then every four weeks)
BP↑   Hypertension
CC   Date of any case conference
CVA   Stroke
dis   Expected/planned date of discharge
FAC   Functional Ambulation Category (in physiotherapy)
FAST   Frenchay Aphasia Screening Test
       E = Expression (out of 10)
       C = Comprehension (out of 10)
HI   Head injury
Hod   Hodkinson Mental Test score
MMS   Mini-Mental State score
NHPT   Nine-hole Peg Test (in seconds, *or* number of pegs in 50 sec)
PTA   Post-traumatic amnesia
RBMT   Rivermead Behavioural Memory Test (normal = 10–12/12)
RTA   Road Traffic Accident (Motor Vehicle Injury)
Rx   Any drug medication
TCT   Trunk Control Test
WCh   Wheelchair

Table 12.2 (*cont.*)

%	Score on Motricity Index (arm and leg)
#	Fracture

10m xs = time in seconds to walk 10 m

---

and Ritchie Russell House but also when seeing referrals as out-patients and on other wards.

Motor impairment

For any patient with upper motor neuron loss the Motricity Index and Trunk Control Test are recorded. The measurements are simple, and of practical prognostic importance. They can be used when assessing patients on other wards—for example, other team members can be given an idea of the severity of motor loss when discussing possible admission of a patient referred to Rivermead.

Cognitive impairment

Until recently the author has used the Hodkinson Mental Test almost exclusively, primarily because he can remember the ten questions! However, the author is starting to use the short orientation–memory–concentration test. It is probably more sensitive, particularly in younger patients after head injury (i.e. those who are not severely demented). The author uses the modified scoring system given in Section 4.

Many of Rivermead's patients are referred from distant hospitals and it is impractical to see them before transfer. Therefore, standard forms are sent to obtain information. Referring doctors are unlikely to be familiar with any measures, and are unlikely to complete anything requiring much time or effort. Extensive use is made of the Mini-Mental State, when obtaining information about patients referred from other hospitals. It provides much useful information (provided the original forms are returned).

Once patients have arrived, the Frenchay Aphasia Screening Test, the short OMC test, and the Star-cancellation Test are used. These detect aphasia, problems with attention and memory, and perceptual problems.

Disability

The Barthel ADL Index is the main measure of ADL the author uses in all circumstances. The 10-m walking time is recorded routinely in most out-patients who have mobility problems, whatever the diagnosis (MS,

Table 12.3   Routine 'Audit' information collected at Rivermead

---

Demography

____   Age
____   Sex
____   Marital status
____   Employment status
____   Carer status
____   Responsible Health Authority   Post code _____
____   Reason for admission

Pathology

____   Main diagnosis
____   Diagnosis 2

History

____   Onset–referral (weeks)
____   Referral–admission (weeks)
____   Length of stay

Impairment

Admission   Discharge

____   Motricity right arm   ____
____   Motricity right leg   ____
____   Motricity left arm   ____
____   Motricity left leg   ____
____   Trunk Control Test   ____

____   Hodkinson Mental Test   ____
____   FAST—Comprehension   ____
____   FAST—Expression   ____
____   Dysarthria   ____
____   Post-traumatic amnesia   ____

Disability

____   Barthel   ____
____   NHPT—right arm   ____
____   NHPT—left arm   ____
____   Functional Ambulation Category   ____
____   10-m time (seconds)   ____

Follow up

____   Discharge destination
____   Discharge rehabilitation

Table 12.4 An example of a patient summary sheet

	GENERAL	
PATIENT (DoB 5.6.41)	PRACTITIONER	HOSPITAL (No: 000000)
Wesley, Jean	Dr F. R. Herbert,	Dr D. T. Wade,
45 Rissington Rd.,	The Health Centre	Ritchie Russell House
Eynsham,	High St., Witney,	Churchill Hospital,
Oxon OX4 5FT	Oxon OX5 3QS	Oxford OX3 7LJ
Tel: 93–78423	Tel: 94–675656	Tel: 0865–225480

History
Ventriculo-septal defect from birth. On 4th Nov. 1968, after birth 3rd child, had subarachnoid haem. Developed Rt hemiplegia and focal epilepsy of left side. Coma 6/52; investigations NAD. Rivermead 1970. Radiation menopause May and Oct. 1971. Referred RRH 1978. Screaming caused trouble 1981; pain Rt knee April 1990, patella dislocated laterally; pain left knee July 90, transfers worse—needed a hoist.

Pathology
Subarachnoid haemorrhage; stroke (cerebral infarction); ventriculo-septal defect; epilepsy; contractures Rt arm; osteoporosis Rt knee

Impairments
Right hemiparesis, ataxia on Rt., aphasia (mild), anarthria (severe), Rt arm fixed, pain in knees Rt > Lt

Disability
General: Barthel 7/20; Domestic ADL 0
Mobility: Electric WCh indep, FAC 0; RMI 1/15
Dexterity: NHPT Rt 0
Behaviour/mood: Demanding, odd behaviour. Eats odd material
Cognitive: No problem (probably poor)   Nursing hours: 3.5
Communication: FAST C 4/10, E 0   Day-care load: 26/33

Handicap (social situation)
Family: Husband (stopped work Sept. 87), 3 children
Occupation: Mother/housewife
Social integration: Limited to family

Environment
House: Bungalow, warden-controlled
Family: Husband only at home

Table 12.4 (*cont.*)

| | GENERAL | |
| PATIENT (DoB 5.6.41) | PRACTITIONER | HOSPITAL (No: 000000) |

Support and treatment given
RRH: IP 1/52 every 2/12; OP Tue & Fri
Other: Home Care Assistants, Nursing Auxiliary; total 22 hours/week

Drugs and equipment
Rx: Night sedation, analgesia
Equip: Hoist; Electric Wheelchair; orthotic shoes; lower leg calipers

Current problems and aims
Problems: Pain Rt knee, & not transferring; Behaviour, physical care needs increasing
One year: Maintain at home if possible
Five year: Maintain at home, or find suitable institutional care

Other information
Strong-willed, rarely becomes involved in activities, knows own wishes, usually sits by windows alone at RRH. Increased dependency April–August 1990. For orthopaedic review of knees.

Summary completed: 12th September 1990   Derick T. Wade

Parkinson's disease, motor neuron disease, neuropathies, etc.). It is also used for in-patients. With out-patients the author has recently started using the Rivermead Mobility Index, finding it very useful. The Functional Ambulation Categories is used only to monitor progress in therapy. The Nine-hole Peg Test is used frequently, particularly in out-patients with Parkinson's disease or ataxia (of any cause). For in-patients at Rivermead extensive use is made of the Rivermead Behavioural Memory Test. It has been found to be very useful.

Conclusions

It is possible to use measures in daily clinical practice and they have proved useful. Hopefully, there will slowly develop a consensus among professionals as to which measures should be used. We should aim for recommendations which allow some individual choice of measure from a limited basket of allowable measures. The proof of a test's worth is that it should continue to be used by practising clinicians for months after its initial introduction. Unfortunately, few measures achieve this.

Section 4
Measures for use in neurological disability

Section 4 shows in detail the measures mentioned in the previous chapters. To help the reader, the measures have been divided into groups which, as far as possible, include all measures likely to be considered as alternatives. Further, the chapters generally follow the same order as the chapters in the second section. However, there are inevitably some inconsistencies and some measures are difficult to fit in anywhere. Each chapter starts with a list of the measures included (in order), as well as a brief introduction. If the reader wishes to find a specific measure, it will usually be quicker to look in the index.

As far as possible each measure is shown in its standard (published) form with any published guide-lines also given. After each measure some key references are noted. These will usually include the reference to the original publication (or that for the most recent modification), provided that it is known. (Some measures the author has been given, but he has never found an original reference.) There will also be a selection of references to articles, the authors of which have either evaluated the measure, used it, or made significant comment on it. The list is rarely exhaustive, and nor is it intended to be. However, it should introduce the reader to the relevant literature. Finally, there are some brief comments, which are only intended to make a few points, and obviously should nöt be taken as an in-depth, critical review.

The reader should bear two cautions in mind when choosing a measure from this book.

1. Although the author hopes to have included most measures likely to be useful, it is still necessary to be aware that there may be a better measure available which is not shown in this book.
2. Although the author has tried to give a rough review of the virtues and vices of each measures, it is important that the reader conducts his or her own evaluation, both in clinical (or research) practice and by searching through the literature.

Inclusion of a measure within this book does not imply that it is necessarily a good measure and indeed the author has included (deliberately) some he considers to be bad.

13 Measures of cognitive impairment and disability

Summary

1. Glasgow Coma Scale
2. Children's Coma Score
3. Edinburgh-2 Coma Scale
4. Digit span
5. 'Logical memory' (paragraph recall)
6. Blessed Dementia Rating Scales
   Information–Concentration–Memory Test
   Dementia Scale
7. Hodkinson Mental Test
8. Short Orientation–Memory–Concentration Test
9. Mini-Mental State Examination (MMSE)
10. Modified MMSE
11. Clifton Assessment Procedures for the Elderly (CAPE)
    Information/orientation
    Behaviour rating scale
12. Everyday Memory Questionnaire
13. Cognitive Failures Questionnaire (CFQ)
14. CFQ-for-others
15. Hachinski Ischaemia Score
16. The Speech Questionnaire

Introduction

This chapter groups measures which measure cognitive impairments, and some disabilities arising from cognitive impairments. The main disabilities are those associated with amnesia/dementia and aphasia. The constructs included vary from level of consciousness through to complex measures of intelligence, on to short screening tests for dementia and global cognitive loss.

The most important and useful measures from this section are the Glasgow Coma Scale (GCS), the Hodkinson Mental Test, the Short Orientation–Memory–Concentration Test, and the Mini-Mental State Examination (MMSE). These all focus on cognitive impairment.

There are also some measures of cognitive disability, the behavioural problems commonly seen in patients with severe cognitive impairment.

Most of these disability measures were developed with reference to dementia in the elderly. The CAPE behaviour rating scale and the Cognitive Failures Questionnaires are two examples. The speech questionnaire measures communicative disability. There are a few other measures; for example, one which attempts to diagnose the pathology underlying cognitive failure (Hachinski Ischaemia Score).

Readers requiring further information on neuropsychological assessment are strongly recommended to consult Lezak (1983), an excellent book giving very many tests.

Glasgow Coma Scale

Instructions
Three sections, each scored separately.
Record BEST response observed to command, voice, or pain.
Record as: E = ____, M = ____, V = ____.

Item Response	Score	Details
Eye opening		
None	1	Even to pain (supra-orbital pressure)
To pain	2	Pain from sternum/limb/supra-orbital ridge
To speech	3	Non-specific response, not necessarily to command
Spontaneous	4	Eyes open, not necessarily aware
Motor response		
None	1	To any pain; limbs remain flaccid
Extension	2	'Decerebrate'; shoulder adducted and internally rotated, forearm pronated
Abnormal flexion	3	'Decorticate'; shoulder flexes/adducts
Withdrawal	4	Arm withdraws from pain, shoulder abducts
Localizes pain	5	Arm attempts to remove supraorbital/chest pain
Obeys commands	6	Follows simple commands
Verbal response		
None	1	As stated
Incomprehensible	2	Moans/groans; no words
Inappropriate	3	Intelligible, no sustained sentences
Confused	4	Responds with conversation, but confused
Oriented	5	Aware of time, place, person

References Teasdale and Jennett (1974); Teasdale *et al.* (1978); Teasdale *et al.* (1979)

Comment

The best-known, most widely used scale to assess level of consciousness. It has obvious face validity and well-proven predictive validity, not only after head injury but also in medical coma (Levy *et al.* 1981). Reliability is well established. Simplicity is obvious. It is designed for use by anyone. It is of adequate sensitivity to detect deterioration requiring neurosurgical intervention.

It is best reported as separate scores, but a summed total is commonly used while some have suggested concentrating upon the motor subscale (Jagger *et al.* 1983). A score of 8/15 or less is frequently taken to separate coma from non-coma. The GCS is increasingly being incorporated into other scales.

There is competition, for example from the Edinburgh-2 Coma Scale and the Comprehensive Level of Consciousness Scale (Stanczak *et al.* 1984), but there are at present no reasons for abandoning the GCS.

Children's Coma Score

This scale was designed for use with infants and toddlers aged 0–3 years after head injury.

Item Score	Response
Ocular response	
4	Pursuit
3	Extra-ocular muscles (EOM) intact, and reactive pupils
2	Fixed pupils, *or* EOM impaired
1	Fixed pupils *and* EOM impaired
Verbal response	
3	Cries
2	Spontaneous respirations
1	Apneic
Motor response	
4	Flexes and extends
3	Withdraws from painful stimuli
2	Hypertonic
1	Flaccid

Reference   Raimondi and Hirschauer (1984)

Comment

A scale devised for use with infants. It is more discriminant than the GCS at the lower level of function.

Edinburgh-2 Coma Scale

This scale measures consciousness (awareness) through identifying 'the best response to maximal stimuli.' The patient scores according to his best response.

Stimulation (maximum)	Response (best)	Score
A Two sets of questions:	Answers correctly to both	0
1. Month?	Answers correctly to either	1
2. Age?	Answers incorrectly	2
B Two sets of commands:	Obeys correctly to both	3
1. Close and open hand	Obeys correctly to either	4
2. Close and open eyes	Obeys incorrectly	5
C Strong pain	Localizes	6
	Flexion response	7
	Extension response	8
	No response	9

Reference   Sugiura *et al.* (1983)

Comment

This scale is the only real competitor to the Glasgow Coma Scale, and its use is probably restricted to Japan (despite its name). The study referred to investigated its use after operations (not in head injury). Validity was established both by reference to the GCS and through prediction of outcome. Reliability was not assessed in this study (but has been in a Japanese journal).

In contrast to the GCS, the E-2CS is a single scale, whereas the GCS has three subscales. This might enhance its value. However, its major drawback is simply the lack of experience in its use. As Sugiura *et al.* point out, it needs to be compared with the GCS to determine which is better. Until then, the GCS should be used.

Digit span

Instructions
This is a test of attention span. Score longest series correctly repeated (forwards or backwards as asked).

Digits forwards	Score	Digits backwards	Score
6–4–3–9	4	2–8–3	3
7–2–8–6	4	4–1–5	3
4–2–7–3–1	5	3–2–7–9	4
7–5–8–3–6	5	4–9–6–8	4
6–1–9–4–7–3	6	1–5–2–8–6	5
3–9–2–4–8–7	6	6–1–8–4–3	5
5–9–1–7–4–2–3	7	5–3–9–4–1–8	6
4–1–7–9–3–8–6	7	7–2–4–8–5–6	6
5–8–1–9–2–6–4–7	8	8–1–2–9–3–6–5	7
3–8–2–9–5–1–7–4	8	4–7–3–9–1–2–8	7
Forward score =	_____		
Backward score =	_____		

Comment
One subtest of the Wechsler Memory Scale and Wechsler Adult Intelligence Scale (WAIS). The utility of this test is unclear. Commonly used, probably because it is simple but the clinical significance of abnormal results is not established.

'Logical memory' (paragraph recall)

Instruction
Read the first paragraph to the subject. Then ask the subject what he or she recalls, marking off items as shown in the original. The immediate score is the number of items recalled. Do not warn, that will ask for later recall. Repeat for second paragraph. At a later time (20 min, 30 min, or 60 min) ask for recall again, and score as above.

Paragraph 1
Eliza Thompson/ of North Oxford,/ employed/ as a cleaner/ in a college building/ reported/ at the city/ Police Station/ that she had been held up/ in the High street/ the evening before/ and robbed/ of sixteen pounds./ She had five/ little children,/ the rent/ was due/ and they had not eaten/ for two days./ The policemen,/ touched by the woman's story,/ made a collection/ for her.

Paragraph 2
The British/ liner/ Queen Anne/ struck a mine/ near Liverpool/ on Sunday/ night./ In spite of a blinding/ snowstorm/ and darkness/ the seventy/ passengers including 19/ women/ were all rescued/ although the lifeboats/ were tossed about/ like corks/ in the heavy sea./ They were brought into port/ the next morning/ by a French/ steamer.

Immediate recall score (para 1)	____/24
Immediate recall score (para 2)	____/23
Total Immediate	____ Average Immediate ____
Delayed recall score (para 1)	____/24
Delayed recall score (para 2)	____/23
Total Delayed	____ Average Delayed ____

Comment
A second subtest from the Wechsler Memory Scale but widely used in other tests, such as the Rivermead Behavioural Memory Test (RBMT) and in many studies. There is evidence that verbal memory is closely related to actual memory problems (i.e. that this impairment is related to disability), supporting its validity as a measure of memory problems (Sunderland *et al.* 1983). Interpretation is difficult in the presence of significant aphasia or deafness.

Blessed Dementia Rating Scales

These are a pair of scales first published in 1968 and widely used and adapted since. Although later research has led to probable improvements, the original tests are shown here first: the 'Information–Memory–Concentration' Test (of impairment) and the 'Dementia Scale' (of disability).

Information-Memory-Concentration Test

Instructions
One point for each correct answer unless otherwise indicated.

Information
Name
Age
Time (hour)
Time of day
Day of week
Date
Month
Season
Year
Place: name
      street
      town
Type of place (for example, home, hospital, etc.)
Recognition of two persons (*one point for each*)

Memory
Personal
   Date of birth
   Place of birth
   School attended
   Occupation
   Name of siblings/name of spouse
   Name of any town where patient worked/lived
   Name of employers

Non-personal
   Date of First World War (½ if within 3 years)
   Date of Second World War (½ if within 3 years)
   Monarch
   Prime Minister

Five-minute recall (score 0–5 points)
   Mr John Brown
   42 West Street
   Gateshead

Concentration (all scored 0–1–2)
Months of year backwards
Counting 1–20
Counting 20–1

Dementia Scale

Instructions
Information is obtained as far as possible from a relative in close and continual contact with the patient. Inquiries are directed towards defining changes in capacity, habits, and personality. Allowance should be made in scoring for physical disabilities that would restrict activities. Score 1 for each positive, unless otherwise stated.

Preceding letters A,B,C, or D indicates four factors (see under 'Comment')
* = item not contributing to any factor

Changes in performance of everyday activities (½ if minor).
A Inability to perform household tasks
A Inability to cope with small sums of money
A Inability to remember shortlist of items; for example, in shopping list
A Inability to find way about indoors
A Inability to find way about familiar streets
A Inability to interpret surroundings; for example, to recognize whether in hospital, or at home; to discriminate between patients, doctors, nurse, relatives, other hospital staff, etc.
A Inability to recall recent events; for example, recent outings, visits of relatives or friends to hospital, etc.
* Tendency to dwell in the past

Changes in habits
D Eating
    (0) = cleanly, with proper utensils
    (1) = messily, with spoon only
    (2) = simple solids (for example, biscuits)
    (3) = has to be fed

D Dressing
    (0) = unaided
    (1) = occasionally misplaced buttons etc.
    (2) = wrong sequence, commonly forgetting items
    (3) = unable to dress

D Sphincter control
    (0) = complete control
    (1) = occasional wet bed
    (2) = frequent wet bed
    (3) = doubly incontinent

Changes in personality, interests, drive
B Increased rigidity
B Increased egocentricity
B Impairment of regard of feeling for others
B Coarsening of affect
B Impairment of emotional control
    (for example, increased petulance and irritability)
B Hilarity in inappropriate situations
C Diminished emotional responsiveness
* Sexual misdemeanour (arising *de novo* in old age)
C Hobbies relinquished
C Diminished initiative or growing apathy
* Purposeless hyperactivity

References Blessed *et al.* (1968); Stern *et al.* (1990); Zillmer *et al.* (1990)

Comment
A widely used pair of scales, with good research credentials, validated against neuropathology but not tested for reliability. For the functional section, four factors have been identified (Stern *et al.* 1990).

A cognition
B personality change
C apathy/withdrawal
D self-care

The tests of impairment do probably form a single construct (Zillmer *et al.* 1990) measuring memory and attention. They are now probably redundant as shorter tests of almost equal sensitivity have been derived from the original test (see next few pages). The disability scale may still be useful; there are few genuine competitors. The Mini-Mental State Exam is possibly a more sensitive diagnostic test in patients with possible Alzheimer's disease (Zillmer *et al.* 1990).

Hodkinson Mental Test

Instruction
Score one point for each question answered correctly.

Score	Question
____	Age of patient
____	Time (to nearest hour)
____	Address given, for recall at end of test:
	42 West Street (alternative: 92 Columbia Road)
____	Name of hospital (or area of town if at home)
____	Year
____	Date of birth of patient
____	Month
____	Years of First World War
____	Name of monarch (President in USA)
____	Count backwards from 20–1 (no errors, but may correct self)

References Hodkinson (1972); Qureshi and Hodkinson (1974); Stonier (1974); Wade *et al.* (1989)

Comment
Derived from the Blessed Information–Memory–Concentration tests, this has been devised and validated for use with the elderly. It measures (briefly) fixed knowledge, new learning, and concentration. Inter-rater reliability studies are not available. Its advantages include brevity, relative lack of culture-specific knowledge, and wide-spread use. A score of 6/10 or less is abnormal in the elderly, but little has been published on its use in younger people. Essentially, it is a very crude, basic test of memory and/or orientation, which is only able to detect severe disorientation ('dementia'). It is useful as a screening test, not least because the tester can usually remember it, and it does not need a special form! It is likely to be adopted in the UK for community screening of the elderly.

Short Orientation-Memory-Concentration Test

Instruction
Score 1 error for each incorrect response, to maximum for item.

No.	Question	Maximum error	Score ×	Weight	
1.	What year is it now?	1	___ ×	4	= ___
2.	What month is it now?	1	___ ×	3	= ___
	Repeat this phrase: John Brown, 42 Market Street, Chicago *or* (UK): John Brown, 42 West Street, Gateshead				
3.	About what time is it? (within one hour)	1	___ ×	3	= ___
4.	Count backwards 20 to 1	2	___ ×	2	= ___
5.	Say the months in reverse order	2	___ ×	2	= ___
6.	Repeat the phrase just given	5	___ ×	2	= ___
		Total error score			= ___/28

Reference   Katzman *et al.* (1983)

Comment
A well-studied test, which is (so far) little used. It has been validated against neuropathology, and was derived from the longer Blessed scale. Reliability not formally tested. The score correlated highly ($r = 0.92$) with the full scale and it was almost as sensitive as the longer test. Any error score of 0–6 is within normal limits.

Scoring is difficult as originally devised and as shown, and it is more easily understood if scored positively, subtracting from maximum (for item) for each error. This gives a 0–28 score, with a higher score being better, scores over 20 being 'normal', as shown below.

Short Orientation–Memory–Concentration Test (alternative version)

Instruction
Subtract error score from maximum to give item score.

No. Question	Maximum score	Subtract per error to maximum (in parentheses)	Score
1. What year is it now? Answer: _____	4	−4 (×1)	____
2. What month is it now? Answer: _____	3	−3 (×1)	____

3. Repeat this phrase:
   John Brown,
   42 Market Street,
   Chicago
   or (UK):
   John Brown,
   42 West Street,
   Gateshead
	Answer (recall score):
	   John / Brown
	   42 / Market street
	   Chicago
	
	   John / Brown
	   42 / West street
	   Gateshead		

4. About what time is it? (within one hour) Answer: _____	3	−3 (×1)	____
5. Count backwards 20 to 1 20 19 18 17 16 15 14 13 12 11 10 9 8 7 6 5 4 3 2 1	4	−2 (×2)	____
6. Say months in reverse order Dec Nov Oct Sept Aug July June May Apr Mar Feb Jan	4	−2 (×2)	____
7. Repeat the address just given (Answer next to address)	10	−2 (×5)	____
	Total score =		____/28

Mini-Mental State Examination (MMSE)

Instructions
Record response to each question.

Domain tested Test	Score

Orientation
   Year, month, day, date, time   ___/5

   Country, town, district, hospital, ward   ___/5

Registration
   Examiner names three objects (for example, apple, table, penny)
   Patient asked to repeat three names—score one for each correct
   answer   ___/3

   Then patient to learn three names (i.e. repeat until correct)

Attention and Calculation
   Subtract 7 from 100, then repeat from result, etc. Stop after 5.
   100, 93, 86, 79, 72, 65.   ___/5

   (Alternative: spell 'world' backwards. D L R O W)

Recall
   Ask for three objects learnt earlier   ___/3

Language
   Name a pencil and watch   ___/2
   Repeat 'No ifs, ands, or buts'   ___/1
   Give a three-stage command. Score one for each stage   ___/3
   (for example, 'Place index finger of right hand on your nose, and
      then on your left ear.')
   Ask patient to read and obey a written command on a piece of   ___/1
      paper stating: 'Close your eyes'
   Ask patient to write a sentence. Score if it is sensible and has a   ___/1
      subject and a verb

Domain tested	Score
Test	

Copying
Ask patient to copy a pair of intersecting pentagons   ___/1

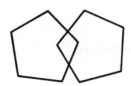

References   Folstein *et al*. (1975); DePaulo *et al*. (1980); Dick *et al*. (1984); Bleecker *et al*. (1988); Galasko *et al*. (1990); Zillmer *et al*. (1990); Beatty and Goodkin (1990).

Comment
The MMSE is now widely used as a brief screening measure of cognitive impairment. A score of 24 is used to distinguish normal from abnormal. Validity (as a test of marked cognitive impairment) and reliability has been tested, but there are problems. The test includes memory, attention, language, etc., making it difficult to interpret any score. Galasko *et al*. (1990) draw attention to difficulties in scoring. Sensitivity and specificity have not been well established, but 'normal' values have (Bleeker *et al*. 1988).

It can be clinically very useful, provided these marked limitations are remembered. It is best to study the actual response to each question, not the total score. It is useful if obtaining information from other hospitals by post. However, on balance, the author would recommend using a simple measure of aphasia, the Frenchay Aphasia Screening Test, with a simple measure of information, orientation, and memory.

Modified Mini-Mental State Examination

Instructions
Record response to each question

Domain-tested 　Test	Score
Orientation (place) 　Country, town, district, hospital, ward	＿＿/5
Registration (not scored) 　Examiner names three objects (for example, apple, table, penny) 　*then patient to learn three names (i.e. repeat until correct)*	
Attention and Calculation 　Spell 'world' backwards. D L R O W	＿＿/5
Subtract 7 from 100, then repeat from result etc. Stop after 5. 　100, 93, 86, 79, 72, 65	＿＿/5
Recall 　Ask for three objects learnt earlier	＿＿/3
Abbreviated total (= Recall + Orientation for Place)	＿＿/8

Reference Galasko *et al.* (1990)

Comment
Recently, Galasko *et al.* identified the items from the MMSE most useful in detecting early dementia. These are:

1. Recall
2. Recall and orientation for place
3. A 'serial 7' score less than a 'world backwards' score

They recommend adding scores for recall and orientation for place, with a score of 3 or less being almost as specific as the whole MMSE in detecting early Alzheimer's disease.

Clifton Assessment Procedures for the Elderly (CAPE)

Information/orientation

Instructions
Questions may be rephrased once or twice where necessary, for example 'What is your date of birth?' could be 'When were you born'?, or 'When is your birthday'? followed by 'And what year were you born'?. No assistance or cues should be given, and excessive repetition is not recommended. Each correct response is given one point.

Question
   Guidelines

1. What is your name/full name?
   First name and surname are both required.

2. How old are you?
   Present age in years or predicted age next birthday; for example, 79 next August.

3. What is your date of birth?
   The date, month, and year must all be correctly given.

4. What is this place/Where are you now?
   The name of the hospital ward, or recognition that it is a hospital ward is required for hospital patients.
   Recognition that they are in their own home, social services accommodation, or whatever, for non-hospital subjects.

5. What is the name of this hospital? *or*
   What is the address of this place?
   Name of the hospital is required.
   Address of the home or, if in their own home, number and street name as appropriate.

6. What is the name of this town/city?
   The correct name of the town or city in which they are currently located.

7. Who is the Prime Minister?
   Surname of the current PM is sufficient.

8. Who is the President of the USA?
   Surname of the current president.

9. What are the colours of the national flag/Union Jack?
   Red, white, and blue.

10. What day is it?
   The day of the week, not the date, is required. (This can be explained once if the date is given.)

11. What month is it?
    Current month.

12. What year is it?
    Current year.

Reference   Pattie and Gilleard (1975, 1978)

Comment
The various CAPE assessments are quite widely used in geriatric practice
and in dementia studies, although not much in neurological rehabilitation.
This test measures impairment of orientation. The author is unaware
of major studies of reliability. The similarity to other tests of cognitive
impairment is obvious.

Clifton Assessment Procedures for the Elderly (CAPE)

Behaviour rating scale

Item Scoring	Score

When bathing or dressing, he/she requires: ____
  0 = no assistance
  1 = some assistance
  2 = maximum assistance

With regard to walking, he/she: ____
  0 = shows no signs of weakness
  1 = walks slowly without aid, or uses a stick
  2 = is unable to walk, or if able to walk needs frame, crutches or
      someone by his/her side

He/she is incontinent of urine and/or faeces (day or night):   ____
  0 = never
  1 = sometimes (once or twice per week)
  2 = frequently (3 times per week or more)

He/she is in bed during the day: ____
(bed does **not** include couch, settee, etc.)
  0 = never
  1 = sometimes
  2 = almost always

CAPE, Behaviour rating scale (*cont.*)

Item	Score
Scoring	

He/she is confused: _____
(unable to find way around, loses possessions, etc.)
   0 = almost never confused
   1 = sometimes confused
   2 = almost always confused

When left to his/her own devices, his/her appearance is: _____
(clothes and/or hair)
   0 = almost never disorderly
   1 = sometimes disorderly
   2 = almost always disorderly

If allowed outside, he/she would: _____
   0 = never need supervision
   1 = sometimes need supervision
   2 = always need supervision

He/she helps out in the home/ward: _____
   0 = often helps out
   1 = sometimes helps out
   2 = never helps out

He/she keeps him/herself occupied in a constructive or useful activity
(works, reads, plays games, has hobbies etc):   _____
   0 = almost always occupied
   1 = sometimes occupied
   2 = almost never occupied

He/she socializes with others: _____
   0 = does establish good relationship with others
   1 = has some difficulty in establishing good relationships
   2 = has a great deal of difficulty establishing good relationships

He/she is willing to do things suggested or asked of him/her: _____
   0 = often goes along
   1 = sometimes goes along
   2 = almost never goes along

He/she understands what you communicate to him/her: _____
(you may use speaking, writing, or gesturing)
   0 = understands almost everything you communicate
   1 = understands some of what you communicate
   2 = understands almost nothing of what you communicate

CAPE, Behaviour rating scale (*cont.*)

Item Scoring	Score

He/she communicates in any manner: ____
(by speaking, writing, or gesturing)
   0 = well enough to make him/herself easily understood at all times
   1 = can be understood sometimes or with some difficulty
   2 = can rarely or never be understood for whatever reason

He/she is objectionable to others during the day: ____
(loud or constant talking, pilfering, soiling furniture)
   0 = rarely or never
   1 = sometimes
   2 = frequently

He/she is objectionable to others during the night: ____
(loud or constant talking, pilfering, soiling furniture, interfering with
affairs of others, wandering about, etc.)
   0 = rarely or never
   1 = sometimes
   2 = frequently

He/she accuses others of doing him/her bodily harm or stealing
his/her personal possessions: ____
(rate 0 if accusations are true)
   0 = never
   1 = sometimes
   2 = frequently

He/she hoards apparently meaningless items: ____
(wads of paper, string, scraps of food, etc.)
   0 = never
   1 = sometimes
   2 = frequently

His/her sleep pattern at night is: ____
   0 = almost never awake
   1 = sometimes awake
   2 = often awake

References   Gilleard and Pattie (1977); Pattie and Gilleard (1975, 1978)

Comment

A second CAPE assessment, this is designed to measure the behavioural
problems (disabilities) seen in elderly people with dementia. It was designed

for use predominantly with patients in institutional care. It is derived from an earlier scale, the Stockton Geriatric Rating Scale (Meer and Baker 1966). It is probably not suitable for younger people with acquired cognitive impairments, for example after head injury.

Everyday Memory Questionnaire

Instructions

The 28 statements set out below are about forgetting things, something everyone does to an extent. Please indicate how frequently the examples given have happened to you, (or to the subject) over the last three months, using the following scale:

0 = Not at all in the last three months

1 = About once in the last three months

2 = More than once in the last three months, but less than once a month

3 = About once a month

4 = More than once a month but less than once a week

5 = About once a week

6 = More than once a week but less than once a day

7 = About once a day

8 = More than once a day

1__   Forgetting where you have put something. Losing things around the house.

2__   Failing to recognize places that you are told you have been to before.

3__   Finding a television story difficult to follow.

4__   Not remembering a change in your daily routine, such as a change in the place where something is kept or a change in the time something happens. Following your old routine by mistake.

5__   Having to go back to check whether you have done something you meant to do.

6__   Forgetting when it was that something happened; for example, whether it was yesterday or last week.

7__   Completely forgetting to take things with you, or leaving things behind and having to go back and fetch them.

8__   Forgetting you were told something yesterday or a few days ago, and maybe having to be reminded about it.

9__   Starting to read something (a book or an article in a newspaper or magazine) without realizing you have already read it before.

10__   Letting yourself ramble on, to speak about unimportant or irrelevant things.

11__   Failing to recognize, by sight, close friends or relatives who you meet frequently.

12__   Having difficulty in picking up a new skill; for example, finding it hard to learn a new game, or to work some new gadget after you have practised it once or twice.

13— Finding that a word is 'on the tip of your tongue'. You know what it is but cannot quite find it.

14— Completely forgetting to do things you said you would do and you planned to do.

15— Forgetting important details of what you did or what happened to you the day before.

16— When talking to someone, forgetting what you have just said. Maybe saying 'What was I just talking about'?

17— When reading a newspaper or magazine being unable to follow the thread of a story; losing track of what it is about.

18— Forgetting to tell someone something important. Perhaps forgetting to pass on a message or remind someone of something.

19— Forgetting important details about yourself; for example, your birthdate, or where you live.

20— Getting the details of what someone has told you mixed up and confused.

21— Telling someone a story or joke that you have told them once already.

22— Forgetting details of things you do regularly, whether at home or at work. For example, forgetting details of what to do, or forgetting at what time to do it.

23— Finding that the faces of famous people seen on television or in photographs look unfamiliar.

24— Forgetting where things are normally kept or looking for them in the wrong place.

25— Getting lost or turning in the wrong direction on a journey, on a walk or in a building where you have *often* been before.

26— Getting lost or turning in the wrong direction on a journey, on a walk or in a building where you have *only been once or twice* before.

27— Doing some routine thing twice by mistake. For example, putting two lots of tea in the teapot or going to brush/comb your hair when you have just done so.

28— Repeating to someone what you have just told them or asking the same question twice.

References Sunderland *et al.* (1983); Sunderland *et al.* (1984); Sunderland *et al.* (1986); Tinson and Lincoln (1987); Lincoln and Tinson (1989)

Comment

This measure of memory disability (the behavioural consequences of poor memory) was initially developed from a larger questionnaire in the context of patients with head injury. There is reasonable evidence of validity (compared with standard tests of memory). Reliability is reasonable but not excellent, but the very nature of the problem makes reliability difficult in severely impaired patients. The questionnaire can be used by relatives, and has been used with stroke patients.

Cognitive Failures Questionnaire

Instructions
The following questions are about minor mistakes which everyone makes from time to time, but some of which happen more often than others. We want to know how often these things have happened to you in the last six months. Please put in the number of your answer.

Answers
0 = Never   3 = Quite often
1 = Very rarely   4 = Very often
2 = Occasionally

ANSWER	No.	QUESTION
____	1.	Do you read something and find that you haven't been thinking about it and must read it again?
____	2.	Do you find you forget why you went from one part of the house to another?
____	3.	Do you fail to notice signposts on the road?
____	4.	Do you find you confuse right and left when giving instructions?
____	5.	Do you bump into people?
____	6.	Do you find you forget whether you've turned off a light or fire or locked the door?
____	7.	Do you fail to listen to people's names when you are meeting them?
____	8.	Do you say something and realize afterwards that it might be taken as insulting?
____	9.	Do you fail to hear people speaking to you when you are doing something else?
____	10.	Do you lose your temper and regret it?
____	11.	Do you leave important letters unanswered for days?
____	12.	Do you find you forget which way to turn on a road you know well but rarely use?
____	13.	Do you fail to see what you want in a supermarket (although it's there)?
____	14.	Do you find yourself suddenly wondering whether you've used a word correctly?
____	15.	Do you have trouble making up your mind?
____	16.	Do you find you forget appointments?
____	17.	Do you forget where you put something like a newspaper or book?

___   18.   Do you find you accidentally throw away the thing you want and keep what you meant to throw away—as in the example of throwing away the matchbox and putting the used match in your pocket?

___   19.   Do you daydream when you ought to be listening to something?

___   20.   Do you find you forget people's names?

___   21.   Do you start doing one thing at home and get distracted into something else (unintentionally)?

___   22.   Do you find you can't quite remember something although it's on the tip of your tongue?

___   23.   Do you find you forget what you came to the shops to buy?

___   24.   Do you drop things?

___   25.   Do you find you can't think of anything to say?

CFQ-for-others

Instructions

The questions given below are about mistakes and difficulties which everybody has from time to time. We want to know how often, in your opinion, your relative or partner has shown any of these troubles during the past six months. After each question, please tick only one of the five possible answers.

Please make sure you read them carefully because for some questions 'very often' is on the left side of the page and 'never' is on the right, but for other questions 'never' is on the left and 'very often' on the right.

During the last six months has your relative or partner seemed to be:

1. Absent-minded; that is, making mistakes in what he/she is doing because he/she is thinking of something else?

    Very often   Quite often   Occasionally   Very rarely   Never

2. Finding it difficult to concentrate upon anything because his/her attention tends to wander from one thing to another?

    Never   Very rarely   Occasionally   Quite often   Very often

3. Forgetful, such as forgetting where he/she has put things, or about appointments, or about what he/she has done

    Very often   Quite often   Occasionally   Very rarely   Never

4. Busy thinking about his/her own affairs and so not noticing what is going on around him/her?

    Never   Very rarely   Occasionally   Quite often   Very often

5. Clumsy, for example, dropping things or bumping into people?

   Very often   Quite often   Occasionally   Very rarely   Never

6. Having difficulty making up his/her mind?

   Never   Very rarely   Occasionally   Quite often   Very often

7. Disorganized, that is, getting into a muddle when doing something because of lack of planning or concentration?

   Very often   Quite often   Occasionally   Very rarely   Never

8. Getting unduly cross about minor matters?

   Never   Very rarely   Occasionally   Quite often   Very often

---

Reference   Broadbent *et al.* (1982)

Comment

Two measures of cognitive disability, the behavioural consequences of general cognitive failures. The original paper gives evidence for validity and reliability. One is for the patient, the other for the relative. The author is unaware of any published studies using these questionnaires since their original publication.

Hachinski Ischaemia Score

Feature	Score	Feature	Score
Abrupt onset	2	Emotional incontinence	1
Stepwise deterioriation	1	History of hypertension	1
Fluctuating course	2	History of strokes	2
Nocturnal confusion	1	Evidence of associated	
Relative preservation of		atherosclerosis	1
personality	1	Focal neurological symptoms	2
Depression	1	Focal neurological signs	2
Somatic complaints	1		

References   Hachinski *et al.* (1975); Molsa *et al.* (1985)

Comment

A widely used index supposed to distinguish dementia arising from vascular disease from that due to Alzheimer's disease; a score of 7 or more is taken as indicating multi-infarct dementia, and 0–4 suggests a non-ischaemic cause. Its validity as a method of separating Alzheimer's dementia from vascular dementia is not adequately proven, the sensitivity and specificity not adequately established, and the reliability of scoring untested.

The Speech Questionnaire

Instructions

This questionnaire is given to the relatives (or other carers) of someone with language difficulties.

Please tick the most appropriate description of this person's behaviour at the moment, based on your own experience with them.

Speech

1. Does he/she produce appropriate spoken responses to familiar serial phrases produced by you, such as 'Hello', 'Good morning', and 'Goodbye'.

   __ Often   __ Sometimes   __ Rarely   __ Never

2. Does he/she say any single words spontaneously (without any help from you)?

   __ Often   __ Sometimes   __ Rarely   __ Never

3. Does he/she say any single words in response to your questions?

   __ Never   __ Rarely   __ Sometimes   __ Often

4. Does he/she say 'yes' or 'no' spontaneously?

   __ Never   __ Rarely   __ Sometimes   __ Often

5. Does he/she say 'yes' and 'no' the right way round?

   __ Often   __ Sometimes   __ Rarely   __ Never

6. Does he/she say any common everyday phrases such as 'Hello', 'Goodbye', 'Please', and 'Thank you' spontaneously?

   __ Never   __ Rarely   __ Sometimes   __ Often

7. Does he/she say common everyday phrases appropriately?

   __ Often   __ Sometimes   __ Rarely   __ Never

8. Is his/her conversation appropriate?

   __ Often   __ Sometimes   __ Rarely   __ Never

9. Does he/she say phrases spontaneously?

   __ Never   __ Rarely   __ Sometimes   __ Often

10. Does he/she say phrases in response to your questions?

    __ Never   __ Rarely   __ Sometimes   __ Often

11. Does he/she initiate spoken conversation with you?

    __ Never   __ Rarely   __ Sometimes   __ Often

12. Does he/she say sentences spontaneously?

    __ Never   __ Rarely   __ Sometimes   __ Often

13. Does he/she say sentences in response to your questions?

    __ Often   __ Sometimes   __ Rarely   __ Never

14. Is his/her speech slow or hesitant?

    __ Often   __ Sometimes   __ Rarely   __ Never

Understanding

1. Does he/she understand simple instructions given by you using gestures (signs with your hands such as pointing) if necessary?

    __ Often   __ Sometimes   __ Rarely   __ Never

2. Does he/she understand simple spoken instructions without use of gestures?

    __ Never   __ Rarely   __ Sometimes   __ Often

3. Does he/she understand general conversation with you about everyday topics?

    __ Never   __ Rarely   __ Sometimes   __ Often

4. Does he/she understand rapid conversation with more than one person?

    __ Often   __ Sometimes   __ Rarely   __ Never

5. Does he/she understand complicated ideas and explanations?

    __ Often   __ Sometimes   __ Rarely   __ Never

Reference   Lincoln (1982)

Scoring
It was scored as '1' for 'Often' or 'Sometimes', and '0' for 'Rarely' or 'Never'; this is reversed for question 14. A 0–3 scale could be used (reversed for Q.14).

Comment
This is a measure of communicative disability designed for use with patients who have aphasia (usually after stroke). Validity, reliability, and scalability were all established in the original study and it has been used once in a trial of speech therapy. The author is unaware of any use since.

14 Measures of motor impairment

Summary

1. Motor Club Assessment
2. Rivermead Motor Assessment
3. Motricity Index
4. Trunk Control Test
5. Motor Assessment Scale
6. Modified Ashworth Scale for grading spasticity
7. Tufts Quantitative Neuromuscular Exam (TQNE)
8. Dynanometry

Introduction

This chapter illustrates measures of voluntary muscle power and use. Other measures of motor impairment can be found in Chapter 23, which covers measures in Parkinson's disease and movement disorders. All measures are reasonable, and the choice will depend upon what the measure is wanted for. In routine practice, especially after stroke, the Motricity Index and Trunk Control Test are probably sufficient. Dynanometry should be used whenever possible.

One major assessment is not shown, the Brunnstrom–Fugl-Meyer (BFM) assessment. The original publication (Fugl-Meyer *et al.* 1975) gives long details, but the author finds them difficult to understand or abbreviate. Given that there are other, shorter, simpler measures available, it has been omitted.

Motor Club Assessment

MOTOR SECTION

Scale
   0 = No movement
   1 = Limited range of movement (add − or + for further detail)
   2 = Completed range of movement (compared with other side). Coordination need not be normal, but range should be full.

Positions
  a = Good side lying
  b = Lying
  c = Sitting
  d = Standing

Movements—arm

Position/score

Shoulder shrugging
  Elevation of the shoulder girdle

a____
b____
c____

Arm thrusting
  Forward extension of the arm from the flexed position

a____
b____
c____
d____

Arm lifting
  Upward extension of the arm from the flexed position

a____
b____
c____
d____

Forearm supinating
  Supination of the forearm from the prone position (elbow at
  right angles in front of the body)

c____

Wrist cocking, forearm supported
  Extend wrist from mid-position

c____

Wrist cocking, with arm raised straight in front
  Extend wrist from mid-position
  Straight arm raised in front

c____

Pinch grip, forearm supported
  Pick up 1 cm marble between index finger and thumb
  (pass = 2, fail = 0)

c____

Pinch grip, with arm raised straight in front
  Pick up 1 cm marble between index finger and thumb
  (pass = 2, fail = 0)

c____

Movements—leg

Hip and knee bending
   Bend (flex) hip and knee from straight position; combined
   movement

a ____
b ____
d ____

Knee flexion
   Isolated knee flexion, thigh immobilized

a ____
b ____
d ____

Ankle dorsiflexion; leg straight
   Dorsiflex from the mid-position

b ____
d ____

Ankle dorsiflexion; hip and knee bent
   Dorsiflex from the mid-position

c ____

Motor Club Assessment: functional movement activities

Scoring
0 = Impossible (no co-operation, help from two or more people)
1 = Assistance (patient co-operates; help of only one person required)
2 = Independent with use of aid
3 = Independent
X = Not tested (state why)

Grade	Activity	Notes
____	Supine to left side sitting	Pulling on edge of bed = aid
____	Supine to right side sitting	Pulling on edge of bed = aid
____	Bridging	Using unaffected leg to help affected/bad leg straighten = aid
____	Sitting balance (60 sec)	Use of hands for support = aid
____	Sitting, touch floor and return	Use of hands for support going down or up = aid
____	Sitting to standing	Use of hands to push down on chair for standing = aid

Grade	Activity	Notes
____	Standing balance (30 sec)	Must have both feet on the floor. Use of chair, stick, etc. = aid
____	Standing on left leg (5 sec)	Use of chair, stick, etc. = aid
____	Standing on right leg (5 sec)	Use of chair, stick, etc. = aid
____	Standing, get down on floor	Use of chair, stick, etc. = aid
____	Kneel standing balance (10 sec)	Use of stool, etc. = aid
____	½ kneel standing, left (5 sec)	Use of stool, etc. = aid
____	½ kneel standing, right (5 sec)	Use of stool, etc. = aid
____	Get up from floor to standing	Use of stool, etc. = aid
____	Transfer sitting on chair to lying on bed	Use of tripod/stick = aid Support on bed/chair = 1
____	Transfer lying on bed to sitting on chair	Use of tripod/stick = aid Support on bed/chair = 1
____	Walking (15 m)	Also record time and aid used
____	Stairs (up and down 10 steps)	Also record time and aid used
____	Total	

Reference   Ashburn (1982); Turton and Fraser (1986); Sunderland *et al.* (1989)

Comment
A good assessment put together by consensus by a group of specialist physiotherapists. Validity is obvious (but not formally tested). The author is unaware of formal reliability studies. It was initially presented as an easily completed form (see Ashburn 1982). Although parts of this assessment are used, it has not become widely used. The first section covers impairment, the second mobility disability. It probably deserves more widespread use.

Rivermead Motor Assessment

General instructions
Go through the items in order of difficulty. Score 1 if patient can perform activity, 0 if he cannot. Three tries are allowed. After three consecutive failures, stop that section and proceed to the next. Give no feedback of whether correct or incorrect, just give general encouragement. Repeat instructions and demonstrate them to the patient if necessary. All exercises to be carried out independently unless otherwise stated. All arm tests refer to the affected arm unless otherwise stated.

Section Item	Score

Gross function

1. Sit unsupported
   Without holding on, on edge of bed, feet unsupported.   ____

2. Lying to sitting on side of bed
   Using any method.   ____

3. Sitting to standing
   May use hands to push up. Must stand up in 15 sec and stand for
   15 sec, with an aid if necessary.   ____

4. Transfer from wheelchair to chair towards unaffected side
   May use hands.   ____

5. Transfer from wheelchair to chair towards affected side
   May use hands.   ____

6. Walk 10 m indoors with an aid
   Any walking aid. No stand-by help.   ____

7. Climb stairs independently
   Any method. May use bannister and aid—must be a full flight of
   stairs.   ____

8. Walk 10 m indoors without an aid
   No stand-by help. No caliper, splint or walking aid.   ____

9. Walk 10 m, pick up bean bag from floor, turn and carry back
   Bend down any way, may use aid to walk if necessary. No stand-by
   help. May use either hand to pick up bean bag.   ____

10. Walk outside 40 m
    May use walking aid, caliper or splint. No stand-by help.   ____

11. Walk up and down four steps
    Patient may use an aid if he would normally use one, but may not
    hold on to rail. This is included to test ability to negotiate curb or
    stairs without a rail.   ____

12. Run 10m
    Must be symmetrical.   ____

13. Hop on affected leg five times on the spot
    Must hop on ball of foot without stopping to regain balance. No
    help with arms.   ____

Gross function total   ____

Section	
Item	Score

Leg and trunk

1. Roll to affected side   ____
   Starting position should be lying, not crook lying.

2. Roll to unaffected side   ____
   Starting position should be lying, not crook lying.

3. Half-bridging   ____
   Starting position—half-crook lying. Patient must put some weight
   through affected leg to lift hip on affected side. Therapist may
   position leg, but patient must maintain position even after movement
   is completed.

4. Sitting to standing   ____
   May not use arms—feet must be flat on floor—must put weight
   through both feet.

5. Half-crook lying: lift affected leg over side of bed and return it to same
   position   ____
   Affected leg in half-crook position. Lift leg off bed on to support;
   for example, box, stool, floor, so that hip is in neutral and knee at
   90 degrees while resting on support. Must keep affected knee flexed
   throughout movement. Do not allow external rotation at hip. This
   tests control of knee and hip.

6. Standing, step unaffected leg on and off block   ____
   Without retraction of pelvis or hyperextension of knee. This tests
   knee and hip control while weight bearing through the unaffected
   leg.

7. Standing, tap ground lightly five times with unaffected foot   ____
   Without retraction of pelvis or hyperextension of knee. Weight must
   stay on affected leg. This again tests knee and hip control while
   weight bearing through the affected leg but is more difficult than
   in 6.

8. Lying, dorsiflex affected ankle with leg flexed   ____
   Physiotherapist may hold affected leg in position, knee at 90 degrees.
   Do not allow any inversion. Must have half range of movement of
   unaffected foot.

9. Lying, dorsiflex affected ankle with leg extended   ____
   Same conditions as in 8, with leg extended. Do not allow any
   inversion or knee flexion. Foot must reach plantigrade (90).

10. Stand with affected hip in neutral position, flex affected knee   ____
    Therapist may not position leg. This is extremely difficult for most
    hemiplegic patients, but is included to assess minimal dysfunction.

Section Item	Score

Arm

1. Lying, protract shoulder girdle with arm in elevation
    Arm may be supported.   ____

2. Lying, hold extended arm in elevation (some external rotation) for at
    least 2 sec   ____
    Therapist should place arm in position and patient must maintain
    position with some external rotation. Do not allow pronation. Elbow
    must be held within 30 degrees of full extension.

3. Flexion and extension of elbow, with arm as in 2 above   ____
    Elbow must extend to at least 20 degrees full extension. Palm should
    not face outward during any part of movement.

4. Sitting, elbow into side, pronation and supination   ____
    Three-quarters range is acceptable, with elbow unsupported and at
    right angles.

5. Reach forward, pick up large ball with both hands and place down
    again   ____
    Ball should be on table so far in front of patient that he has to extend
    arms fully to reach it. Shoulders must be protracted, elbows
    extended, wrists neutral or extended, and fingers extended through-
    out movement. Palms should be kept in contact with the ball.

6. Stretch arm forward, pick up tennis ball from table, release on mid-
    thigh on affected side, return to table, then release again on table.
    Repeat five times   ____
    Shoulder must be protracted, elbow extended and wrist neutral or
    extended during each phase.

7. Same exercise as in 6 above with pencil   ____
    Patient must use thumb and fingers to grip.

8. Pick up a piece of paper from table in front and release five times   ____
    Patient must use thumb and fingers to pick up paper and not pull it
    to edge of table. Arm position as in 6 above.

9. Cut putty with a knife and fork on plate with non-slip mat and put
    pieces into container at side of plate   ____
    Bite-size pieces.

10. Stand on spot, maintain upright position, pat large ball on floor with
    palm of hand for 5 continuous bounces   ____

11. Continuous opposition of thumb and each finger more than 14 times in
    10 sec   ____
    Must do movements in consistent sequence. Do not allow thumb to
    slide from one finger to the other.

Section Item	Score

12. Supination and pronation on to palm of affected hand 20 times in 10 sec   ——

    Arm must be away from body, the palm and dorsum of hand must touch palm of good hand. Each tap counts as one. This is similar to 4 above, but introduces speed.

13. Standing, with affected arm abducted to 90 degrees with palm flat against wall. Maintain arm in position. Turn body towards wall and as far as possible towards arm, i.e. rotate body beyond 90 degrees   ——

    Do not allow flexion at elbow, and wrist must be extended with palm of hand fully in contact with wall.

14. Place string around head and tie bow at back   ——

    Do not allow neck to flex. Affected hand must be used for more than just supporting string. This tests function of hand without help of sight.

15. 'Pat-a-cake' seven times in 15 sec   ——

    Mark crosses on wall at shoulder level. Clap both hands together (both hands touch crosses—clap—one hand touches opposite cross). Must be in correct order. Palms must touch. Each sentence counts as one. Give patient three tries. This is a complex pattern which involves co-ordination, speed, and memory, as well as good arm function.

References   Lincoln and Leadbitter (1979); Collen *et al.* (1990)

Comment

A widely used measure of motor 'function' after stroke. The scale mixes impairments (arm, and leg and trunk) and disabilities (gross function), but has reasonable validity and reliability. It forms a hierarchy in patients recovering from stroke, which greatly reduces time to administer and simplifies interpretation of a score. Too long for routine use, but the Gross Function section can be assessed simply by asking, which makes it a rapid measure (Collen *et al.* 1990).

Motricity Index

TESTS (in sitting position)

Arm
1. Pinch grip; 2.5 cm cube between thumb and forefinger
2. Elbow flexion; from 90 degrees, voluntary contraction/movement
3. Shoulder abduction; from against chest

Leg
4. Ankle dorsiflexion; from plantar flexed position
5. Knee extension; from 90 degrees, voluntary contraction/movement
6. Hip flexion; usually from 90 degrees

Scoring

Test 1 (pinch grip)
  0 No movement
 11 Beginnings of prehension (any movement of finger or thumb)
 19 Grips cube, but unable to hold against gravity
 22 Grips cube, held against gravity, but not against weak pull
 26 Grips cube against pull, but weaker than other side
 33 Normal pinch grip

Tests 2–6
  0 No movement
  9 Palpable contraction in muscle, but no movement
 14 Movement seen, but not full range/not against gravity
 19 Movement; full range against gravity, not against resistance
 25 Movement against resistance, but weaker than other side
 33 Normal power

Arm score = scores (1) + (2) + (3) + 1 (to make 100)

Leg score = scores (4) + (5) + (6) + 1 (to make 100)

Side score = (ARM + LEG)/2

Trunk Control Test

TESTS (on bed)
1. Rolling to weak side
2. Rolling to strong side
3. Sitting up from lying down
4. Balance in sitting position (on side of bed)

Scoring
  0 Unable to do on own
 12 Able to do, but only with non-muscular help—for example, pulling on bed clothes, using arms to steady self when sitting, pulling up on rope or monkey pole, etc.
 25 Able to complete normally

Trunk score = score (1) + (2) + (3) + (4)

Motricity Index: guidelines

The patient should be sitting in a chair or on the edge of the bed, but can be tested lying if necessary. The grading is derived from the Medical Research Council (MRC) grades, but weighted scores are used. Six limb movements are tested.

Pinch grip
Ask patient to grip a 2.5-cm object (cube) between his thumb and forefinger. Object should be on a flat surface (for example, a book). Monitor any *forearm* or *small hand* muscles.

    19 = drops object when lifted (examiner may need to lift wrist)
    22 = can hold in air, but easily dislodged

Elbow flexion
Elbow flexed to 90 degrees, forearm horizontal and upper arm vertical. Patient asked to bend elbow so that hand touches the shoulder. Examiner resists with hand on wrist. Monitor *biceps*.

    14 = *If* no movement seen, may hold elbow out so that arm is *horizontal*.

Shoulder abduction
With elbow fully flexed and against chest, patient asked to abduct arm. Monitor contraction of *deltoid*; movement of shoulder girdle does not count—there must be movement of humerus in relation to scapula.

    19 = abducted more than 90 degrees beyond horizontal.

Ankle dorsiflexion
Foot relaxed in plantar flexed position. Patient asked to dorsiflex foot ('As if standing on your heels'). Monitor *tibialis anterior*.

    14 = less than full range of dorsiflexion

Knee extension
Foot unsupported, knee at 90 degrees. Patient asked to extend (straighten) knee to touch examiner's hand held level with the knee. Monitor contraction of the *quadriceps*.

    14 = less than 50 per cent of full extension (i.e. 45 degrees only)
    19 = knee fully extended, but easily pushed down

Hip flexion
Sitting with hip bent at 90 degrees. Patient asked to lift knee towards chin. Check for associated (trick) movement of leaning back, by placing hand behind back and asking patient not to lean back. Monitor contraction of *ilio-psoas* (hip flexors).

    14 = less than full range of possible flexion (check passive movement)
    19 = fully flexed, but easily pushed down

Trunk Control Test: guidelines

Four movements/functions are tested, with the patient lying on the bed.

Rolling to weak side
From lying on back, rolling over on to weak side. May push/pull on bed with good arm.

Rolling to strong side
From lying on back, bringing weak limbs over
12 if uses good limbs to help

Sitting up from lying down
From lying on back—may use arm(s) to push or pull
12 if pulls on pole, rope, sheets, etc.

Sitting balance
Sitting on edge of bed, feet off ground—balance for 30 sec
12 if needs to touch anything with hands to stay upright
0 if unable to stay up (any way) for 30 sec

References   Demeurisse *et al.* (1980); Parker *et al.* (1986); Wade, Langton, and Hewer (1987*b*); Sunderland *et al.* (1989); Collin and Wade (1990); Collen *et al.* (1990)

Comment
A short simple measure of motor loss primarily developed for use after stroke but probably useful in any patient with upper motor neuron weakness. Validity and reliability proven, and sensitive to change seen in recovery after stroke. Although not popular with traditional physiotherapists (and not intended to guide therapy), it is very useful in routine clinical practice. Strongly recommended.

Motor Assessment Scale

General instructions
1. The test should preferably be carried out in a quiet private room or curtained-off area.
2. The test should be carried out when the patient is maximally alert and not when under the influence of hypnotic or sedative drugs. Record if the patient is under the influence of sedative drugs.
3. Patient should be dressed in suitable street clothes with sleeves rolled up and without shoes and socks. Items 1 to 3 inclusive may be scored if necessary with the patient in his right clothes.

4. Each item is recorded on a scale of 0 to 6.

5. All items are to be performed independently by the patient unless otherwise stated. 'Stand-by help' means that the physical therapist stands by and may steady patient but must not actively assist.

6. Items 1 to 8 are recorded according to the patient's responses to specific instructions. General Tonus (item 9) is scored from continuous observations and handling throughout the assessment.

7. Patient should be scored on best performance. Repeat three times unless other specific instructions are given.

8. Because the scale is designed to score the patient's best performance, the physical therapist should give general encouragement but should not give specific feedback on whether response is correct or incorrect. Sensitivity to the patient is necessary to enable him to produce his best performance.

9. Instructions should be repeated and demonstrations given to the patient if necessary.

10. The order of administration of the items can be varied according to convenience.

11. If the patient becomes emotionally labile at any stage during scoring, the physical therapist should wait 15 sec before attempting the following procedures:
    • ask the patient to close his mouth and take a deep breath; and
    • hold the patient's jaw closed and ask the patient to stop crying.

    If patient is unable to control behaviour, the examiner should cease testing him and re-score this item and any other items unscored at a more suitable time.

12. If performance is scored differently on left and right side, the physical therapist may indicate this with an 'L' in one box and an 'R' in another box.

13. The patient should be informed when being timed.

14. You will need: a low, wide plinth, a stopwatch, a polystyrene cup, eight jellybeans, two teacups, a rubber ball 14 cm (5-in) diameter, a stool, a comb, a top of a pen, a table, a dessert spoon and water, a pen, a prepared sheet for drawing lines, and a cylindrical object such as a jar.

A. *Supine to side lying on to intact side*

1. Pulls himself into side lying.
   Starting position must be supine lying, not knees flexed. Patient pulls himself into side lying with intact arm, moves affected leg with intact leg.

2. Moves leg across actively and lower half of body follows.
   Starting position as above. Arm is left behind.

3. Arm is lifted across body with other arm. Leg is moved actively and body follows in a block.
   Starting position as above.

4. Moves arm across body actively and rest of body follows in a block.
   Starting position as above.

5. Moves arm and leg and rolls to side but overbalances.
   Starting position as above. Shoulder protracts and arm flexes forward.

6. Rolls to side in 3 sec.
   Starting position as above. Must not use hands.

B. *Supine to sitting over side of bed*

1. Side lying, lifts head sideways but cannot sit up.
   Patient assisted to side lying.
2. Side lying to sitting over side of bed.
   Therapist assists patient with movement. Patient controls head position throughout.
3. Side lying to sitting over side of bed.
   Therapist gives stand-by help by assisting legs over side of bed.
4. Side lying to sitting over side of bed.
   With no stand-by help.
5. Supine to sitting over side of bed.
   With no stand-by help.
6. Supine to sitting over side of bed within 10 sec.
   With no stand-by help.

C. *Balanced sitting*

1. Sits only with support.
   Therapist should assist patient into sitting.
2. Sits unsupported for 10 sec.
   Without holding on, knees and feet together, feet can be supported on floor.
3. Sits unsupported with weight well forward and evenly distributed.
   Weight should be well forward at the hips, head and thoracic spine extended, weight evenly distributed on both sides.
4. Sits unsupported, turns head and trunk to look behind.
   Feet supported and together on floor. Do not allow legs to abduct or feet to move. Have hands resting on thighs, do not allow hands to move on to plinth.
5. Sits unsupported, reaches forward to touch floor, and returns to starting position.
   Feet supported on floor. Do not allow patient to hold on. Do not allow legs and feet to move, support affected arm if necessary. Hand must touch floor at least 10 cm (4 in) in front of feet.
6. Sits on stool unsupported, reaches sideways to touch floor, and returns to starting position.
   Feet supported on floor. Do not allow patient to hold on. Do not allow legs and feet to move, support affected arm if necessary. Patient must reach sideways, not forward.

D. *Sitting to standing*

1. Gets to standing position with help from therapist.
   Any method.

2. Gets to standing position with stand-by help.
   Weight unevenly distributed, uses hands for support.

3. Gets to standing position.
   Do not allow uneven weight distribution or help from hands.

4. Gets to standing position and stands for 5 sec with hips and knees extended.
   Do not allow uneven weight distribution.

5. Sitting to standing with no stand-by help.
   Do not allow uneven weight distribution. Full extension of hips and knees.

6. Sitting to standing with no stand-by help three times in 10 sec.
   Do not allow uneven weight distribution.

E. *Walking*

1. Stands on affected leg and steps forward with other leg.
   Weight-bearing hip must be extended. Therapist may give stand-by help.

2. Walks with stand-by help from one person.

3. Walks 3 m (10 ft) alone or uses any aid but no stand-by help.

4. Walks 5 m (16 ft) with no aid in 15 sec.

5. Walks 10 m (33 ft) with no aid, turns around, picks up a small sandbag from floor, and walks back in 25 sec.
   May use either hand.

6. Walks up and down four steps with or without an aid but without holding on to the rail three times in 35 sec.

F. *Upper-arm function*

1. Lying, protract shoulder girdle with arm in elevation.
   Therapist places arm in position and supports it with elbow in extension.

2. Lying, hold extended arm in elevation for 2 sec.
   Therapist should place arm in position and patient must maintain position with some external rotation. Elbow must be within 20 degrees of full extension.

3. Flexion and extension of elbow to take palm to forehead with arm as in 2 above.
   Therapist may assist supination of forearm.

4. Sitting, hold extended arm in forward flexion at 90 degrees to body for 2 sec.
   Therapist should place arm in position and patient must maintain position with some external rotation and elbow extension. Do not allow excess shoulder elevation.

5. Sitting, patient lifts arm to above position, holds it there for 10 seconds, and then lowers it.
   Patient must maintain position with some external rotation. Do not allow pronation.

6. Standing, hand against wall. Maintain arm position while turning body towards wall.
   Have arm abducted to 90 degrees with palm flat against the wall.

G. *Hand movements*

1. Sitting, extension of the wrist.
   Therapist should have patient sitting at table with forearm resting on the table. Therapist places cylindrical object in palm of patient's hand. Patient is asked to lift object off the table by extending the wrist. Do not allow elbow flexion.

2. Sitting, radial deviation of wrist.
   Therapist should place forearm in midpronation–supination (i.e. resting on ulnar side, thumb in line with forearm and wrist in extension, fingers around a cylindrical object). Patient asked to lift hand off table. Do not allow elbow flexion or pronation.

3. Sitting, elbow into side, pronation and supination.
   Elbow unsupported and at a right angle. Three-quarter range is acceptable.

4. Reach forward, pick up large ball of 14 cm (5-in) diameter with both hands and put it down.
   Ball should be on table so far in front of patient who has to extend arms fully to reach it. Shoulders must be protracted, elbows extended, wrist neutral or extended. Palms should be kept in contact with the ball.

5. Pick up a polystyrene cup from table and put it on table across other side of body.
   Do not allow alteration in shape of cup.

6. Continuous opposition of thumb and each finger more than 14 times in 10 sec.
   Each finger in turn taps the thumb, starting with index finger. Do not allow thumb to slide from one finger to the other, or to go backwards.

H. *Advanced hand activities*

1. Picking up the top of a pen and putting it down again.
   Patient stretches arm forward, picks up pen top, releases it on table close to body.

2. Picking up one jellybean from a cup and placing it in another cup.
   Teacup contains eight jellybeans. Both cups must be at arms' length. Left hand takes jellybean from cup on right and releases it in cup on left.

3. Drawing horizontal lines to stop at a vertical line 10 times in 20 sec.
   At least five lines must touch and stop at the vertical line.

4. Holding a pencil, making rapid consecutive dots on a sheet of paper.
   Patient must do at least two dots a second for 5 sec. Patient picks pencil up and positions it without assistance. Patient must hold pen as for writing. Patient must make a dot and not a stroke.

5. Taking a dessert spoon of liquid to the mouth.
   Do not allow head to lower towards spoon. Do not allow liquid to spill.

6. Holding a comb and combing hair at back of head.

I. *General tonus*

1. Flaccid, limp, no resistance when body parts are handled.
2. Some response felt as body parts are moved.
3. Variable, sometimes flaccid, sometimes good tone, sometimes hypertonic.
4. Consistently normal response.
5. Hypertonic 50 per cent of the time.
6. Hypertonic at all times.

References   Carr *et al.* (1985); Poole and Whitney (1988); Loewen and Anderson (1988)

Comment
Eight hierarchical measures largely focused on disability (the assessment of tone is of impairment, but it is unreliable). Although well studied, with good support for validity and reliability, it is a long test. Gaining some popularity in research protocols.

Modified Ashworth Scale for grading spasticity

Grade	Description
0	No increase in muscle tone.
1	Slight increase in muscle tone, manifested by a catch and release, or by minimal resistance at the end of the range of motion when the affected part(s) is moved in flexion or extension.
2	Slight increase in muscle tone, manifested by a catch, followed by minimal resistance throughout the remainder (less than half) of the range of movement (ROM).
3	More marked increase in muscle tone through most of ROM, but affected part(s) easily moved.
4	Considerable increase in muscle tone, passive movement difficult.
5	Affected part(s) rigid in flexion or extension.

Reference   Bohannon and Smith (1987)

Comment
The only assessment of abnormal tone caused by upper motor neuron damage to have been formally evaluated. It has face validity, but the

Isometric Muscle Strength

Tufts Quantitative Neuromuscular Exam (TQNE)

Instructions
Use a hand-held dynamometer to measure maximum voluntary contraction at the sites detailed below.

Muscle group	Position of patient	Position of limb	Position of strap	Stabilization
Shoulder flexion	Supine	Shoulder at 90 degrees	Proximal to olecranon	At thorax
Shoulder extension	Supine	Shoulder at 90 degrees	Proximal to olecranon	Over the acromion
Elbow flexion	Supine	Elbow at 90 degrees, forearm in neutral	At the wrist	Under epicondyles
Elbow extension	Supine	Elbow at 90 degrees, forearm in neutral	At the wrist	Over biceps belly
Hip extension	Trunk at 20 degrees, supported on pillows	Hip at 20 degrees, knee at 90 degrees	Proximal to knee	Over both ant. sup. iliac spines
Hip flexion	Trunk at 20 degrees, supported on pillows	Hip at 20 degrees, knee at 90 degrees	Proximal to knee	Supporting opposite hip and knee at 90 degrees
Knee extension	Sitting up, towel roll under distal thigh	Knee at 90 degrees	Proximal to lateral malleolus	Over both shoulders
Knee flexion	Sitting up, towel roll under distal thigh	Knee at 90 degrees	Proximal to lateral malleolus	Over anterior thigh
Ankle dorsiflexion	Supine, towel roll under ankle	Ankle in plantar flexion	Around metatarsals	Over proximal calf

validity (reality) and importance of disturbance of tone as a specific impairment needs further testing. Reliability has been proven at the elbow, but not otherwise. Patient variability is a major source of unreliability. It is simple.

Therefore it is the only available clinical measure of tone, **if** assessment is thought necessary (but is it ever?). It should not be used in dystonia and other movement disorders (for example, Parkinson's disease).

Motor neuron disease/Amyotrophic lateral sclerosis

Tufts Quantitative Neuromuscular Exam (TQNE)

Pulmonary function
  1. Forced Vital Capacity (FVC); best of two trials
  2. Maximum Voluntary Ventilation (MVV)

Oropharyngeal
  1. Time (seconds) to say 'pa' 20 times
  2. Time (seconds) to say 'pata' 15 times

Timed motor activities
  1. Dialling 764–7172 on spring-loaded dial phone
  2. Number of pegs placed on Purdue peg board in 30 sec
  3. Time (seconds) taken to walk 15 ft (5 m) with any aid or assistance needed

Isometric muscle strength, as detailed in Table, p. 163.

Reference   Andres *et al.* (1986)

Comment
The TQNE is a well-developed measure of motor impairments in MND/ALS, tested for redundancy (i.e. each item contributes information) and reliability. It takes 45–60 min to complete, and so is restricted to research applications.

Dynanometry

The measurement of isometric strength using hand-held dynanometers has been studied by various groups. One set of positions has been illustrated already; here an alternative group is shown (Wiles and Karni 1983).

Muscle group	Subject position	Myometer position
Shoulder abduction	Subject sitting; shoulder abducted to 90 degrees; forearm pronated (also done with subject prone)	Just proximal to lateral epicondyle of humerus
Elbow flexors	Subject supine; shoulder abducted 30 degrees from trunk, upper arm supported; elbow flexed to 90 degrees; forearm supinated	Just proximal to wrist crease (flexor surface).
Elbow extensors	As above; upper arm stabilized by examiner. May also be done with subject in position for shoulder abduction (sitting), forearm supinated.	Just proximal to wrist crease (extensor surface).
Wrist extensors	Subject supine or sitting; forearm supported and pronated; wrist extended; fingers flexed.	Just proximal to 2nd/3rd metacarpal heads.
Hip flexors	Subject supine; hip and knee flexed to 90 degrees; ankle supported by examiner	Just proximal to patella.
Hip abductors	Subject lying on side; hip and knee extended; lifting against gravity. **or** supine, knee extended, ankle supported by examiner so that hip flexed 10–20 degrees.	Lateral condyle of femur.
Knee flexors	Subject seated on high chair/couch; hip and knee flexed to 90 degrees; knee held by examiner to prevent hip flexion	Just proximal to malleoli of ankle posterior surface of leg
Knee extensors	As for flexors	As for knee flexors, but anterior surface of leg
Neck flexion	Patient supine, neck flexed to 40–60 degrees	Forehead, centrally

References Wiles and Karni (1983); also Bohannon and Andrews (1987*a b*), Agre *et al.* (1987)

Comment
Reliability is reasonable, but limited and small changes cannot be considered significant. Other standard positions for testing strength exist, and the main point is to use the same technique on each occasion.

15 Measures of 'focal' disability

Summary

1. Standing Balance
2. Functional Ambulation Categories
3. 'Hauser' Ambulation Index
4. Timed Walking Tests
5. Rivermead Mobility Index
6. Nine-hole Peg Test
7. Action Research Arm Test
8. Frenchay Arm Test

Introduction

This chapter shows five measures related to mobility, and three measures which concentrate upon arm function. All are reasonably well studied. The last two require equipment and may be better suited to research, but the remainder can easily be used in clinical practice without too much difficulty. Timed walking tests and the Rivermead Mobility Index are recommended for routine measurement of mobility, and the Nine-hole Peg Test as a routine measure of dexterity.

There is obviously a need for a simple clinical measure of the help needed in transfers. Unfortunately, the author is unaware of any good measures of the ability to transfer (or the difficulty of helping with transfer). Having recently tried to develop an index, the author now understands why no such index exists!

There is also scope for the development of a manual dexterity or arm function index similar to the Rivermead Mobility Index. Most clinicians will have their own questions related to arm function, often asking about cutting up food, writing, and fastening buttons.

Standing Balance

An ordinal scale to grade bilateral static standing performance while subjects stand with their eyes open.

Grade	Description
0	Unable to stand (i.e. worse than next grade)
1	Able to stand with feet apart, but less than 30 sec
2	Stand with feet apart for 30 sec, but not with feet together
3	Stand with feet together, but less than 30 sec
4	Stand with feet together, 30 sec or more

Reference Bohannon (1989*b*)

Comment
A simple categorical scale, said to be reliable (in unpublished research). Possibly useful, but not widely reported yet.

Functional Ambulation Categories

No.	Category	Guidance
0	Nonfunctional (unable)	Patient cannot walk, or requires help of two or more people.
1	Dependent—level 2	Patient requires firm continuous support from one person who helps carrying weight and with balance.
2	Dependent—level 1	Patient needs continuous or intermittent support of one person to help with balance or co-ordination.
3	Dependent—supervision	Patient requires verbal supervision or stand-by help from one person without physical contact.
4	Independent—on level ground	Patient can walk independently on level ground, but requires help on stairs, slopes or uneven surfaces.
5	Independent	Patient can walk independently anywhere.

Note: This classification does not take account of any aid used.

References Holden *et al.* (1984); Holden *et al.* (1986); Collen *et al.* (1990)

Comment
This categorization is designed to give detail on the physical support needed by patients who are walking, particularly in a physiotherapy department.

Therefore it is most useful in active rehabilitation rather than as measure of actual disability. Validity and reliability established; simple to use and sensitive to change during the transition from being immobile to walking.

'Hauser' Ambulation Index

0 Asymptomatic; fully active.

1 Walks normally, but reports fatigue that interferes with athletic or other demanding activities.

2 Abnormal gait or episodic imbalance; gait disorder is noticed by family and friends; able to walk 25 ft (8 m) in 10 sec or less.

3 Walks independently; able to walk 25 ft in 20 sec or less.

4 Requires unilateral support (cane or single crutch) to walk; walks 25 ft in 20 sec or less.

5 Requires bilateral support (canes, crutches or walker) and walks 25 ft in 25 sec or less; *or* requires unilateral support but needs more than 20 sec to walk 25 ft.

6 Requires bilateral support and more than 20 sec to walk 25 ft; may use wheelchair on occasion.

7 Walking limited to several steps with bilateral support; unable to walk 25 ft; may use wheelchair for most activities.

8 Restricted to wheelchair; able to transfer self independently.

9 Restricted to wheelchair; unable to transfer self independently.

Note. The use of a wheelchair may be determined by life-style and motivation. It is expected that patients in grade 7 will use a wheelchair more frequently than those in Grades 5 or 6. Assignment of a grade in the range of 5 to 7, however, is determined by the patient's ability to walk a given distance, and not by the extent to which the patient uses a wheelchair.

Reference   Hauser *et al.* (1983)

Comment

This index was specifically designed for use in a study of immunosuppressive treatment in patients with multiple sclerosis. It has been used in other studies, and seems able to detect expected differences. No study on reliability has been reported. Has face validity as a measure of mobility disability, but it mixes information about the use of aids, which can be determined by many factors, with mobility.

Timed Walking Tests

Timing of walking can be carried out in several ways. These either test speed over a short distance, or endurance.

Short distance speed
5 m walk
10 m walk
20 m (10 m and return)

Endurance tests
—2-, 6-, or 12-min walk

Instructions for short distance speed
In general the patient is asked to walk at his or her own preferred speed, using whatever aid needed (including personal support if wanted). If a turn is required, instructions are given on where to turn. They are then asked to walk the specified distance in a straight line, turning as needed.

The patient is timed over the distance in seconds. The result can be reported as the number of seconds taken, or as speed (metres/second). Any aid or assistance should be recorded.

Instructions for endurance tests
The patient is asked to walk at his or her own preferred speed, using any aid or assistance, up and down a fixed distance, usually 20 m, until told to stop. They are warned of the time (2, 6, or 12 min), and are told that they may stop earlier if they feel unable to continue. Six minutes is probably best.

The total distance walked should be recorded. If the patient stops before the end of the endurance test, the time and distance walked should be recorded.

References   Butland *et al*. (1982); Bradstater *et al*. (1983); Lipkin *et al*. (1986); Wade *et al*. (1987*a*); Wolfson *et al*. (1990)

Comment
These tests are all very simple, have obvious face validity, and are reliable. They can detect change seen after stroke, in motor neuron disease and in Parkinson's disease. (There is further discussion in Chapter 8.)

Rivermead Mobility Index

Instructions

The patient is asked the following 15 questions, and observed (for item 5). A score of 1 is given for each 'yes' answer.

Qu. No.	Question	Comment
1 ___	Turning over in bed Do you turn over from your back to your side without help?	_____
2 ___	Lying to sitting From lying in bed, do you get up to sit on the edge of bed on your own?	_____
3 ___	Sitting balance Do you sit on the edge of the bed without holding on for 10 seconds?	_____
4 ___	Sitting to standing Do you stand up (from any chair) in less than 15 seconds, and stand there for 15 seconds (using hands, and with an aid if necessary)?	_____
5 ___	Standing unsupported Observe standing for 10 seconds without any aid.	_____
6 ___	Transfer Do you manage to move from bed to chair and back without any help?	_____
7 ___	Walking inside, with an aid if needed Do you walk 10 metres, with an aid if necessary, but with no standby help?	_____
8 ___	Stairs Do you manage a flight of stairs without help?	_____
9 ___	Walking outside (even ground) Do you walk around outside, on pavements without help?	_____
10 ___	Walking inside, with no aid Do you walk 10 metres inside with no caliper, splint, or aid, and no standby help?	_____
11 ___	Picking off floor If you drop something on the floor, do you manage to walk 5 metres, pick it up and then walk back?	_____

12 ____	Walking outside (uneven ground)	_____
	Do you walk over uneven ground (grass, gravel, dirt, snow, ice, etc.) without help?	
13 ____	Bathing	_____
	Do you get in/out of bath or shower unsupervised and wash self?	
14 ____	Up and down four steps	_____
	Do you manage to go up and down four steps with no rail, but using an aid if necessary?	
15 ____	Running	_____
	Do you run 10 metres without limping in four seconds (fast walk is acceptable)?	

Reference   Collen *et al.* (1991)

Comment
This index has been developed, and should be published soon. It is simple to use, clinically relevant, and reliable within 1 point.

Nine-hole Peg Test (NHPT)

Equipment
• 9 wooden dowels; 9 mm diameter, 32 mm long.
• Wood base with 9 holes (10 mm diam, 15 mm deep) spaced 15 mm apart in three rows of three holes.
• Lid to base, with tray 100 mm square and 100 mm deep to hold pegs.

Instructions. Patient to sit at table, and asked to place pegs in holes. Observer times from start to end, but can stop at 50 sec and record number of pegs placed.

Results. Best presented as number of seconds taken to place each peg.

References   Mathiowetz *et al.* (1985); Parker *et al.* (1986); Heller *et al.* (1987); Goodkin *et al.* (1988); Sunderland *et al.* (1989)

Comment
One of several peg tests. It is sometimes used by timing the patient both placing and removing pegs. It has been tested for validity and reliability. Its advantages include simplicity, portability, and brevity. It is sensitive to change at the upper levels of performance, but not useful when impairment is severe. Most normal people complete the test in 18 sec. It has been used in a major randomized controlled trial of therapy after acute stroke (Sunderland *et al.* 1991).

Action Research Arm Test

Instructions
There are four subtests: Grasp, Grip, Pinch, Gross movement. Items in each are
ordered so that:

- if the subject passes the first, no more need to be administered and he scores top
  marks for that subtest;
- if the subject fails the first *and* fails the second, he scores zero, and again no more
  tests need be performed in that subtest;
- otherwise he needs to complete all tasks within the subtest.

Grasp
1 ____   Block, wood, 10-cm cube (If score = 3, total = 18 and go to *Grip*)
        Pick up a 10-cm block
2 ____   Block, wood, 2.5-cm cube (If score = 0, total = 0 and go to *Grip*)
        Pick up 2.5-cm block
3 ____   Block, wood, 5-cm cube
4 ____   Block, wood, 7.5-cm cube
5 ____   Ball (Cricket), 7.5-cm diameter
6 ____   Stone $10 \times 2.5 \times 1$ cm

Coefficient of reproducibility = 0.98
Coefficient of scalability   = 0.94

Grip
1 ____   Pour water from glass to glass.
        (If score = 3, total = 12 and go to *Pinch*)
2 ____   Tube 2.25 cm
        (If score = 0, total = 0 and go to *Pinch*)
3 ____   Tube 1 cm $\times$ 16 cm
4 ____   Washer (3.5 cm diameter) over bolt

Coefficient of reproducibility = 0.99
Coefficient of scalability   = 0.94

Pinch
1 ____   Ball bearing, 6 mm, 3rd finger and thumb
        (If score = 3, total = 18 and go to *Grossmt*)
2 ____   Marble, 1.5 cm, index finger and thumb
        (If score = 0, total = 0 and go to *Grossmt*)
3 ____   Ball bearing 2nd finger and thumb
4 ____   Ball bearing 1st finger and thumb
5 ____   Marble 2nd finger and thumb
6 ____   Marble 1st finger and thumb

Coefficient of reproducibility = 0.99
Coefficient of scalability   = 0.98

Grossmt (Gross movement)
1 ____ Place hand behind head
      (If score = 3, total = 9 and finish)
2 ____ (If score = 0, total = 0 and finish)
3 ____ Place hand on top of head
4 ____ Hand to mouth

Coefficient of reproducibility = 0.98
Coefficient of scalability   = 0.97

References   Carroll (1965); Lyle (1981); De Weerdt and Harrison (1985); Crow *et al.* (1989)

Comment
The original long and comprehensive test (Carroll 1965) has been abbreviated so that it usually takes only 8–10 min to complete. It has good validity and reliability, and has been compared with other tests. However, it does require some equipment and (potentially) 30 min in a recovering patient. Probably most useful in research studies (for example, Crow *et al.* 1989).

Frenchay Arm Test

Instructions
The patient sits at a table with his hands on his lap. Each task starts from this position. The patient scores one for each task completed successfully (and nought if he fails), and asked to use his affected hand to:

1. Stabilize a ruler while drawing a line with a pencil held in the other hand. To pass, the ruler must be held firmly.

2. Grasp a cylinder (12 mm diameter, 5 cm long) set on its end approximately 15 cm from the table edge, lift it about 30 cm and replace it without dropping.

3. Pick up a glass half-full of water positioned 15–30 cm from the table edge, drink some water and replace the glass without spilling any water.

4. Remove and replace a sprung clothes peg from a 10 mm diameter dowel, 15 cm long, set in a 10 cm square base, placed 15–30 cm from the table edge. He is not to drop the peg or to knock the dowel over.

5. Comb his hair (or imitate); he must comb across the top, down the back and down each side of the head.

References   De Souza *et al.* (1980); Wade *et al.* (1983); Parker *et al.* (1986); Berglund and Fugl-Meyer (1986); Heller *et al.* (1987); Sunderland *et al.* (1989); Sunderland *et al.* (1991)

Comment
This test was originally derived from a 25-item test, shortened to 7 and then 5 times. It is designed primarily for use in research studies. Validity and reliability have been demonstrated. Sensitivity is reasonable, but patients tend to either pass or fail all tests. It is simple and quick, but requires some equipment, and is not portable. It has been used in randomized controlled trial of physiotherapy.

16 Activities of daily living (ADL) and extended ADL tests

Summary

1. Barthel ADL Index
2. Katz ADL Index
3. Nottingham Ten-point ADL Index
4. Rivermead ADL Scales
5. Northwick Park Index of Independence in ADL
6. Kenny Self-care Evaluation
7. Health Assessment Questionnaire (HAQ)
8. Nottingham Extended ADL Index
9. Frenchay Activities Index

Introduction

There are many ADL scales and these have been reviewed many times (Donaldson *et al.* 1973; Deyo 1984; Feinstein *et al.* 1986; McDowell and Newell 1987; Law and Letts 1989; Eakin 1989; Applegate *et al.* 1990) including briefly in Chapter 8 of this book. This chapter simply shows nine indices, six that are purely ADL and two which cover extended ADL, and the Rivermead ADL Index which spans both.

All ADL indices are similar, and the author strongly recommends the use of the Barthel ADL Index shown here not because it is intrinsically much better but primarily because it is now the best known and we must start to standardize measurement (Wade 1988). The Nottingham Extended ADL Index and the Frenchay Activities Index should both be considered when we are concerned with how patients actually function within their wider community at home.

Barthel ADL Index

Bowels
0 = incontinent (or needs to be given enemata)
1 = occasional accident (once a week)
2 = continent

Bladder
0 = incontinent, or catheterized and unable to manage alone
1 = occasional accident (maximum once per 24 hours)
2 = continent

Grooming
0 = needs help with personal care
1 = independent face/hair/teeth/shaving (implements provided)

Toilet use
0 = dependent
1 = needs some help, but can do something alone
2 = independent (on and off, dressing, wiping)

Feeding
0 = unable
1 = needs help cutting, spreading butter, etc.
2 = independent

Transfer (bed to chair and back)
0 = unable, no sitting balance
1 = major help (one or two people, physical), can sit
2 = minor help (verbal or physical)
3 = independent

Mobility
0 = immobile
1 = wheelchair independent, including corners
2 = walks with help of one person (verbal or physical)
3 = independent (but may use any aid; for example, stick)

Dressing
0 = dependent
1 = needs help but can do about half unaided
2 = independent (including buttons, zips, laces, etc.)

Stairs
0 = unable
1 = needs help (verbal, physical, carrying aid)
2 = independent

Bathing
0 = dependent
1 = independent (or in shower)

Total   0–20

The Barthel ADL Index: guidelines

1. The index should be used as a record of what a patient does, *not* as a record of what a patient could do.
2. The main aim is to establish degree of independence from any help, physical or verbal, however minor and for whatever reason.
3. The need for supervision renders the patient *not* independent.
4. A patient's performance should be established using the best available evidence. Asking the patient, friends/relatives and nurses are the usual sources, but direct observation and common sense are also important. However direct testing is not needed.
5. Usually the patient's performance over the preceding 24–48 hours is important, but occasionally longer periods will be relevant.
6. Middle categories imply that the patient supplies over 50 per cent of the effort.
7. Use of aids to be independent is allowed.

Bowels (preceding week)
- If needs enema from nurse, then 'incontinent'
- Occasional = once a week

Bladder (preceding week)
A catheterized patient who can completely manage the catheter alone is regarded as 'continent'.

Grooming (preceding 24–48 hours)
Refers to personal hygiene: doing teeth, fiting false teeth, doing hair, shaving, washing face. Implements can be provided by helper.

Toilet use
- Should be able to reach toilet/commode, undress sufficiently, clean self, dress and leave
- With help = can wipe self and do some of above

Feeding
- Able to eat any normal food (not only soft food). Food cooked and served by others but not cut up
- Help = food cut up, patient feeds self

Transfer
- From bed to chair and back
- Dependent = *no* sitting balance (unable to sit); two people to lift
- Major help = one strong/skilled, or two normal people—can sit up
- Minor help = one person easily, *or* needs any supervision

Mobility
- Refers to mobility about house or ward, indoors. May use aid. If in wheelchair, must negotiate corners/doors unaided
- Help = by one untrained person, including supervision and moral support

Dressing
- Should be able to select and put on all clothes, which may be adapted
- Half = help with buttons, zips, etc. (check!), but can put on some garments alone

Stairs
- Must carry any walking aid used to be independent

Bathing
- Usually the most difficult activity
- Must get in and out unsupervised and wash self
- Independent in shower = 'independent' if unsupervised and unaided

---

References   Wade and Collin (1988); Collin *et al*. (1988); Roy *et al*. (1988); Loewen and Anderson (1988)

Comment
This index is reviewed in Chapter 8 and by Wade and Collin (1988), and is now very widely used.

Katz Activities of Daily Living (ADL) Index

Instructions
For each area of functioning listed below, check (score) description that applies. The word 'assistance' means supervision, direction, or personal assistance.
   '*' indicates that the performance counts as independent in the classification given later.

Number	Item
____	*Bathing* Either sponge bath, bath tub, or shower.
2*	Receives no assistance: gets in and out of tub by self if tub is usual means of bathing.
1*	Receives assistance in bathing only one part of the body, such as back or leg.
0	Receives assistance in bathing more than one part of body, or not bathed.

Number	Item

Dressing

_____ Gets clothes from closets and drawers, including underclothes, outer garments and using fasteners (and braces if worn).

2* Gets clothes and completely dresses without assistance.

1* Gets clothes and gets dressed without assistance, except assistance in tying shoes.

0 Receives assistance in getting clothes, or in getting dressed, or stays partly or completely undressed.

Toileting

_____ Going to the 'toilet room', for bowel and bladder elimination, cleaning self after elimination, and arranging clothes.

2* Goes to 'toilet room', cleans self, and arranges clothes without assistance. May use object for support, such as cane (walking stick), walker, or wheelchair and may manage night bedpan or commode, emptying same in the morning.

1 Receives assistance in going to 'toilet room', or in cleansing self, or in arranging clothes after elimination, or in use of night bedpan or commode.

0 Doesn't go to room termed 'toilet' for the elimination process.

Transfer

2* Moves in and out of bed as well as in and out of chair without assistance. May be using object for support, such as a cane (walking-stick) or walker.

1 Moves in and out of bed or chair with assistance.

0 Doesn't get out of bed.

Continence

2* Controls urination and bowel movement completely by self.

1 Has occasional accidents.

0 Supervision helps keep urine or bowel control; catheter is used; or is incontinent.

Number	Item

Feeding

2*   Feeds self without assistance.

1*   Feeds self, except for getting assistance in cutting meat or buttering bread.

0   Receives assistance in feeding, or is fed partly or completely by using tubes or intravenous fluids.

Scoring—categorization

Seven different categories can be described (used), depending upon independence defined as scoring at levels marked by star (*).

A   Independent in all six activities.

B   Independent in all but one of the activities.

C   Independent in all but *bathing*, and one additional function.

D   Independent in all but *bathing*, *dressing*, and one additional function.

E   Independent in all but *bathing*, *dressing*, *going to toilet*, and one additional function.

F   Independent in all but *bathing*, *dressing*, *going to toilet*, *transferring*, and one additional function.

G   Dependent in all six functions.

O   Dependent in at least two functions, but not classifiable as C, D, E, or F.

Reference   Katz *et al.* (1963)

Comment
A long-established, widely used index of ADL for use with any condition. It is based upon the premise that abilities return (or are lost) in a predictable order. This hierarchy has been established, but seems to offer little advantage over simply scoring (except that the use of letters reminds the user that it is not an interval or ratio scale). Reliability has only been established once. It does not include walking in contrast to most other ADL indices. Although it was once the best ADL index, the Barthel ADL Index is now superior.

Nottingham Ten-point ADL Index

Instructions
Check ability to perform each item independently. Score '1' for pass. Score is obtained by adding number passed.

Number	Item
1 ____	Drink from cup
2 ____	Eat
3 ____	Wash face and hands
4 ____	Transfer from bed to chair
5 ____	Walk (or use wheelchair) indoors
6 ____	Use toilet
7 ____	Undress
8 ____	Dress
9 ____	Make a hot drink
10 ____	Get in and out of a bath

Reference   Ebrahim *et al.* (1985)

Comment
A very simple ADL index designed originally for use with stroke patients. It forms a valid hierarchy with stroke patients, meaning that scores can be compared with confidence. It is simple, reliable, and has been tested for postal use. It does not include any measure of continence. It does include an activity usually considered as domestic (making a hot drink). There are no published guidelines, but the guidelines used in the Rivermead ADL Index should be applicable.

Rivermead Activities of Daily Living (ADL) Scales

Instructions
1. Decide where to start. If the patient can do that item, go back three to make sure that the patient can do these as well, and forward until three consecutive failures—then stop. This applies to each section.
2. All aids supplied or recommended to be stated on form.
3. Guidelines are given on next page.

Scoring
3 = Independent with/without aid
2 = Verbal assistance only
1 = Dependent (i.e. if unfit, unassessable, unsafe or time taken is beyond practical bounds)

Item	Score	Equipment
Self-care		
Drinking	———	———
Clean teeth	———	———
Comb hair	———	———
Wash face/hands	———	———
Make up or shave	———	———
Eating	———	———
Undress	———	———
Indoor mobility	———	———
Bed to chair	———	———
Lavatory	———	———
Outdoor mobility	———	———
Dressing	———	———
Wash in bath	———	———
In/out bath	———	———
Overall wash	———	———
Floor to chair	———	———
Household 1		
Preparation of hot drink	———	———
Preparation of snack	———	———
Cope with money	———	———
Get in/out car	———	———
Prepare meal	———	———
Carry shopping	———	———
Crossing roads	———	———
Transport self to shop	———	———
Public transport	———	———
Household 2		
Washing	———	———
Ironing	———	———
Light cleaning	———	———
Hang out washing	———	———
Bed-making	———	———
Heavy cleaning	———	———

Rivermead ADL Index: guidelines

Self-care
- Drinking
  A full cup of hot liquid, not spilling more than $1/8$ of the contents.
- Clean teeth
  Unscrewing toothpaste, putting toothpaste on brush, managing tap (faucet).
- Comb hair
  To be presentable on completion.
- Wash face and hands
  At basin (not with bowl), including putting in plug and managing taps and patient drying him/herself. (All materials to hand.)
- Make up or shave
  Shaving to be done by patient's preferred method.
- Eating
  A slice of cheese on toast eaten with a knife and fork.
- Undress
  Dressing gown, pyjamas, socks and shoes to be taken off.
- Indoor mobility
  Moving from one room to another. Turns must be to the left. Distance of 10 m.
- Bed to chair
  From lying covered, to chair with arm, within reach.
- Lavatory
  Mobility to WC (less than 10 m). To include managing pants and trousers, cleaning self and transferring.
- Outdoor mobility
  To cover a distance of 50 m, and to include going up a ramp and through a door.
- Dressing
  Does not involve fetching clothes. Clothes to be within reach in a pile, but not in any specific order. All essential fastenings to be done up by patient.
- Wash in bath
  Showing movements, i.e. ability to wash all over. Ability to manage taps (faucets) and plugs.
- In and out of bath
  A dry bath.
- Overall wash
  Not in bath—at basin (not with bowl). Patient must be able to wash good arm, stand up and touch toes from sitting in order to be able to wash all over.
- Floor to chair
  From lying to upholstered chair without arms, seat 15 inches (45 cm) high.

Household 1

- Preparation of hot drink
  Fill electric kettle, everything to be ready on working surface.

- Preparation of snack
  Cheese on toast—materials to be easily reached. Washing and cleaning work surface to be done afterwards.

- Cope with money
  Match coins to packet of sugar, cornflakes, and margarine. Ask for change of 34p from 50p; 72p from £1.00; £3.21 from £5.00.

- Get in and out of car
  Front seat of any car except sports model.

- Preparation of meal
  Peel one potato, fry sausage. Frozen vegetables from fridge. Open tin.

- Carry shopping
  Half-pound (250 g) butter, 14 oz (500 g) tin, and money.

- Crossing roads
  Cross at traffic lights with kerbs—no pedestrian crossing.

- Transport self to shop and back
  Distance of ½ mile (1 km).

- Public transport
  Travel on bus (not Park-and-Ride). Distance at least 1 mile (2 km) with minimum three stops before destination.

Household 2

- Washing
  Handwash underwear at sink

- Ironing
  Not with steam iron. Organize surface (board or table).

- Light cleaning
  Cleaning and tidying surface—height 13–37 inches (30–90 cm).

- Hang out washing
  On rail indoors, away from sink, no pegs.

- Bed making
  Putting on sheet and blanket, straightening and tucking in. Bed 21 inches (50 cm) high.

- Heavy cleaning
  Hoover (vacuum), sweep and dustpan/brush in 11-ft (3-m) square room, moving dining room chairs only.

References   Whiting and Lincoln (1980); Lincoln and Edmans (1990)

Comment

The original (1980) scale is given here; the 1990 scale has the same items, but (a) scores each item simply as independent (= 1) or needs help (= 0), (b) has amalgamated the two household sections, and (c) has a different order of items.

It was developed for use with the stroke patients in a specialist rehabilitation centre. Recent evidence shows that the order of the hierarchy changes, either with time (10 years) or with location (Nottingham vs. Oxford) and the associated differences in physical surroundings and approach of therapists. The recent version (Lincoln and Edmans 1990) has increased reliability by simply using each item as a pass–fail item (i.e. without an intermediate grade).

This index is valid and reliable and for stroke, probably forms a hierarchy. The ADL section does not include continence, and this is a major deficit given the importance of incontinence in causing stress.

Northwick Park Index of Independence in ADL

Instructions

The patient is assessed in a room, and is observed undertaking each activity as described. General guidelines are given at the end.

Transfer: bed to chair
In and out of bed to a chair beside bed.

  0 = Cannot get out of bed
  1 = Moves in and out of bed with assistance
  2 = Independent

Dressing
Patient asked to undress and dress again.

  0 = Unable to put on any clothes
  1 = Gets fully dressed and undressed with assistance
  2 = Independent

Bathing: in and out
Patient is asked to get in and out of a bath using bath seat and bath board if needed.

  0 = Cannot get into bath, or needs more than one assistant
  1 = Gets in and out of bath with assistance
  2 = Independent

Bathing: washing
Patient asked to simulate washing of back, arms, and feet (either in bath tub or in front of wash basin).

  0 = Unable to wash himself
  1 = Needs assistance with washing
  2 = Independent

Lavatory
Patient is asked to use or mime use of lavatory.

  0 = Cannot use lavatory
  1 = Goes to and uses lavatory with assistance for cleaning, and/or clothes
  2 = Independent in reaching lavatory, cleaning, and clothes

Continence
Enquiry is made of the patient/nursing staff/relatives as to continence of bowels and bladder.

  0 = Incontinent, or only able to keep control with help
  1 = Has 'occasional' accidents
  2 = Continent

Grooming: teeth
Patient asked to demonstrate cleaning of teeth.

  0 = Cannot clean teeth
  2 = Cleans teeth

Grooming: other
Patient asked to demonstrate brushing and combing hair (women only), shaving (men only).

  0 = Cannot brush and comb hair/shave
  2 = Independent shaving/brushing and combing hair

Transfer off floor
Patient is asked to lie (or is put to lie) on floor. A chair is placed by his side and he is asked to seat himself in his chair by any method he chooses.

  0 = Cannot get off floor without more than one person helping
  1 = Gets from floor to chair with assistance
  2 = Independent

Preparation of tea
Patient is asked to make a pot of tea. This requires him to collect items from a high and low cupboard and refrigerator and to manipulate cooker. He makes and serves tea using a trolley if necessary.

  0 = Cannot prepare tea
  1 = Gets ingredients and prepares tea with assistance
  2 = Independent

Use of taps
Patient is asked to turn on and off normal four-pronged taps.

  0 = Cannot turn any taps
  1 = Turns specially adapted taps on and off
  2 = Independent with standard taps

Cooking
Patient is asked to fill and lift a kettle on and off a cooker without using adjacent work surfaces.

  0 = Cannot lift/fill kettle
  1 = Fills/lifts kettle on and off cooker with assistance
  2 = Independent

Feeding
Patient is asked to cut and eat a piece of food/simulated food, using a knife and fork or adapted cutlery if necessary.

  0 = Cannot feed himself even with assistance
  1 = Feeds with assistance
  2 = Independent

Mobility (indoors)
Patient is asked to move from assessment room to stairs, negotiating doors, carpet and polished surfaces. Wheelchair-bound patients are rated according to their independence.

  0 = Unable to move between rooms
  1 = Moves between rooms with assistance
  2 = Independent

Stairs: up
Patient is asked to go up and down a flight of stairs. (Ten stairs, maximum depth 19 cm, minimum tread 24 cm. The banister rail may be used.)

  0 = Cannot climb stairs
  1 = Climbs stairs with assistance
  2 = Independent

Stairs: down

  0 = Cannot descend stairs
  1 = Descends stairs with assistance
  2 = Independent

Mobility (outdoors)
Patient is asked to negotiate a kerb, uneven ground and a slope. Wheelchair-bound patients are rated according to their independence.

  0 = Cannot move about outdoors even with assistance
  1 = Moves about outdoors with assistance
  2 = Independent

General guidelines

Total independence—This means the ability to perform an activity without supervision, direction or active personal assistance. A patient who refuses to perform is scored 'totally dependent' even though he is deemed able. The patient may use any method or aid to perform the activity.

Partial dependence—The patient can perform the greater part of the activity himself, but needs assistance (verbal or physical), or supervision to complete the activity.

Total dependence—The activity is carried out for the patient or assistance is required from more than one person.

Scoring

Originally:
   1 = total independence
   2 = partial dependence
   3 = total dependence
   Range = 17–55 (good–bad)

Recommended (and shown above):
   2 = total independence
   1 = partial dependence
   0 = total dependence
   Range = 0–34 (bad–good)

References   Benjamin (1976); Sheikh *et al.* (1979); Smith *et al.* (1981)

Comment

Developed for use in a large randomized controlled trial of therapy late after stroke, this ADL index has never gained much popularity. It includes more items and activities than most, including domestic activities. It requires actual observation. The original scoring gave an inelegant scale ranging from 17 (good) to 55 (bad). None the less it has been well studied for validity and reliability. It has nothing specific to commend it now.

Kenny Self-care Evaluation

For each item, the patient is rated:
   0 = Completely dependent
   1 = Extensive assistance
   2 = Moderate assistance
   3 = Minimal assistance and/or supervision
   4 = Independent

Main area			Main area		
	Grade	Component items		Grade	Component items

Main area			Main area		
Bed			*Dressing*		
	____	Move in bed		____	Upper trunk and arms
	____	Rise and sit		____	Lower trunk and legs
				____	Feet
Transfers					
	____	Sitting	*Personal hygiene*		
	____	Standing		____	Face, hair, arms
	____	Toilet		____	Trunk, perineum
				____	Lower extremities
				____	Bowel programme
Locomotion				____	Bladder programme
	____	Walking			
	____	Stairs			
	____	Wheelchair	*Other*		
				____	Feeding
	____	*Total score*			

References   Schoening *et al.* (1965); Schoening and Iversen (1968); Donaldson *et al.* (1973); Gresham *et al.* (1980)

Comment

This ADL index has reasonable credentials but has not gained widespread use. Its apparent increase in sensitivity (covering more areas and with finer gradations) is probably countered by a loss in reliability.

Health Assessment Questionnaire

We are interested in learning how your illness affects your ability to function in daily life. Please feel free to add any comments at the end of this form. Please choose from the answers given.

Answers
   0 = without *any* difficulty
   1 = with *some* difficulty
   2 = with *much* difficulty
   3 = unable to do

Item	Answer (score)

1. *Dressing and grooming*
Are you able to:
- dress yourself, including tying shoelaces and doing-up buttons?   ____
- shampoo your hair?   ____

2. *Rising*
Are you able to:
- stand up from an armless straight chair?   ____
- get in and out of bed?   ____

3. *Eating*
Are you able to:
- cut your meat?   ____
- lift a full cup or glass to your mouth?   ____
- open a new carton of milk (or soap powder)?   ____

4. *Walking*
Are you able to:
- walk outdoors on flat ground?   ____
- climb up five steps?   ____

5. *Hygiene*
Are you able to:
- wash and dry your entire body?   ____
- take a bath?   ____
- get on and off the toilet?   ____

6. *Reach*
Are you able to:
- reach and get down a 5 lb (2 kg) object from above your head (for example, a bag of potatoes)?   ____
- bend down and pick up clothing from the floor?   ____

7. *Grip*
Are you able to:
- open car doors?   ____
- open jars which have been previously opened?   ____
- turn taps (faucets) on and off?   ____

8. *Activities*
Are you able to:
- run errands and go shopping?   ____
- get in and out of the car?   ____
- do chores such as vacuuming, housework, or light gardening?   ____

Comment

This questionnaire is primarily used in the rehabilitation of patients with rheumatic diseases. Some of the items (for example, turning taps) are specific disabilities faced frequently by patients with joint disease, but most apply equally well in neurological rehabilitation. It is included to illustrate how a simple yet useful questionnaire can be completed. It includes both ADL and extended ADL items. It gives a 0–60 score. The author is unaware of studies on reliability or validity, and he does not think it has been used in neurologically based studies.

Nottingham Extended ADL Index

ANSWERS:	Not at all	With help	Alone with difficulty	Alone easily

QUESTIONS:

Mobility
  Do you:
  • walk around outside? | ___ | ___ | ___ | ___ |
  • climb stairs? | ___ | ___ | ___ | ___ |
  • get in and out of the car? | ___ | ___ | ___ | ___ |
  • walk over uneven ground? | ___ | ___ | ___ | ___ |
  • cross roads? | ___ | ___ | ___ | ___ |
  • travel on public transport? | ___ | ___ | ___ | ___ |

In the kitchen
  Do you:
  • manage to feel yourself? | ___ | ___ | ___ | ___ |
  • manage to make yourself a hot drink? | ___ | ___ | ___ | ___ |
  • take hot drinks from one room to another? | ___ | ___ | ___ | ___ |
  • do the washing up? | ___ | ___ | ___ | ___ |
  • make yourself a hot snack? | ___ | ___ | ___ | ___ |

Domestic tasks
  Do you:
  • manage your own money when you are out? | ___ | ___ | ___ | ___ |
  • wash small items of clothing? | ___ | ___ | ___ | ___ |
  • do your own shopping? | ___ | ___ | ___ | ___ |
  • do a full clothes wash? | ___ | ___ | ___ | ___ |

ANSWERS:	Not at all	With help	Alone with difficulty	Alone easily

Leisure activities
Do you:
- read newspapers or books? ____ ____ ____ ____
- use the telephone? ____ ____ ____ ____
- write letters? ____ ____ ____ ____
- go out socially? ____ ____ ____ ____
- manage your own garden? ____ ____ ____ ____
- drive a car? ____ ____ ____ ____

Scoring
0 = Not at all; with help.
1 = On my own with difficulty; alone easily.

Reference   Nouri and Lincoln (1987)

Comment
A simple extended ADL index in four sections, each of which was found to form an hierarchical scale with stroke patients. Little published evidence concerning validity, reliability, utility, or sensitivity but can be used as postal questionnaire. No published guide-lines. Scoring might be more useful if scored 0–3 in line with potential answers. None the less, an attractive EADL index.

Frenchay Activities Index

Score	Activity	Code (score)

In the last three months

		0 = Never
____	Preparing main meals	1 = Under once weekly
____	Washing up	2 = 1–2 times/week
		3 = Most days
____	Washing clothes	
____	Light housework	
____	Heavy housework	0 = Never
____	Local shopping	1 = 1–2 times in three months
____	Social occasions	2 = 3–12 times in three months
____	Walking outside > 15 mins	3 = At least weekly
____	Actively pursuing hobby	
____	Driving car/going on bus	

Score	Activity	Code (score)
		In the last six months
____	Travel outings/car rides	0 = never 1 = 1–2 times in 6 months 3 = 3–12 times in 6 months 4 = At least twice weekly
____ ____	Gardening Household/car maintenance	0 = Never 1 = Light 2 = Moderate 3 = All necessary
____	Reading books	0 = None 1 = One in 6 months 2 = Less than one in a fortnight 3 = Over one each fortnight
____	Gainful work	0 = None 1 = Up to 10 hours/week 2 = 10–30 hours/week 3 = Over 30 hours/week

Frenchay Activities Index: guidelines

General

The aim is to record activities which require some initiative from the patient. It is important to concentrate upon the patient's actual frequency of activity over the recent past, not distant past performance nor potential performance. One activity can only score on one item.

Specific items

1. Needs to play a substantial part in the organization, preparation and cooking of main meal. Not just making snacks.

2. Must do it all or share equally; for example, washing or wiping and putting away. Not just rinsing an occasional item.

3. Organization of washing and drying of clothes, whether in washing machine, by hand wash, or at launderette.

4. Dusting; polishing; tidying small objects. Anything heavier is included in item 5.

5. All housework including making beds, cleaning floors and fires, moving chairs, etc.

6. Playing a substantial role in organizing and buying shopping, whether small or large amounts. Must go to shops and not just push a trolley.

7. Going out to clubs, church activities, cinema, theatre, drinking, to dinner with friends, etc. May be transported there, provided patient takes an active part once arrived. The common factor is activity, not travel.

8. Sustained walking for at least 15 min (allowed short stops for breath). About one mile. Can include walking to do shopping, provided walks far enough.

9. Must require some 'active' participation and thought; for example, propagating plants in the house, knitting, painting, games, sports. Not just watching sport on television.

10. Must drive a car (not just be a passenger in a car) or get to a bus/coach and travel on it.

11. Coach or rail trips, or car rides, to some place for pleasure. Not for a routine 'social outing' (i.e. shopping, going to local friends). Must involve some organization and decision-making by the patient. Excludes trips organized passively by institution unless patient exercises choice on whether to go. The common factor is travel for pleasure.

12. Gardening outside.
    • light; occasional weeding
    • moderate; regular weeding, pruning, etc.
    • heavy; all necessary work, including heavy digging

13. Household maintenance:
    • Light: repairing small items
    • Moderate: some painting/decorating, routine car maintenance
    • Heavy: most necessary household/car maintenance and repairs

14. Must be full length books; not magazines, periodicals, papers.

15. Work for which the patient is paid; not voluntary work.

References   Holbrook and Skilbeck (1983); Wade *et al.* (1985)

Comment
This index was devised initially by a social worker (Mrs Holbrook) in order to help her in her clinical service. It has since been revised but its reliability needs further testing. However, it is clinically relevant and easy to perform and has been used in clinical research.

17   Global measures of disability

Summary

1. OPCS Disability Scales
2. OPCS Disability Scales: severity categories
3. OPCS Questionnaire
4. Functional Limitations Profile (Sickness Impact Profile)
5. Lambeth Disability Screening Questionnaire
6. Functional Independence Measure
7. Functional Status Questionnaire
8. Rand Functional Limitations Battery
9. Rand Physical Capacities Battery
10. PULSES profile

Introduction

There are several measures which are intended to cover all aspects of disability to a greater or lesser extent. The WHO categorization, not included in this chapter, is one example. In general, global measures of disability are designed to be used with any disease. They are sometimes used to measure 'quality of life'.

The shortest measure which is none the less designed to encompass all consequences of disease is the PULSES profile. Most measures are much longer. The measures shown have not been used in any large-scale specifically neurological study. The best two are probably the OPCS scales, which could be used separately if required, and the Sickness Impact Profile. Also shown is the Functional Independence Measure which is intended to be a standard method for recording outcome in rehabilitation centres. There are two postal questionnaires that have been well tested for use in community screening.

Most of these measures are reviewed by McDowell and Newell (1987) who discuss many other similar measures. Few have been used specifically in neurological rehabilitation.

OPCS Disability Scale: locomotion

Code	Description	Severity score
L1	Cannot walk at all.	11.5
L2	Can only walk a few steps without stopping or severe discomfort; cannot walk up and down one step.	9.5
L3	Has fallen 12 or more times in the last year.	7.5
L4	Always needs to hold on to something to keep balance.	7.0
L5	Cannot walk up and down a flight of 12 stairs.	6.5
L6	Cannot walk 50 yards (metres) without stopping or severe discomfort.	5.5
L7	Cannot bend down far enough to touch knees and straighten up again.	4.5
L8	Cannot bend down and pick something up from the floor and straighten up again.	4.0
L9	Cannot walk 200 yards (metres) without stopping or severe discomfort; *or* can only walk up and down a flight of 12 stairs if holds on and takes a rest; *or* often needs to hold on to something to keep balance; *or* has fallen three or more times in the last year.	3.0
L10	Can only walk up and down a flight of 12 stairs if holding on (doesn't need a rest).	2.5
L11	Cannot bend down to sweep up something from the floor and straighten up again.	2.0
L12	Can only walk up and down a flight of stairs if going sideways or one step at a time.	1.5
L13	Cannot walk 400 yards (metres) without stopping or severe discomfort.	0.5

OPCS Disability Scale: reaching and stretching

Code	Description	Severity score
RS1	Cannot hold out either arm in front to shake hands.	9.5
RS2	Cannot put either arm up to the head to put a hat on.	9.0
RS3	Cannot put either hand behind the back to put a jacket on or to tuck his shirt in.	8.0
RS4	Cannot raise either arm above the head to reach for something.	7.0
RS5	Has difficulty holding either arm in front to shake hands with someone.	6.5
RS6	Has difficulty putting either arm to his or her head to put a hat on.	5.5
RS7	Has difficulty putting either hand behind the back to put a jacket on or to tuck his shirt in.	4.5
RS8	Has difficulty raising either arm above the head to reach for something.	3.5
RS9	Cannot hold one arm out in front or up to the head (but can with the other arm).	2.5
RS10	Cannot put one arm behind the back to put on a jacket or to tuck his shirt in (but can with the other arm); *or* has difficulty putting one arm behind the back to put a jacket on, or to tuck his shirt in; or putting one arm out in front, or up to the head (but no difficulty with the other arm).	1.0

OPCS Disability Scale: dexterity

Code	Description	Severity score
D1	Cannot pick up and hold a mug of coffee with either hand.	10.5
D2	Cannot turn a tap (faucet) or control knobs on a cooker with either hand.	9.5
D3	Cannot pick up and carry a pint of milk or squeeze the water from a sponge with either hand.	8.0
D4	Cannot pick up a small object such as a safety pin with either hand.	7.0
D5	Has difficulty picking up and pouring from a full kettle, or serving food from a pan using a spoon or ladle.	6.5
D6	Has difficulty unscrewing the lid of a coffee jar or using a pen or pencil.	5.5
D7	Cannot pick up and carry a 5 lb (2 kg) bag of potatoes with either hand.	4.0
D8	Has difficulty in wringing out light washing or using a pair of scissors.	3.0
D9	Can pick up and hold a mug of tea or coffee with one hand but not with the other.	2.0
D10	Can turn a tap or control a knob with one hand but not with the other; *or* can squeeze the water from a sponge with one hand but not with the other.	1.5
D11	Can pick up a small object such as a safety pin with one hand but not with the other, *or* can pick up and carry a pint of milk with one hand but not with the other; *or* has difficulty in tying a bow in laces or strings.	0.5

OPCS Disability Scale: personal care

Code	Description	Severity score
PC1	Cannot feed self without help; *or* cannot go to and use the toilet without help.	11.0
PC2	Cannot get into and out of bed without help; *or* cannot get into and out of a chair without help.	9.5
PC3	Cannot wash hands and face without help; *or* cannot dress and undress without help.	7.0
PC4	Cannot wash all over without help.	4.5
PC5	Has difficulty feeding self; *or* has difficulty getting to and using the toilet.	2.5
PC6	Has difficulty getting in and out of bed; *or* has difficulty getting in and out of a chair.	1.0

OPCS Disability Scale: continence

Code	Description	Severity score
CO1	No voluntary control over bowels.	11.5
CO2	No voluntary control over bladder.	10.5
CO3	Loses control of bowels at least once every 24 hours.	10.0
CO4	Loses control of bladder at least once every 24 hours.	8.0
CO5	Loses control of bowels at least once a week.	8.0
CO6	Loses control of bowels at least twice a month.	6.5
CO7	Loses control of bladder at least once a week.	5.5
CO8	Loses control of bowels at least once a month.	5.0
CO9	Loses control of bladder at least twice a month; *or* loses control of bowels occasionally.	4.0
CO10	Loses control of bladder at least once a month.	2.5
CO11	Loses control of bladder occasionally; *or* uses a device to control bowels or bladder.	1.0

OPCS Disability Scale: seeing

Code	Description	Severity score
S1	Cannot tell by the light where the windows are.	12.0
S2	Cannot see the shapes of furniture in a room.	11.0
S3	Cannot see well enough to recognize a friend if close to his face.	10.0
S4	Cannot see well enough to recognize a friend who is an arm's length away.	8.0
S5	Cannot see well enough to read a newspaper headline.	5.5
S6	Cannot see well enough to read a large print book.	5.0
S7	Cannot see well enough to recognize a friend across a room.	4.5
S8	Cannot see well enough to recognize a friend across a road.	1.5
S9	Has difficulty seeing to read ordinary newspaper print.	0.5

OPCS Disability Scale: hearing

Code	Description	Severity score
H1	Cannot hear at all.	11.0
H2	Cannot follow a TV programme with the volume turned up.	8.5
H3	Has difficulty hearing someone talking in a loud voice in a quiet room.	6.0
H4	Cannot hear a doorbell, alarm clock, or telephone bell.	5.5
H5	Cannot use the telephone.	4.0
H6	Cannot follow a TV programme at a volume others find acceptable.	2.0
H7	Difficulty hearing someone talking in a normal voice in a quiet room.	1.5
H8	Difficulty in following a conversation against background noise.	0.5

OPCS Disability Scale: communication

Code	Description	Severity score
C1	Is impossible for people who knew him/her well to understand; *or* finds it impossible to understand people who know him/her well.	12.0
C2	Is impossible for strangers to understand; *or* is very difficult for people who know him/her well to understand; *or* finds it impossible to understand strangers; *or* finds it very difficult to understand people who know him/her well.	8.5
C3	Is very difficult for strangers to understand; *or* is quite difficult for people who know him/her well to understand; *or* finds it difficult to understand strangers; *or* finds it quite difficult to understand people who know him/her well.	5.5
C4	Is quite difficult for strangers to understand; *or* finds it quite difficult to understand strangers.	2.0
C5	Other people have some difficulty in understanding him/her; *or* has some difficulty understanding what other people say or what they mean.	1.0

OPCS Disability Scale: behaviour

Code	Description	Severity score
B1	Gets so upset that he or she hits other people, or injures him/herself.	10.5
B2	Gets so upset that he or she breaks or rips up things.	7.5
B3	Feels the need to have someone present all the time.	7.0
B4	Finds relationships with members of the family very difficult.	6.0
B5	Often has outbursts of temper at other people with very little cause.	4.0
B6	Finds relationships with people outside the family very difficult.	2.5
B7	Sometimes sits for hours doing nothing.	1.5
B8	Finds it difficult to stir him/herself to do things; *or* often feels aggressive or hostile towards other people.	0.5

OPCS Disability Scale: eating, drinking, and digestion

Code	Description	Severity score
EDD1	Suffers from problems with eating, drinking, or digestion which severely affects the ability to lead a normal life.	0.5

OPCS Disability Scale: disfigurement

(scars, blemishes, and deformities)

Code	Description	Severity score
DF1	Suffers from a scar, blemish, or deformity which severely affects the ability to lead a normal life.	0.5

OPCS Disability Scale: intellectual functioning

Code	No. of problems	Severity score	**Number of problems from the following list:**
I1	11	13.0	Often forgets what he or she was supposed to be doing in the middle of something.
I2	10	12.0	Often loses track of what is being said in the middle of a conversation.
I3	9	10.5	Thoughts tend to be muddled and slow.
I4	8	9.5	Often gets confused about what time of day it is.
I5	7	8.0	Cannot watch a half-hour TV programme all the way through and tell someone what it was about.
I6	6	7.0	Cannot remember and pass on a message correctly.
I7	5	6.0	Often forgets to turn off things such as fires, cookers, or taps (faucets).
I8	4	4.5	Often forgets names of people in the family or friends seen regularly.
I9	3	3.5	Cannot read a short article in newspaper.
I10	2	2.0	Cannot write a short letter to someone without help.
I11	1	1.0	Cannot count well enough to handle money.

OPCS Disability Scale: consciousness

Code	'Fit' score	Severity score	Add scores for the following items relating to epileptic fits:
CS1	13.8	12.5	Frequency of fits: 0 = less than once a year
CS2	12.8–13.0	11.5	1 = once a year but fewer than four times a year 2 = four times/year but less than once a month
CS3	11.8	10.5	3 = once a month but less than once a week 4 = once a week but less than every day
CS4	10.8	10.0	5 = every day
CS5	9.8–10.0	9.0	Timing of fits:
CS6	8.8–9.0	8.0	1 = only has fits during the night
CS7	7.8–8.0	7.0	3.8 = only has fits at night or on awakening
CS8	6.8–7.0	6.0	5.8 = only has fits at night, on awakening or in the evening
CS9	5.8–6.0	5.0	6.8 = has fits during the daytime
CS10	4.8–5.0	4.0	
CS11	4.0	3.0	Warning of fit:
CS12	3.0	2.0	0 = always has a warning before a fit
CS13	2.0	1.0	1 = has fits without warning
CS14	1.0	0.5	Consciousness in fit: 0 = does not lose consciousness 1 = loses consciousness during fit

OPCS Disability Scales: severity categories

It is possible to derive an overall 'severity of disability' score or category from the ten individual disability measures. To do this, calculate:
An overall weighted severity score =
$$\text{worst score} + (0.4 \times \text{second worst score}) + (0.3 \times \text{third worst score})$$

Then look up the category in the table below:

Weighted severity score	Severity category
0.5–2.95	1
3–4.95	2
5–6.95	3
7–8.95	4
9–10.95	5
11–12.95	6
13–14.95	7
15–16.95	8
17–18.95	9
19–21.40	10

Reference   Martin *et al.* (1988)

Comment

The OPCS disability scales were developed for use in a national survey designed to investigate the prevalence and severity of all forms of disability in the population. They represent a coherent attempt to assess all disabilities, and in addition the scales have been weighted so that different disabilities can be compared. A version of the scale suitable for use with children is also available. This measure deserves further trials in clinical circumstances.

OPCS Questionnaire

A. Does anyone in your household have the following difficulties due to long-term health problems or disabilities, either physical or mental?

____ (a) Difficulty walking for a quarter of a mile on the level?
____ (b) Great difficulty walking up or down steps or stairs?
____ (c) Difficulty bending down and straightening up, even when holding on to something?
____ (d) Falling, or having great difficulty keeping balance?
____ (e) Difficulty using arms to reach and stretch for things?
____ (f) Great difficulty holding, gripping or turning things?
____ (g) Difficulty recognizing a friend across the road, even if glasses or contact lenses are worn?

_____ (h) Difficulty reading ordinary newspaper print, even if glasses or contact lenses are worn?

_____ (i) Difficulty hearing someone talk in a quiet room?

_____ (j) Suffering severely from noises in the head or ears?

_____ (k) Difficulty going outside the house or garden without help?

_____ (l) Great difficulty following a conversation if there is background noise, for example a TV, radio, or children playing?

B.   Is there anyone in your household who is affected by the following health problems or disabilities?

_____ (a) Severe and frequent bouts of breathlessness, wheezing, or coughing which limit daily activities?

_____ (b) Severe difficulties with eating, drinking, or digestion which limit daily activities?

_____ (c) Severe pain or irritation which limits daily activities?

_____ (d) A scar, blemish, or deformity which limits daily activities?

_____ (e) Lack of control of bladder at least once a day or night?

_____ (f) Lack of control of bowels at least once a month?

C.   Does anyone in your household have the following long-term health problems or disabilities?

_____ (a) A fit or convulsion in the past two years?

_____ (b) Difficulty in being understood by others?

_____ (c) Difficulty understanding what others say or what they mean?

_____ (d) Frequently getting confused or disorientated?

_____ (e) Severe depression or anxiety?

_____ (f) Difficulty getting on with people, so that family work or leisure is severely affected?

_____ (g) Mental handicap or other severe learning difficulties?

_____ (h) Mental illness or phobias which limit daily activities?

D.   In the last twelve months has anyone in your household seen a psychiatrist or other specialist because of a mental, nervous, or emotional problem?

_____

E.   In the last twelve months has anyone in your household attended a day centre, taken sheltered work, or lived in sheltered housing because of a health problem or disability?

_____

F.   Has anyone in your household attended a special school because of a long-term health problem or disability?

_____

G.   Is there anyone in your household who, because of a long-term health problem or disability:

____ (a) Would find it difficult to live alone without help?
____ (b) Is dependent on life-sustaining equipment?
____ (c) Is limited in the type or amount of paid work they can do?

H.   Is there any child aged under 16 in your household:

____ (a) Who is unable to do things which most children of the same age can do, because of a health, development, or behaviour problem?
____ (b) Who needs more help than usual for children of the same age with feeding, dressing, toileting, walking, going up and down stairs, or other daily activities?
____ (c) Who attends a special school, or special or remedial unit of an ordinary school because of health or behaviour problems, disabilities, or learning difficulties?
____ (d) Who attends an ordinary school but is limited in taking part in school activities because of health or behaviour problems or disabilities?
____ (e) Whose health behaviour, or development causes worry that he or she may have a long term health problem, physical, or mental disability or handicap?

I.   Does anyone (including any child) in your household have other difficulties with daily activities because of disabilities or long-term health or behaviour problems not mentioned above?

____

Reference   Martin *et al.* (1988)

Comment

This questionnaire was developed for use in the recent national British survey of disability. It has been validated and field tested. The postal questionnaire should be considered for any community survey aiming to establish the prevalence of disability (for example, to establish the need for statutory services).

Functional Limitations Profile

Each question refers to your function today, and refers to limitations arising due to your health.

Number	Question/statement	Weight
Ambulation items		
1 __	I walk shorter distances or often stop for a rest.	54
2 __	I do not walk up or down hills.	64
3 __	I only use stairs with a physical aid; for example a handrail, stick, or crutches.	82
4 __	I only go up and down stairs with assistance from someone else.	87
5 __	I get about in a wheelchair.	121
6 __	I do not walk at all.	126
7 __	I walk by myself but with some difficulty; for example I limp, wobble, stumble, or I have a stiff leg.	
8 __	I only walk with help from someone else.	98
9 __	I go up and down stairs more slowly; for example, one step at a time or I have to stop.	62
10 __	I do not use stairs at all.	106
11 __	I get about only by using a walking frame, crutches, stick, walls, or hold on to furniture.	96
12 __	I walk more slowly.	39
	Total ambulation items (max = 1006)	___

Functional Limitations Profile

Each question refers to your function today, and refers to limitations arising due to your health.

Number	Question/statement	Weight
Body care and movement items		
13 __	I make difficult movements with help; for example, getting in and out of the bath or a car.	82
14 __	I do not get in and out of bed or chairs without the help of a person or mechanical aid.	100
15 __	I only stand for short periods of time.	67
16 __	I do not keep my balance.	93
17 __	I move my hands or fingers with some difficulty or limitation.	66
18 __	I only stand up with someone's help.	93
19 __	I kneel, stoop or bend down only by holding on to something.	61
20 __	I am in a restricted position all the time.	124
21 __	I am very clumsy.	47
22 __	I get in and out of bed or chairs by grasping something for support or by using a stick or walking frame.	79
23 __	I stay lying down most of the time.	120
24 __	I change position frequently.	53
25 __	I hold on to something to move myself around in bed.	82
26 __	I do not bathe myself completely; for example, I need help with bathing.	85
27 __	I do not bathe myself at all but am bathed by someone else.	100
28 __	I use the bedpan with help.	107
29 __	I have trouble putting on my shoes, socks, or stockings (tights).	54
30 __	I do not have control of my bladder.	122
31 __	I do not fasten my clothing; for example, I require help with buttons, zips, or shoelaces.	68
32 __	I spend most of the time partly dressed or in pyjamas.	75
33 __	I do not have control of my bowels.	124
34 __	I dress myself but do so very slowly.	43
35 __	I only get dressed with someone's help.	82
	Total body care and movement (max = 1927)	____

Functional Limitations Profile

Each question refers to your function today, and refers to limitations arising due to your health.

Number	Question/statement	Weight
Mobility items		
36 __	I only get about in one building.	76
37 __	I stay in one room.	101
38 __	I stay in bed more.	91
39 __	I stay in bed most of the time.	114
40 __	I do not use public transport now.	52
41 __	I stay at home most of the time.	79
42 __	I only go out if there is a lavatory nearby.	64
43 __	I do not go out into town.	47
44 __	I only stay away from home for short periods.	46
45 __	I do not get about in the dark or in places that are not lit unless I have someone to help.	57
	Total mobility items (max = 727)	____

Functional Limitations Profile

Each question refers to your function today, and refers to limitations arising due to your health.

Number	Question/statement	Weight
Household management items		
46 __	I only do housework or work around the house for short periods of time, or I rest often.	50
47 __	I do less of the daily household chores than I would usually do.	37
48 __	I do not do any of the usual household chores that I would usually do.	90
49 __	I do not do any of the maintenance or repair work that I would usually do in my home or garden.	75
50 __	I do not do any of the shopping that I would usually do.	84
51 __	I do not do any of the cleaning that I would usually do.	78
52 __	I have difficulty using my hands; for example turning taps (faucets), using kitchen gadgets, sewing, or doing repairs.	78
53 __	I do not do any of the clothes washing that I would usually do.	75
54 __	I do not do any heavy work around the house.	59
55 __	I have given up taking care of personal or household business affairs; for example, paying bills, banking, or doing household accounts.	69
	Total household management items (max = 685)	____

Functional Limitations Profile

Each question refers to your function today, and refers to limitations arising due to your health.

Number	Question/statement	Weight
Recreation and pastime items		
56 __	I spend shorter periods of time on my hobbies and recreation.	32
57 __	I go out less often to enjoy myself.	27
58 __	I am cutting down on some of my usual inactive pastimes; for example, I watch TV less, play cards less, or read less.	50
59 __	I am not doing any of my usual inactive pastimes; for example, I do not watch TV, play cards, or read.	91
60 __	I am doing more inactive pastimes instead of my other usual activities.	43
61 __	I take part in fewer community activities.	25
62 __	I am cutting down on some of my usual physical recreation or more active pastimes.	34
63 __	I am not doing any of my usual physical recreation or more active pastimes.	81
	Total recreation and pastime items (max = 383)	____

Functional Limitations Profile

Each question refers to your function today, and refers to limitations arising due to your health.

Number	Question/statement	Weight

Social interaction items

Number	Question/statement	Weight
64 __	I go out less often to visit people.	31
65 __	I do not go out at all to visit people.	91
66 __	I show less interest in other people's problems; for example I don't listen when they tell me about their problems, I don't offer to help.	50
67 __	I am often irritable with those around me; for example, I snap at people or criticize easily.	64
68 __	I show less affection.	44
69 __	I take part in fewer social activities than I used to; for example, I go to fewer parties or social events.	25
70 __	I am cutting down the length of visits with friends.	31
71 __	I avoid having visitors.	73
72 __	My sexual activity is decreased.	64
73 __	I often express concern over what might be happening to my health.	44
74 __	I talk less with other people.	44
75 __	I make many demands on other people; for example I insist that they do things for me or tell them how to do things.	76
76 __	I stay alone much of the time.	91
77 __	I am disagreeable with my family; for example, I act spitefully or stubbornly.	86
78 __	I frequently get angry with my family; for example, I hit them, scream, or throw things at them.	103
79 __	I isolate myself as much as I can from the rest of the family.	100
80 __	I pay less attention to the children.	59
81 __	I refuse contact with my family; for example, I turn away from them.	109
82 __	I do not look after my children or family as well as I usually do.	66
83 __	I do not joke with members of my family as much as I usually do.	38

Total social interaction items (max = 1289)   ____

Functional Limitations Profile

Each question refers to your function today, and refers to limitations arising due to your health.

Number	Question/statement	Weight
Emotion		
84 __	I say how bad or useless I am; for example that I am a burden on others.	89
85 __	I laugh or cry suddenly.	58
86 __	I often moan or groan because of pain or discomfort.	67
87 __	I have attempted suicide.	141
88 __	I behave nervously or restlessly.	48
89 __	I keep holding or rubbing areas of my body that hurt or are uncomfortable.	59
90 __	I am irritable or impatient with myself; for example, I run myself down, I swear at myself, I blame myself for things that happen.	79
91 __	I talk hopelessly about the future.	96
92 __	I get sudden frights.	56
	Total for emotion (max = 693)	____

Functional Limitations Profile

Each question refers to your function today, and refers to limitations arising due to your health.

Number	Question/statement	Weight
Alertness		
93 __	I am confused and start to do more than one thing at a time.	74
94 __	I have more minor accidents; for example, I drop things, I trip and fall, I bump into things.	90
95 __	I react slowly to things that are said or done.	52
96 __	I do not finish things I start.	45
97 __	I have difficulty reasoning and solving problems; for example, making plans, making decisions, learning new things.	78
98 __	I sometimes get confused; for example, I do not know where I am, who is around, or what day it is.	115
99 __	I forget a lot; for example, things that happened recently, where I put things, or to keep appointments.	85
100 __	I do not keep my attention on any activity for long.	52
101 __	I make more mistakes than usual.	49
102 __	I have difficulty in doing things which involve thought and concentration.	71
	Total score alertness (max = 711)	____

Functional Limitations Profile

Each question refers to your function today, and refers to limitations arising due to your health.

Number	Question/statement	Weight
Sleep and rest items		
103 __	I spend much of the day lying down to rest.	96
104 __	I sit for much of the day.	62
105 __	I sleep or doze most of the time, day and night.	111
106 __	I lie down to rest more often during the day.	72
107 __	I sit around half asleep.	84
108 __	I sleep less at night; for example, I wake up easily, I don't fall asleep for a long time, or I keep waking up.	86
109 __	I sleep or doze more during the day.	80
	Total sleep and rest (max = 591)	____

Functional Limitations Profile

Each question refers to your function today, and refers to limitations arising due to your health.

Number	Question/statement	Weight

Eating items

Number	Question/statement	Weight
110 __	I eat much less than usual.	34
111 __	I feed myself, but only with specially prepared food or special utensils.	76
112 __	I eat special or different food; for example, I follow a soft food, bland, low salt, low fat, or low sugar diet.	52
113 __	I eat no food at all, but only take liquids.	113
114 __	I just pick or nibble at my food.	39
115 __	I drink less fluids.	33
116 __	I feed myself with help from someone else.	95
117 __	I do not feed myself at all but have to be fed.	121
118 __	I eat no food at all except by tubes or intravenous infusion.	143

Total eating items (max = 706)   ____

Functional Limitations Profile

Each question refers to your function today, and refers to limitations arising due to your health.

Number	Question/statement	Weight

Communication items

Number	Question/statement	Weight
119 __	I have trouble writing or typing.	50
120 __	I communicate mostly by nodding my head, pointing or using sign language.	127
121 __	My speech is understood only by a few people who know me well.	94
122 __	I often lose control of my voice when I speak; for example, my voice gets louder or softer, or changes unexpectedly.	59
123 __	I don't write except to sign my name.	84
124 __	I carry on a conversation when very close to other people or looking directly at them.	59
125 __	I speak with difficulty; for example, I get stuck for words, I stutter, I stammer, I slur my words.	76
126 __	I am understood with difficulty.	89
127 __	I do not speak clearly when I am under stress.	47

Total communication items (max = 685)   ____

Functional Limitations Profile

Each question refers to your function today, and refers to limitations arising due to your health.

Number	Question/statement	Weight

Work items

- If not working at all (retired, unemployed) due to health, answer question 128 'yes' and leave remaining questions.
- If not working for other reasons (for example, retired for other reasons, unemployed, looking after home), leave this section.

Number	Question/statement	Weight
128 __	I do not work at all (includes retired due to health).	361
129 __	I do part of my job at home.	40
130 __	I am not getting as much work done as usual.	41
131 __	I often get irritable with my workmates; for example, I snap at them or criticize them easily.	42
132 __	I work shorter hours.	52
133 __	I only do light work.	56
134 __	I only work for short periods of time or often stop to rest.	65
135 __	I work at my usual job but with some changes; for example, I use different tools or special aids, or I swap jobs with someone else.	36
136 __	I do not do my job as carefully and accurately as usual.	50
	Total work items (max = 520)	____

Total ambulation items (max = 1006)	____
Total body care and movement items (max = 1927)	____
Total mobility items (max = 727)	____
Total household management items (max = 685)	____
Total recreation and pastime items (max = 383)	____
Total social interaction items (max = 1289)	____
Total for emotion items (max = 693)	____
Total score alertness items (max = 711)	____
Total sleep and rest items (max = 591)	____
Total eating items (max = 706)	____
Total communication items (max = 685)	____
Total work items (max = 520)	____
Total for all FLP items (max = 9923)	____

References   Patrick and Peach (1989); Bergner *et al.* (1981); Charlton (1989)

Comment

The Functional Limitation Profile (FLP) is the British version of the Sickness Impact Profile (SIP)—the differences are minor and relate largely to wording. Like the OPCS scales, it has been used in community surveys, and the items have weighted scores. The SIP has been used in several studies. It must be possible to use subsections if one is only interested in one or two specific areas of disability.

Lambeth Disability Screening Questionnaire

Please answer the questions in relation to those living in the household.

1. Who has difficulty with any of the following:
    (a) Walking without help?
    (b) Getting outside the house without help?
    (c) Crossing the road without help?
    (d) Travelling on a bus or train without help?

2. Who has difficulty with any of the following:
    (a) Getting in and out of bed or chair without help?
    (b) Dressing or undressing without help?
    (c) Kneeling or bending over without help?
    (d) Going up or down stairs without help?
    (e) Having a bath or wash all over without help?
    (f) Holding or gripping (for example, a comb or pen) without help?
    (g) Getting to and using the toilet without help?

3. Who has any of the following problems:
    (a) Difficulty with spells of giddiness or fits?
    (b) Frequent falls?
    (c) Weakness or paralysis of arms or legs?
    (d) A stroke?
    (e) Difficulty in seeing newspaper print even with glasses?
    (f) Difficulty seeing people across the road even with glasses?
    (g) Hearing difficulties?
    (h) Loss of whole or significant part of an arm, hand, leg or foot?
    (i) Controlling bowels or bladder?

4. Who is limited in doing any of the following *because of illness or disability*:
    (a) Working at all?
    (b) Doing the job of their choice?
    (c) Doing housework?
    (d) Visiting family or friends?

5. Does anyone else in the household have an illness or disability which affects their activities in any way?

Reference   Patrick and Peach (1989)

Comment

A postal questionnaire designed to detect disability in the community. Its validity has been established. This is an alternative to the OPCS questionnaire.

Functional Independence Measure (FIM)

Independent: another person is not required

4.0 Complete independence
   All components of activity performed safely, without modification or assistive devices within a reasonable time.

3.0 Modified independence
   Needs modification of normal items; needs assistive device (aid); slow; unsafe.

Dependent: another person is required for supervision or assistance

2.0 Modified dependence
   Subject expends at least 50 per cent of effort required:

   2.0 Supervision
      Only needs cueing, coaxing, etc. No physical contact.

   1.7 Minimal assistance
      Only requires slight physical contact (touching); subject expends at least 75 per cent of effort.

   1.3 Moderate assistance
      Subject needs more help than touching; subject expends 50–75 per cent of effort.

1.0 Complete dependence
   Subject expends less than 50 per cent of effort. Needs maximal or total assistance, or activity not performed.

   1.0 Maximal assistance
      Subject expends 25–50 per cent of effort.

   0.5 Total assistance
      Subject expends 0–25 per cent of effort.

Personal care

____ Feeding

   4   Total independence in all aspects of eating and drinking including opening containers, pouring liquids, cutting meat, buttering bread, chewing, and swallowing.

   3   Requires prior preparation of food, or adaptive devices, but reasonable speed and no help *during* mealtime.

2   Chews and swallows, but requires supervision or help during activity of eating or drinking.

1   Requires total assistance and/or relies at least in part on alternative nutritional techniques (for example, enteral feeding).

_____ Grooming

4   Total independence in oral care, hair grooming, washing hands and face, and shaving or applying make-up.

3   Requires prior preparation, adaptive or assistive device, or is unreasonably slow.

2   Requires supervision and/or minimal to moderate assistance.

1   Requires maximal/total assistance, or not performed.

_____ Bathing

4   Total independence in bathing and drying body from neck down, using bath, shower, or bed-bath.

3   Requires adaptive/assistive device, or is very slow, or is unsafe.

2   Requires supervision and/or minimal to moderate assistance.

1   Requires maximum/total assistance, or not performed.

_____ Dressing—upper body

4   Total independence in dressing and undressing, including obtaining clothes from usual storage place; managing all normal garments (for example, bra); managing all fastenings (for example, buttons); and putting on and taking off prostheses and orthoses.

3   Requires prior retrieval and/or arrangement of clothes before dressing, or uses modified clothing, or uses assistive devices or unreasonably slow.

2   Requires supervision and/or minimal to moderate assistance.

1   Requires maximal/total assistance, or not performed.

_____ Toileting

4   Complete independence in toileting, including cleaning self (perineal area) after voiding or bowel evacuation; using sanitary napkins or inserting tampons; adjusting clothes.

3   Needs adaptive equipment, or is slow.

2   Requires supervision and/or minimal to moderate assistance in using toilet paper or in wiping self or in adjusting clothes.

1   Requires maximal or total assistance.

Sphincter control

____ Bladder management

4 Controls bladder completely and intentionally, never incontinent.

3 Requires a catheter, collection device or medication. Controls use of device independently (for example, empties bags).

2 Requires supervision and/or moderate assistance to maintain voiding pattern (i.e. regular toileting) or to use device. Or occasional accident (less than once a day).

1 Requires maximum help, or incontinent despite use of devices.

____ Bowel management

4 Controls bowels completely and intentionally, never incontinent.

3 Requires artificial help—digital evacuation, laxatives, enemata—but does not require help from another person. Maintains colostomy. No accidents.

2 Requires supervision and/or minimal to moderate assistance, such as reminding to evacuate bowels or help with artificial aids. Or occasional accident but not daily.

1 Requires maximal/total assistance, and is regularly incontinent most days.

Mobility

____ Transfers A (bed, chair, wheelchair)

4 If walking, approaches chair, sits down, and gets up without help.
If in wheelchair, approaches chair/bed, locks brakes, moves on to chair/bed and back again safely, moving arm rest if necessary, all without help.

3 As above, but requires adaptive/assistive device (for example, sliding board, special seat); or is slow and/or unsafe. Assistance from another person not required.

2 Requires supervision and/or minimal to moderate assistance.

1 Requires maximal/total assistance.

____ Transfers B (toilet)

4 If walking, approaches, sits down and gets up independently from standard toilet.
If in wheelchair, approaches toilet, locks brakes, and transfers both ways safely.

3 As above, but needs assistive device (for example, grab rails, raised seat), or is unreasonably slow, or is unsafe. Assistance of another person not required.

2 Requires supervision and/or minimal to moderate help.

1 Requires maximum or total help.

____ Transfers C (bath tub or shower)

4 If walking, gets into and out of bath or shower independently. If in wheelchair, approaches bath or shower, locks brakes, and transfers both ways safely.

3 As above, but needs assistive device (for example, grab rails, raised seat), or is unreasonably slow, or is unsafe. Assistance of another person not required.

2 Requires supervision and/or minimal to moderate help.

1 Requires maximum or total help.

Locomotion

____ Walking, or using a wheelchair

4 Once standing, walks 150 ft (50 m) safely without assistive device.

3 If walking 150 ft, needs orthosis (for example, splint) or special shoes, or other device (for example, stick, frame); or is unreasonably slow; or is unsafe.
   If in wheelchair (electric or self-propelled), manoeuvres at least 150 ft (50 m) independently including turns, approaching table/bed/toilet, managing 3 per cent slope, rugs, and door sills.

2 Requires supervision and/or minimal to moderate assistance to go as far as 150 ft (50 m), or can manage 50 ft (15 m) independently—walking or wheelchair.

1 Requires maximal/total help to reach 150 ft (50 m) and cannot achieve 50 ft (15 m) independently.

____ Stairs

4 Goes up and down 12–14 stairs (one flight) safely without any handrail or support.

3 Goes up and down 12–14 stairs using support (stick, rails), or is unsafe, or is unreasonably slow. Does not require assistance of another person.

2 Requires supervision and/or minimal to moderate assistance to go up and down one flight of stairs.

1 Requires maximal/total help, or does not go up stairs.

Communication

____ Comprehension (best mode)

4 Follows spoken *or* written directions (for example, three-step commands) or conversation; comprehends spoken *or* written native language.

3 Has difficulty following spoken or written directions or conversation. Needs a hearing aid or visual aid, or extra time to comprehend information.

2   Does not follow directions or conversation without cues or assistance of another person, including an interpreter for the deaf or a reader for the blind.

1   Does not follow spoken or written directions or conversation.

_____ Expression

4   Expresses complex ideas intelligibly and fluently, verbally or non-verbally, including signing or writing.

3   Expresses complex ideas with mild difficulty, but communicates basic wants and needs without difficulty. May require an augmentative device or system.

2   Expresses thoughts in a telegraphic or confused pattern, or requires prompts, cues, or assistance of another person.

1   Does not express basic needs and wants.

Social cognition

_____ Social interaction

4   Participates appropriately with family members, other patients, authorities (for example, staff) etc. For example, controls temper, accepts criticism.

3   Participates appropriately in suitably structured situations or modified environments. Assistance of another person not required.

2   Unpredictable or uncooperative behaviour, requiring assistance of another person for less than half of the time.

1   Does not function in a group/family setting, or has outbursts of unacceptable behaviour or inappropriate outbursts of crying or laughter. Requires assistance of another person for more than half of the time.

_____ Problem-solving

4   Able, in new or unfamiliar situations to apply previously acquired knowledge, to initiate and carry out a sequence of steps until a task is complete and to correct self if errors are made.

3   Has some difficulty in initiating, sequencing, or self-correcting. Supervision of another person is not required.

2   Problem-solves only with help of another person (supervision, coaxing, cueing) for less than 50 per cent of time.

1   Does not problem-solve.

_____ Memory

4   Recognizes people frequently encountered, remembers daily routines without cueing, prompting, or aids; executes requests of others without need for repetition.

3 Has some difficulty recognizing familiar people, remembering daily routines and requests. Uses self-initiated or environmental cues, prompts, or aids. Reminding by another person not required.

2 Has difficulty recognizing familiar people, remembering daily routines and requests. Requires prompting by another person less than half of the time.

1 Does not recognize other people, remember daily routines and requests of others. Requires supervision over half of the time.

Reference   Granger *et al.* (1986).

Comment
The FIM is being developed as a standard measure of disability for use in specialist rehabilitation centres within the United States. Reliability has been tested for the four levels, but not for the seven levels. The score weights are arbitrary and so different disabilities cannot be compared (unlike the previous two scales).

Functional Status Questionnaire

Physical function
(Basic activities of daily living, and intermediate activities of daily living.)

Responses:
4 = usually did with no difficulty
3 = usually did with some difficulty
2 = usually did with much difficulty
1 = usually did not do because of health
0 = usually did not do for other reasons

During the past month have you had difficulty:
____ • taking care of yourself, that is eating, dressing, or bathing?
____ • moving in and out of a bed or chair?
____ • walking indoors, such as around your home?
____ • walking several blocks?
____ • walking one block or climbing one flight of stairs?
____ • doing work around the house, such as cleaning, light yard work, home maintenance?
____ • doing errands, such as grocery shopping?
____ • driving a car or using public transport?
____ • doing vigorous activities, such as running, lifting heavy objects, or participating in strenuous sports?

Psychological function (Mental health)

Responses:
   1 = all of the time
   2 = most of the time
   3 = a good bit of the time
   4 = some of the time
   5 = a little of the time
   6 = none of the time

During the past month:

____ • have you been a very nervous person?
____* • have you felt calm and peaceful?
____ • have you felt downhearted and blue?
____* • were you a happy person?
____ • did you feel so 'down in the dumps' that nothing could cheer you up?

Social-role function

A. *Work performance* (if employed)

Responses:
   1 = all of the time
   2 = most of the time
   3 = some of the time
   4 = none of the time

If in work, during the past month have you:

____* • done as much work as others in similar jobs?
____ • worked for short periods of time, or taken frequent rests because of your health?
____* • worked your regular number of hours?
____* • done your job as carefully and accurately as others with similar jobs?
____ • worked at your usual job, but with some changes because of your health?
____ • feared losing your job because of your health?

B. *Social activity*

Responses:
   4 = usually did with no difficulty
   3 = usually did with some difficulty
   2 = usually did with much difficulty
   1 = usually did not do because of health
   0 = usually did not do for other reasons

During the past month have you had difficulty:

____ • visiting relatives or friends?

____ • participating in community activities, such as religious services, social activities or volunteer work?

____ • taking care of other people, such as family members?

C. *Quality of interaction*

Responses:
  1 = all of the time
  2 = most of the time
  3 = a good bit of the time
  4 = some of the time
  5 = a little of the time
  6 = none of the time

During the past month did you:

____ • isolate yourself from people around you?

____* • act affectionately towards others?

____ • act irritably towards those around you?

____ • make unreasonable demands on your family and friends?

____* • get along well with other people?

Single-item questions

A. Which of the following statements best describes your work situation during the past month?

____ • working full-time?

____ • working part-time?

____ • unemployed, looking for work?

____ • unemployed, because of my health?

____ • retired because of my health?

____ • retired for some other reason?

B. During the past month, how many days did illness keep you in bed all or most of the day?

____ Reply: 0–31 days

C. During the past month, how many days did you cut down on things you usually do for one-half day or more because of your illness?

____ Reply: 0–31 days

D. During the past month, how satisfied were you with your sexual relationships?

____ • very satisfied?
____ • satisfied?
____ • not sure?
____ • dissatisfied?
____ • very dissatisfied?
____ • did not have any sexual relationships?

E. How do you feel about your own health?

____ • very satisfied?
____ • satisfied?
____ • not sure?
____ • dissatisfied?
____ • very dissatisfied?

F. During the past month, about how often did you socialize with friends or relatives, that is go out together, visit each other's homes or talk on the telephone:

____ • every day?
____ • several times a week?
____ • about once a week?
____ • two or three times a month?
____ • about once a month?
____ • not at all?

____* This indicates that responses are scored in reverse on this item.

References Jette and Clearly (1987); McDowell and Newell (1987)

Comment

This index was designed primarily for use with, or on, a computer (hence reversal of scoring is of little importance) in the setting of a rehabilitation centre. Reliability and validity addressed in original study.

Formula gives 0–100 score:
  score $= ((\text{sum 1 to } n \text{ of valid scores minus } n)/n) \times 100/k$
  $n =$ number of questions with valid answers
      '0' responses are invalid and do not count
  $k =$ max–min valid score

Rand Functional Limitations Battery

Responses (Question 1):
  1 = No, because of my health
  2 = No, for some other reason
  3 = Yes, able to drive a car

Responses (Questions 2–13):
  1 = No, not limited
  2 = Yes, for three months or less
  3 = Yes, for more than three months

No.	Answer	Question
1.	____	Are you able to drive a car?
2.	____	When you travel around your community, does someone have to help you because of your health?
3.	____	Do you have to stay indoors most or all of the day, because of your health?
4.	____	Are you in bed or a chair for most or all of the day, because of your health?
5.	____	Does your health limit the kind of vigorous activity you can do, such as running, lifting heavy objects, or participating in strenuous sports?
6.	____	Do you have any trouble either walking several blocks or climbing a few flights of stairs, because of your health?
7.	____	Do you have any trouble bending, lifting, or stooping because of your health?
8.	____	Do you have any trouble either walking one block or climbing one flight of stairs because of your health?
9.	____	Are you unable to walk unless you are assisted by another person or by a cane (walking stick), crutches, artificial limb(s), or braces (splints)?
10.	____	Are you unable to do certain kinds or amounts of work, housework or schoolwork because of your health?
11.	____	Does your health keep you from working at a job, doing work around the house, or going to school?
12.	____	Do you need help with eating, dressing, bathing, or using the toilet because of your health?
13.	____	Does your health limit you in any way from doing anything you want to?

Reference   Stewart *et al.* (1978)

Comment
Another global measure of disability.

Rand Physical Capacities Battery

Responses
  1 = Yes
  2 = Yes, but only slowly
  3 = No, I can't do this

No.	Answer	Question
1.	____	Can you do hard activities at home, heavy work like scrubbing floors, or lifting or moving heavy furniture?
2.	____	If you wanted to, could you participate in active sports such as swimming, tennis, basketball, volleyball, or rowing a boat?
3.	____	Could you do moderate work at home like moving a chair or table, or pushing a vacuum cleaner?
4.	____	Can you do light work around the house like dusting or washing dishes?
5.	____	If you wanted to, could you run a short distance?
6.	____	Can you walk uphill or up stairs?
7.	____	Can you walk a block or more?
8.	____	Can you walk around inside the house?
9.	____	Can you walk to a table for meals?
10.	____	Can you dress yourself?
11.	____	Can you eat without help?
12.	____	Can you use the bathroom without help?

Reference   Stewart *et al.* (1978)

Comment
A measure of intermediate activities of daily living, spanning higher level personal ADL together with extended ADL items concentrating on physical mobility.

PULSES Profile

P *Physical condition*
Includes diseases of viscera (cardiovascular, gastrointestinal, urologic and endocrine) and neurologic disorders.

1. Medical problems sufficiently stable that medical or nursing monitoring is not required more often that at 3-month intervals.
2. Medical or nurse monitoring is needed more than 3-monthly but not each week.
3. Medical problems are sufficiently unstable as to require regular nursing and/or medical attention at least weekly.
4. Medical problems require intensive medical and/or nursing attention at least daily (excluding personal care assistance only).

U *Upper limb functions*
Self-care activities (drink, feed, dress, brace/prosthesis, groom, wash, perineal care) dependent upon arm function.

1. Independent in self-care without impairment of arms.
2. Independent in self-care with some impairment of arms.
3. Dependent upon assistance or supervision in self-care with or without impairment of arms.
4. Dependent totally in self-care with marked impairment of arms.

L *Lower limb functions*
Mobility (transfer chair/toilet/bath/shower; walk; stairs; wheelchair) dependent mainly upon leg function.

1. Independent in mobility without impairment of legs.
2. Independent in mobility with some impairment in legs, such as needing ambulatory aids, a brace or prosthesis; *or else* fully independent in wheelchair without significant architectural or environmental barriers.
3. Dependent upon assistance or supervision in mobility with or without impairment of legs; *or* partly independent in wheelchair; *or* there are significant architectural or environmental barriers.
4. Dependent totally in mobility with marked impairment in legs.

S *Sensory components*—relating to communication (speech and hearing) and vision.

1. Independent in communication and vision without impairment.
2. Independent in communication and vision with some impairment such as mild dysarthria, mild aphasia, or need for eyeglasses or hearing aid, or needing regular eye medication.
3. Dependent upon assistance, an interpreter, or supervision in communication or vision.
4. Dependent totally in communication or vision.

E. *Excretory functions (bladder and bowel)*

1. Complete voluntary control of bladder and bowel sphincters.
2. Control of sphincters allows normal social activities despite urgency or need for catheter, appliance, suppositories, etc. Able to care for needs without assistance.
3. Dependent upon assistance in sphincter management or else has accidents occasionally.
4. Frequent wetting or soiling from incontinence of bladder or bowel sphincters.

S *Situational factors*
   Consider intellectual and emotional adaptability, support from family unit, financial ability, and social interaction.

1. Able to fulfil usual roles and perform customary tasks.
2. Must make some modification in usual roles and performance of customary tasks.
3. Dependent upon assistance, supervision, encouragement or assistance from a public or private agency due to any of the above considerations.
4. Dependent upon long-term institutional care (chronic hospitalization, nursing home, etc.) excluding time-limited hospital for specific evaluation, treatment or active rehabilitation.

References Granger *et al.* (1979); Gresham and Labi (1984)

Comment
An extremely simple (and limited) measure, first developed for use in the US Army. It forms part of the assessments used by a community rehabilitation network (Carroll *et al.* 1984).

18   Measures of handicap and quality of life

Summary

1. WHO Handicap Scales
2. Karnofsky Performance Status
3. Glasgow Outcome Scale
4. Rankin Scale
5. Rosser's Classification of Illness States
6. Quality of Well-being Scale (index of well-being)
7. Life satisfaction: a measure
8. Quality of life: a measure
9. Life Satisfaction Index
10. Katz Adjustment Scale: relatives
11. Rand Social Health Battery
12. Reintegration to Normal Living Index
13. Environmental Assessment: non-standard

Introduction

This chapter gives measures which assess, to a greater or lesser extent, global outcome. Only the WHO categories and scales are specifically designed to measure handicap. The remaining measures could be used as substitute measures of handicap; some of which include mainly physical disability items, and they could be considered simply as yet further measures of disability. Some are used as measures of 'quality of life', sometimes to allocate resources. At present the wisdom of using such measures must be questioned (Drummond 1987; Smith 1987).

The Glasgow Outcome Scale and the Rankin Scale are the best two for large multicentre research projects: simple, reliable and well-tested. The Karnofsky Index is only included to demonstrate that it should be not used. The Life Satisfaction Index (LSI) is widely used, although of uncertain validity as a measure of quality of life. The other measures are shown so that readers can judge them for themselves.

WHO Handicap Scales

Handicap is discussed in detail in the main text. It is characterized by a discordance between the individual's performance, or status, and the expectations of the individual himself, or of the particular group of which he is a member. The World Health Organization proposed six scales, based on six 'survival roles'.

The scales are intended to classify the circumstances in which individuals find themselves. Each has nine levels, with '0' being the best and '8' the worst. Detailed descriptions are given in the manual. Some general rules are given below.

Rules
1. Occasional difficulty or dependence should not preclude assignment to less disadvantaged category.
2. If in doubt, rate to less favourable category.
3. Rate person as they are at present, do not take into account any future or intended provision of aids or other help.
4. Assign according to actual degree of dependence, not what the assessor things the person should or might be capable of.

Reference   WHO (1980)

Comment
As discussed in the text, these scales have not been tested for validity or reliability. The author's limited clinical experience of their use suggests they can be easy to use when one knows the patient reasonably well, but only relevant once change has stabilized.

WHO Handicap Scale: Orientation

Definition. Orientation is the individual's ability to orient himself in relation to his surroundings.

Scale construct. Orientation to surroundings, including reciprocation or interaction with surroundings.

Includes: reception of signals from surroundings (such as by seeing, listening, smelling, or touching), assimilation of these signals and expression of response to what is assimilated; and
consequences of disabilities of behaviour and communcation, and including the planes of seeing, listening, touching, speaking, and assimilation of these functions by the mind.

Excludes: response to reception and assimilation of signals from the surroundings manifest as handicaps of:
• personal care (physical independence handicap)
• evasion of physical hazard (mobility handicap)
• behaviour in specific situations (occupation handicap)
• and behaviour towards others (social integration handicap)

Scale categories
  0 Fully oriented
  1 Fully compensated impediment to orientation
  2 Intermittent disturbance of orientation
  3 Partially compensated impediment to orientation
  4 Moderate impediment to orientation
  5 Severe impediments to orientation
  6 Orientation deprivation
  7 Disorientation
  8 Unconscious

WHO Handicap Scale: Physical independence

Definition. Physical independence is the individual's ability to sustain a customarily effective independent existence.

Scale construct. Independence in regard to aids and the assistance of others.

Includes: self-care and other activities of daily living.

Excludes: aids or assistance in orientation.

Scale categories
  0 Fully independent
  1 Aided independence
  2 Adapted independence
  3 Situational independence
  4 Long-interval independence (24 + hours)
  5 Short-interval independence (few hours)
  6 Critical-interval independence (unpredictable)
  7 Special-care dependence
  8 Intensive-care dependence

WHO Handicap Scale: Mobility

Definition. Mobility is the individual's ability to move about effectively in his surroundings.

Scale construct. Extent of mobility from a reference point, the individual's bed.

Includes: the individual's abilities augmented, where appropriate, by prostheses or other physical aids, including a wheelchair (all these should have been identified in categories 1 or 2 of physical independence handicap).

Excludes: mobility attainments with the assistance of other individuals (the latter should be identified as 'long-interval dependence', category 4 of physical independence handicap).

Scale categories
   0 Fully mobile
   1 Variable restriction of mobility
   2 Impaired mobility (i.e. slower)
   3 Reduced mobility
   4 Neighbourhood restriction
   5 Dwelling restriction ('housebound')
   6 Room restriction
   7 Chair restriction
   8 Total restriction ('bedbound')

WHO Handicap Scale: Occupation

Definition. Occupation is the individual's ability to occupy his time in the manner customary to his sex, age, and culture.

Scale construct. The ability to sustain appropriate occupation of time for the working day.

Includes: play or recreation, employment, and the elderly pursuing occupations customary to their age group, which in many cultures includes their assuming a more domestic role and fulfilling this after normal retirement age.

Excludes: restriction or loss of the ability to follow an occupation that is not due to an individual's impairment, such as might arise because of changes in employment possibilities.

Scale categories
   0 Customarily occupied
   1 Intermittently occupied
   2 Curtailed occupation
   3 Adjusted occupation
   4 Reduced occupation
   5 Restricted occupation
   6 Confined occupation
   7 No occupation
   8 Unoccupiable

WHO Handicap Scale: Social integration

Definition. Social integration is the individual's ability to participate in and maintain customary social relationships.

Scale construct. Individual's level of contact with a widening circle, from the reference point of self.

Scale categories
   0 Socially integrated
   1 Inhibited participation
   2 Restricted participation
   3 Diminished participation
   4 Impoverished relationships
   5 Reduced relationships
   6 Disturbed relationships
   7 Alienated
   8 Socially isolated

WHO Handicap Scale: Economic self-sufficiency

Definition. Economic self-sufficiency is the individual's ability to sustain customary socio–economic activity and independence.

Scale construct. Fundamentally related to economic self-sufficiency, from the reference point of zero resources but unlike with the other handicap scales, the construct has been extended so as to include possession or command of an unusual abundance of resources; the justification for this extension is the potential that abundant resources provide for ameliorating disadvantage in other dimensions.

Includes:
- the individual's self-sufficiency in regard to obligations to sustain others, such as members of the family;
- economic self-sufficiency sustained by virtue of any compensation or standard disability, invalidity or retirement pension that the individual receives, or to which he or she may be entitled, but excluding any supplementary allowances or benefits to which the individual's poverty may entitle him or her;
- economic self-sufficiency by virtue of income (earned or otherwise) or material possessions such as natural resources, livestock or crops; and
- poverty resulting from, or exacerbated by, impairment or disability.

Excludes:
- economic deprivation due to factors other than impairment or disability.

Scale categories
0 Wealthy
1 Comfortably off
2 Fully self-sufficient
3 Adjusted self-sufficiency
4 Precariously self-sufficient
5 Economically deprived
6 Impoverished
7 Destitute
8 Economically inactive

Rules
Categorize an individual according to the economic self-sufficiency of his/her family unit.

Karnofsky Performance Status

Score	Definition	Criteria
100	Able to carry on normal activity and to work; no special care is needed	Normal; no evidence of disease
90		Able to carry on normal activity; minor signs or symptoms of disease
80		Normal activity with effort; some signs or symptoms of disease
70	Unable to work; able to live at home, care for most personal needs; a varying amount of assistance is needed	Cares for self; unable to carry on normal activity or to do active work

60		Requires occasional assistance and frequent medical care
50		Requires considerable assistance and frequent medical care
40	Unable to care for self; requires equivalent of institutional or hospital care. Disease may be progressing rapidly	Disabled. Requires special care and assistance
30		Severely disabled; hospitalization is indicated, although death not imminent
20		Very sick, hospitalization necessary; active supportive treatment is necessary
10		Moribund, fatal processes progressing rapidly
0		Dead

References   Karnofsky *et al.* (1951); Hutchinson *et al.* (1979)

Comment

This scale was devised for use in early trials of chemotherapeutic agents for carcinoma. At the time it represented a great advance. *Now there is no place for its use*. Its validity has never been demonstrated; it mixes impairments with disabilities (and even pathology) and its reliability has not been established. There are many more far better measures now available.

Glasgow Outcome Scale

Two versions are shown: the five-point and the eight-point version.

1   1   Death

2   2   Vegetative state
Non-sentient, not obeying commands, no verbal response, no meaningful response; may have sleep–wake rhythm, may have spontaneous eye opening and ability to follow moving objects, may swallow food.

3   Severe disability; conscious but dependent
    3   Communication is possible, minimally by emotional response, total or almost total dependency with regards to activities of daily life.

     4   Partial independence in activities of daily life, may require assistance for only one activity, such as dressing; many evident post-traumatic complaints and/or signs; resumption of former life and work not possible.

4   Moderate disability; independent but disabled

     5   Independent in activities of daily life, for instance can travel by public transport; not able to resume previous activities either at work or socially; despite evident post-traumatic signs, resumption of activities at a lower level is often possible.

     6   Post-traumatic signs are present which, however, allow resumption of most former activities either full-time or part-time.

5   Good recovery

     7   Capable of resuming normal occupational and social activities; there are minor physical or mental deficits or complaints.

     8   Full recovery without symptoms or signs.

References   Jennett and Bond (1975); Jennett *et al*. (1981); Maas *et al*. (1983)

Comment

The GOS is the most widely used outcome measure in head injury research. It is very crude (insensitive) and is not very reliable in its eight-point version. Its simplicity means that it can be useful in large multicentre trials but other measures would almost certainly give more useful information (and be more likely to detect a difference between groups). It should be used with these severe limitations in mind.

Rankin Scale

Grade Description

0	No symptoms at all
1	No significant disability, despite symptoms; able to carry out all usual duties and activities
2	Slight disability; unable to carry out all previous activities but able to look after own affairs without assistance
3	Moderate disability; requiring some help, but able to walk without assistance.
4	Moderately severe disability; unable to walk without assistance and unable to attend to own bodily needs without assistance
5	Severe disability; bedridden, incontinent and requiring constant nursing care and attention

---

References   Rankin (1957); Van Swieten *et al*. (1988)

Comment

The stroke research equivalent of the Glasgow Outcome Scale. Well studied for reliability but many different versions exist. Most studies divide patients into two groups (0–3, 4–5), or three groups (0, 1–3, 4–5). The scale mixes impairments and disabilities, and is not really a measure of handicap (as claimed), being strongly based upon mobility. As with the GOS, the Rankin Scale might be useful as an extremely simple outcome measure in large multicentre trials at the cost of low sensitivity.

Rosser's Classification of Illness States

Level	Description

Disability

I	No disability.
II	Slight social disability.
III	Severe social disability and/or slight impairment of performance at work Able to do all housework except very heavy tasks
IV	Choice of work or performance at work very severely limited Housewives and old people able to do light housework only but able to go out shopping
V	Unable to undertake any paid employment Unable to continue any education Old people confined to home except for escorted outings and short walks and unable to do shopping Housewives able only to perform a few simple tasks
VI	Confined to chair or wheelchair or able to move around in the house only with support from an assistant
VII	Confined to bed
VIII	Unconscious

Distress

A None
B Mild
C Moderate
D Severe

Valuation matrix

Distress:	A	B	C	D
Disability:				
I	1.000	0.995	0.990	0.967
II	0.990	0.986	0.973	0.932
III	0.980	0.972	0.956	0.912
IV	0.964	0.956	0.942	0.870
V	0.946	0.935	0.900	0.700
VI	0.875	0.845	0.680	0.000
VII	0.677	0.564	0.000	− 1.486
VIII	− 1.028			

References   Rosser and Watts (1972); Rosser and Kind (1978)

Comment
This scale is the basis of many political and economic decisions relating to
health care, in that QALYs (Quality Adjusted Life Years) are often derived
from the weights given here. The validity (or lack of it) is discussed in the
text. Given the major decisions made on the basis of this and similar
indices, there has been remarkably little critical evaluation of this scale.
Urgent re-evaluation is needed and until the results are published (openly
and widely) the scale should not be used to evaluate services or to allocate
resources.

Quality of Well-being Scale (index of well-being)

Step	Weight	Definition

Mobility (MOB)

3	− 0.000	No limitations in driving or use of public transport (bus, train, plane, subway) for health reasons.
2	− 0.062	Did not drive a car, *or* did not use public transport for health reasons. If aged under 17, did not ride in a car, or had more help to use public transport than usual for age.
1	− 0.090	In hospital (nursing home, hospice, home for the retarded, mental hospital, etc.) as a bed patient overnight.
0	− 0.090	Death.

Physical Activity (PAC)

3	− 0.000	No limitations for health reasons.

2   − 0.060   Found it difficult (or did not try) to lift, stoop, bend over, or use stairs or inclines; *and/or*
Limped, used a cane (walking stick), crutches, or walker; *or*
Had any other physical limitation making it hard (or did not try) to walk as far or as fast as others of the same age, for health reasons; *or*
In wheelchair but controlled its movement without help

1   − 0.077   In bed or couch for most of the day (health related) *or* in wheelchair and did not control movement without help

0   − 0.077   Death

Social activity (SAC)

3   − 0.000   Performed major role (work, home-making, school, retirement, etc.) and other (personal, community, religious, social, recreational) activities, with no limitations for health reasons

2   − 0.061   Limited in, or did not perform major or other role activities for health reasons, but performed self-care (feeding, bathing, dressing, toilet)

1   − 0.106   Did not perform self-care activities (or had more help than usual for age) for health reasons.

0   − 0.106   Death

CPX	Weight	Description

Symptom/problems complexes (CPX)

1   − 0.727   Death

2   − 0.407   Loss of consciousness such as seizure (fits), fainting, coma (out cold or knocked out)

3   − 0.367   Burn over large areas of face, body, arms, or legs

4   − 0.349   Pain, bleeding, itching or discharge (drainage) from sexual organs —does not include normal menstrual (monthly) bleeding

5   − 0.340   Trouble learning, remembering, or thinking clearly

6   − 0.333   Any combination of one or more hands, feet, arms or legs either missing, deformed, crooked, paralysed (unable to move), or broken —including wearing artificial limbs or braces

7   − 0.299   Pain, stiffness, weakness, numbness or other discomfort in chest, stomach (including hernia or rupture), side, neck, back, hips, or any joints of hands, feet, arms, or legs

8   − 0.292   Pain, burning, bleeding, itching, or other difficulty with rectum, bowel movements, or urination (passing water).

CPX	Weight	Description
9	− 0.290	Sick or upset stomach, vomiting or loose bowel movements, with or without fever, chills, or aching all over.
10	− 0.259	General tiredness, weakness, or weight loss.
11	− 0.257	Cough, wheezing, or shortness of breath with or without fever, chills, or aching all over.
12	− 0.257	Spells of feeling upset, being depressed or of crying.
13	− 0.244	Headache, or dizziness, or ringing in ears, or spells of feeling hot or nervous or shaky.
14	− 0.240	Burning or itching rash on large areas of face, body, arms, or legs.
15	− 0.237	Trouble talking, such as lisp, stuttering, hoarseness, or being unable to speak.
16	− 0.230	Pain or discomfort in one or both eyes (such as burning or itching), or any trouble seeing after correction.
17	− 0.186	Overweight for age and height, or skin defect of face, body, arms or legs such as scars, pimples, warts, bruises, or changes in colour.
18	− 0.170	Pain in ear, tooth, jaw, throat, lips, tongue; several missing or crooked permanent teeth—including wearing bridges or false teeth; stuffy, runny nose; or any trouble hearing—including wearing a hearing aid.
19	− 0.144	Taking medication or staying on a prescribed diet for health reasons.
20	− 0.101	Wears eyeglasses or contact lenses.
21	− 0.101	Breathing smog or unpleasant air.
22	− 0.000	No symptoms or problems.
23	− 0.257	Standard symptom/problem.

Weighted score = 1 + MOB(wt) + PAC(wt) + SAC(wt) + CPX(wt)[+ CPX(wt)]

References Kaplan *et al.* (1978); Patrick *et al.* (1973); Kaplan and Bush (1982)

Comment
A well-studied index, with different versions. The author is not aware of its use in neurological rehabilitation. See McDowell and Newell (1987) for more details.

Life satisfaction: a measure

Instructions
Patient is asked to rate life satisfaction on one global and six specific areas, using the following response categories:

6 Very satisfied
5 Satisfied
4 Rather satisfied
3 Rather dissatisfied
2 Dissatisfied
1 Very dissatisfied

Topics
The seven topics are:
• life in general
• self-care activities of daily living
• leisure
• togetherness with friends
• togetherness with family
• marriage
• sexuality

Reference   Viitanen *et al.* (1988)

Comment
Used in only one study on stroke, with no confirmation of reliability.
Validated to an extent against the WHO handicap (social integration) scale.
Simple to use.

Quality of life: a measure

Instructions
Patients are asked to compare their current state in four major domains with
reference to a defined previous state (for example, before their stroke/injury, two
years ago, etc.) and their responses are scored:

− 1 Deterioration
  0 No change
+ 1 Improvement

Working
• Employment
• Work satisfaction
• Attitudes of fellow workers towards patient
• Attitudes of supervisors towards patient
• Patient's attitude towards fellow workers
• Patient's attitude towards supervisors

Activities at home
For self, if living alone; else active participation in:
• Preparation of meals
• Cleaning
• Laundry
• Shopping, major purchases
• Care of family business (financial)
• Child care

Family relationships
Including close personal relationships and sexual patterns:
• Decision making (investments, loans, etc.)
• Participation in important family matters
• Relationships with children
• Role as parent
• Relationships with spouse
• Sexual relationships with spouse/other partner
• Tenderness and emotional expressions between spouses
• Sexual desire
• Considerations of divorce

Leisure-time activities, in and outside home
Participation or interest in:
• Outdoor activities (walking, camping, swimming, games, etc.)
• Family festivities or other occasions arranged by relatives
• Parties arranged by friends or acquaintances
• Going dancing
• Going to movies, theatres, concerts, etc.
• Attending clubs, meetings of charitable or professional groups
• Political activities or occasions
• Activities of church or religious communities
• Visiting exhibitions, museums, libraries, etc.
• Travelling or tours
• Handiwork
• Special cooking or baking
• Reading
• Collecting stamps
• Photography
• Choir, or other musical activity
• Other hobbies

Reference   Niemi *et al.* (1988)

Comment
Only used in one small study on stroke. No validation or reliability studies published.

Life Satisfaction Index (LSI)

Here are some statements about life in general that people feel differently about. Would you read each statement in the list, and if you agree with it put a tick in the space under '*agree*'. If you do not agree with a statement, put a tick in the space under '*disagree*'. If you are not sure one way or the other, put a tick under '?'. *Please be sure to answer every question on the list.*

Agree	Disagree	?	
____	____	____	As I grow older, things seem better than I thought they would be.
____	____	____	I have had more of the breaks in life than most of the people I know.
____*	____	____	This is the dreariest time of my life.
____	____	____	I am just as happy as when I was younger.
____*	____	____	My life could be happier than it is now.
____	____	____	These are the best years of my life.
____*	____	____	Most of the things I do are boring or monotonous.
____	____	____	I expect some interesting and pleasant things to happen to me in the future.
____	____	____	The things I do are as interesting to me as they ever were.
____*	____	____	I feel old and somewhat tired.
____	____	____	I feel my age, but it does not bother me.
____	____	____	As I look back on my life, I am fairly well satisfied.
____	____	____	I would not change my past life even if I could.
____*	____	____	Compared to other people my age, I've made a lot of foolish decisions in my life.
____	____	____	Compared to other people my age, I have a good appearance.
____	____	____	I have made plans for things I'll be doing a month or a year from now.
____*	____	____	When I think back over my life, I didn't get most of the important things I wanted.
____*	____	____	Compared to other people, I get down in the dumps too often.
____	____	____	I've got pretty much what I expected out of life.
____*	____	____	In spite of what people say, the lot of the average person is getting worse, not better.

Scoring
  Score: ? = 1
  If marked '*', score: agree = 0, disagree = 2
  Otherwise score: agree = 2, disagree = 0

References Neugarten *et al.* (1961); Adams (1969); Wood *et al.* (1969); Luker (1979); Hoyt and Creech (1983)

Comment
Primarily devised for use with elderly people, this scale has been used many times, with some evidence to support its validity and reliability. It is brief, lasting about ten minutes. There are many different versions including some shortened ones but the questions may not always be appropriate for all potential subjects.

Katz Social Adjustment Scale: relatives

Please answer all 127 questions, putting a cross (X) in the box which best describes the injured person *as the person was before his/her injury* and a circle (O) in the box which best describes the injured person *as he/she is now*.

If there has been no change following the injury regarding a particular question, please put a circle and a cross in the same box. Do not spend too long on each question; your first impressions are likely to be the most accurate, but please make sure that you answer every question indicating how the injured person was before the injury and as he/she is now.

Remember:
  X = injured person *before* the injury
  O = injured person *now*

	Almost never	Sometimes	Often	Almost always
1. Has trouble sleeping	—	—	—	—
2. Gets very self critical, starts to blame himself or herself for things	—	—	—	—
3. Cries easily	—	—	—	—
4. Feels lonely	—	—	—	—
5. Acts as if s/he has no interest in things	—	—	—	—
6. Is restless	—	—	—	—
7. Has periods where s/he stops moving or doing something	—	—	—	—
8. Just sits	—	—	—	—
9. Acts as if s/he doesn't have much energy	—	—	—	—
10. Looks worn out	—	—	—	—
11. Feelings get hurt easily	—	—	—	—
12. Feels that people don't care about him/her	—	—	—	—
13. Does the same thing over and over again without reason	—	—	—	—
14. Passes out	—	—	—	—
15. Gets very sad, blue	—	—	—	—
16. Tries too hard	—	—	—	—
17. Needs to do things very slowly to do them right	—	—	—	—
18. Has strange fears	—	—	—	—
19. Afraid something terrible is going to happen	—	—	—	—

	Almost never	Sometimes	Often	Almost always
20. Gets nervous easily	___	___	___	___
21. Jittery	___	___	___	___
22. Worries or frets	___	___	___	___
23. Gets sudden fright for no reason	___	___	___	___
24. Has bad dreams	___	___	___	___
25. Acts as if s/he sees people or things that aren't there	___	___	___	___
26. Does strange things without reason	___	___	___	___
27. Attempts suicide	___	___	___	___
28. Gets angry and breaks things	___	___	___	___
29. Talks to himself or herself	___	___	___	___
30. Acts as if s/he has no control over his/her emotions	___	___	___	___
31. Laughs or cries at strange things	___	___	___	___
32. Has mood changes without reason	___	___	___	___
33. Has temper tantrums	___	___	___	___
34. Gets very excited for no reason	___	___	___	___
35. Gets very happy for no reason	___	___	___	___
36. Acts as if s/he doesn't care about other people's feelings	___	___	___	___
37. Thinks only of himself or herself	___	___	___	___
38. Shows his/her feelings	___	___	___	___
39. Generous	___	___	___	___
40. Thinks people are talking about him/her	___	___	___	___
41. Complains of headaches, stomach trouble and other physical ailments	___	___	___	___
42. Bossy	___	___	___	___
43. Acts as if s/he's suspicious of people	___	___	___	___
44. Argues	___	___	___	___
45. Gets into fights with people	___	___	___	___
46. Is not cooperative	___	___	___	___
47. Does the opposite of what is asked	___	___	___	___
48. Stubborn	___	___	___	___
49. Answers when talked to	___	___	___	___
50. Curses at people	___	___	___	___
51. Deliberately upsets routine	___	___	___	___
52. Resentful	___	___	___	___
53. Envious of other people	___	___	___	___
54. Friendly	___	___	___	___
55. Gets annoyed easily	___	___	___	___

56. Critical of other people   ___   ___   ___   ___
57. Pleasant   ___   ___   ___   ___
58. Gets along well with people   ___   ___   ___   ___
59. Lies   ___   ___   ___   ___
60. Gets into trouble with the law   ___   ___   ___   ___
61. Gets drunk   ___   ___   ___   ___
62. Is dependable   ___   ___   ___   ___
63. Is responsible   ___   ___   ___   ___
64. Doesn't argue (talk) back   ___   ___   ___   ___
65. Obedient   ___   ___   ___   ___
66. Shows good judgement   ___   ___   ___   ___
67. Stays away from people   ___   ___   ___   ___
68. Takes drugs other than recommended by hospital or clinic   ___   ___   ___   ___
69. Shy   ___   ___   ___   ___
70. Quiet   ___   ___   ___   ___
71. Prefers to be alone   ___   ___   ___   ___
72. Needs a lot of attention   ___   ___   ___   ___
73. Behaviour is childish   ___   ___   ___   ___
74. Acts helpless   ___   ___   ___   ___
75. Is independent   ___   ___   ___   ___
76. Moves about very slowly   ___   ___   ___   ___
77. Moves about in a hurried way   ___   ___   ___   ___
78. Clumsy; keeps bumping into things or dropping things   ___   ___   ___   ___
79. Very quick to react to something you say or do   ___   ___   ___   ___
80. Very slow to react   ___   ___   ___   ___
81. Gets into peculiar positions   ___   ___   ___   ___
82. Makes peculiar movements   ___   ___   ___   ___
83. Hands tremble   ___   ___   ___   ___
84. Will stay in one position for a long period   ___   ___   ___   ___
85. Loses track of day, month or year   ___   ___   ___   ___
86. Forgets own address or names of people s/he knows well   ___   ___   ___   ___
87. Remembers names of people s/he knows well   ___   ___   ___   ___
88. Acts as if s/he doesn't know where s/he is   ___   ___   ___   ___
89. Remembers important things   ___   ___   ___   ___
90. Acts as if s/he's confused about things, in a daze   ___   ___   ___   ___
91. Acts as if s/he can't get certain thoughts out of his/her mind   ___   ___   ___   ___
92. Acts as if s/he can't concentrate on one thing   ___   ___   ___   ___

	Almost never	Sometimes	Often	Almost always
93. Acts as if s/he can't make decisions	——	——	——	——
94. Talks without making sense	——	——	——	——
95. Hard to understand his/her words	——	——	——	——
96. Speaks clearly	——	——	——	——
97. Refuses to speak at all for periods of time	——	——	——	——
98. Speaks so low you cannot hear him/her	——	——	——	——
99. Speaks very loudly	——	——	——	——
100. Shouts or yells for no reason	——	——	——	——
101. Speaks very fast	——	——	——	——
102. Speaks very slowly	——	——	——	——
103. Acts as if s/he wants to speak but can't	——	——	——	——
104. Keeps repeating the same idea	——	——	——	——
105. Keeps changing from one subject to another for no reason	——	——	——	——
106. Talks too much	——	——	——	——
107. Says that people are talking about him/her	——	——	——	——
108. Says that people are trying to make him/her do or think things s/he doesn't want to	——	——	——	——
109. Talks as if s/he committed the worst sins	——	——	——	——
110. Talks about how angry s/he is at certain people	——	——	——	——
111. Talks about people or things s/he's very afraid of	——	——	——	——
112. Threatens to injure certain people	——	——	——	——
113. Threatens to tell people off	——	——	——	——
114. Says s/he is afraid that s/he will injure somebody	——	——	——	——
115. Says s/he is afraid that s/he will not be able to control him/herself	——	——	——	——
116. Talks about strange things that are going on inside his/her body	——	——	——	——
117. Says how bad or useless s/he is	——	——	——	——
118. Braggs about how good s/he is	——	——	——	——
119. Says the same thing over and over again	——	——	——	——

120.	Complains about people and things in general	___	___	___	___
121.	Talks about big plans s/he has for the future	___	___	___	___
122.	Says or acts as if people are after him/her	___	___	___	___
123.	Says that something terrible is going to happen	___	___	___	___
124.	Believes in strange things	___	___	___	___
125.	Talks about suicide	___	___	___	___
126.	Talks about strange sexual ideas	___	___	___	___
127.	Gives advice without being asked	___	___	___	___

References Katz and Lyerly (1963); Hogarty and Katz (1971)

Comment

This index measures the changes seen in 'personality' within an illness. Note that not all changes necessarily arise from brain damage; some reflect psychological responses to such factors as the experience of an acute life-threatening event, loss of a job, or persistent physical disability. Has been used in some studies on head injury.

Rand Social Health Battery

1. About how many families in your neighbourhood are you well enough acquainted with that you visit each other in your homes?

___ families

2. About how many *close* friends do you have—people you feel at ease with and can talk about what is on your mind? (You may include relatives.)

___ close friends

3. Over a year's time, about how often do you get together with friends or relatives, like going out together or visiting in each other's homes? (Circle one)

1. Every day
2. Several days a week
3. About once a week
4. 2 or 3 times a month
5. About once a month
6. 5 to 10 times a year
7. Less than 5 times a year

4. During the past month, about how often have you had friends over to your home? (Do not count relatives.) (Circle one)

1. Every day
2. Several days a week
3. About once a week
4. 2 or 3 times in past month
5. Once in past month
6. Not at all in past month

5. About how often have you visited with friends at their homes during the past month? (Do not count relatives.) (Circle one)

1. Every day
2. Several days a week
3. About once a week
4. 2 or 3 times in past month
5. Once in past month
6. Not at all in past month

6. About how often were you on the telephone with close friends or relatives during the past month? (Circle one)

1. Every day
2. Several times a week
3. About once a week
4. 2 or 3 times
5. Once
6. Not at all

7. About how often did you write a letter to a friend or relative during the past month? (Circle one)

1. Every day
2. Several times a week
3. About once a week
4. 2 or 3 times in past month
5. Once in past month
6. Not at all in past month

8. In general, how well are you getting along with other people these days—would you say better than usual, about the same, or not as well as usual? (Circle one)

1. Better than usual
2. About the same
3. Not as well as usual

9. How often have you attended a religious service during the past month?
   (Circle one)

1. Every day
2. More than once a week
3. Once a week
4. 2 or 3 times in past month
5. Once in past month
6. Not at all in past month

10. About how many voluntary groups or organizations do you belong to—like church groups, clubs or lodges, parent groups, etc. ('Voluntary' means because you want to.)
    (Write in number. If none, enter '0'.)

__ groups or organizations.

11. How active are you in the affairs of these groups or clubs you belong to? (If you belong to a great many, just count those you feel closest to. If you don't belong to any, circle 4.)
    (Circle one)

1. Very active, attend most meetings
2. Fairly active, attend fairly often
3. Not active, belong but hardly ever go
4. Do not belong to any groups or clubs

Scoring rules

Item	Scoring		Item	Scoring	
1	0–4	= as number	7	1	= 3
	5–10	= 5		2	= 2
	11 +	= 6		3	= 1
2	0–4	= as number	8	1, 2	= 5
	5–9	= 5		3	= 4
	10–20	= 6		4	= 3
	21–25	= 7		5	= 2
	26–35	= 8		6	= 1
	36 +	= 9			
3	1–3	= 4	9	0–4	= as number
	4	= 3		5 +	= 5
	5, 6	= 2			
	7	= 1			

4	1–4	= 3	10	1	= 4
	5	= 2		2	= 3
	6	= 1		3	= 2
				4	= 1
5	1–3	= 3	11	As number	
	4, 5	= 2			
	6	= 1			
6	1	= 5			
	2	= 4	*Grouping*		
	3, 4	= 3	3–5	Social contacts	
	5	= 2	10, 11	Group participation	
	6	= 1	1–6, 9–11	Social support index	

Reference   Donald *et al.* (1978)

Comment

This is a measure of social interaction and social integration. It is intended for use in population surveys, but its utility is as yet unproven. See McDowell and Newell (1987) for further discussion.

Reintegration to Normal Living Index

The patient is asked to rate their agreement with the eleven statements shown below. The rating is made using 10 cm visual analogue scales (VAS), the two anchor points are:

- 'Does not describe my situation.'
- 'Fully describes my situation'.

Each statement was originally scored from 1 to 10, and the total score adjusted to give a 0–100 scale. An alternative is to score each statement between 0 and 9, giving a 0–99 scale.

1. I move around my living quarters as I feel is necessary.
   (Wheelchairs, other equipment or resources may be used.)

2. I move around my community as I feel necessary.
   (Wheelchairs, other equipment or resources may be used.)

3. I am able to make trips out of town as I feel necessary.
   (Wheelchairs, other equipment or resources may be used.)

4. I am comfortable with how my self-care needs are met (i.e. dressing, feeding, toileting, bathing).
   (Adaptive equipment, supervision, and/or assistance may be used.)

5. I spend most of my days occupied in a work activity that is necessary or important to me.
(Work activity could be paid employment, housework, volunteer work, school, etc.)
(Adaptive equipment, supervision, and/or assistance may be used.)

6. I am able to participate in recreational activities as I want (i.e. hobbies, crafts, sports, reading, television, games, computers, etc.)
(Adaptive equipment, supervision, and/or assistance may be used.)

7. I participate in social activities with family, friends, and/or business acquaintances as is necessary or desirable to me.
(Adaptive equipment, supervision, and/or assistance may be used.)

8. I assume a role in my family which meets my needs and those of other family members. (Family means people with whom you live and/or relatives with whom you do not live but see on a regular basis.)
(Adaptive equipment, supervision, and/or assistance may be used.)

9. In general, I am comfortable with my personal relationships.

10. In general, I am comfortable with myself when I am in the company of others.

11. I feel that I can deal with life events as they happen.

Reference   Wood-Dauphinee *et al.* (1988)

Comment

This index seems to measure the extent to which someone has 'adapted' to the limitations imposed by disease. It is therefore a measure of handicap. It has been used in a study on stroke patients.

Environmental Assessment: non-standard

This is a check-list intended to identify broad problem areas, and not a measure. It has not been tested, and is only relevant to Britain.

Personal support
- In house/home
  - __ Spouse
  - __ Younger family (son, daughter, etc.)
  - __ Older family (parents, etc.)
  - __ Other adult (any generation)
  - __ Dependent child (10 years or less)

- Local (within 15 minutes)
  __ Friends prepared to help
  __ Family prepared to help
  __ Neighbours (emergency only)

- 'Organized' support given at home
  __ Meals-on-wheels
  __ Home help
  __ Home care assistant
  __ District Nursing service
  __ Voluntary agency

House

- Ownership
  __ Own house
  __ Living with relatives
  __ Housing Association
  __ Council
  __ Private rented
  __ Nursing home
  __ Institutional

- Structure
  __ Two or more stories
  __ Bungalow
  __ Flat, ground floor
  __ Flat, not ground floor, no lift
  __ Flat, not ground floor, has lift
  __ Caravan/mobile home
  __ Institution

Use of house

- From the patient's bed, can he/she reach a:
  __ Toilet seat (not simply the room)
  __ Basin
  __ Bath or shower
  __ Kitchen (kettle)
  __ Sitting room/other rest room
  __ Front gate/outside roadway

Equipment, aids, and adaptations

Note. Also consider if equipment needs checking or replacing, or if patient needs instruction on use. Any response 1, 2, or 3 should precipitate an appropriate referral.

Scored as:

   0 = Not got *and* not needed (use judgement)
   1 = Not got, *but* might be needed
   2 = Has got, *not* used
   3 = Has got, is used, needs check (or instructions)
   4 = Has got, is used, satisfactory

- ___ For getting out of bed
- ___ For incontinence
- ___ For toileting
- ___ For bathing/showering
- ___ For cooking
- ___ For getting about in house (exclude walking stick)
- ___ For getting about outside house

Finance
The financial support available varies continuously, and up-to-date leaflets should always be used. Some indicated (*) are *not* means tested. Responses to be used are:

   0 = Not received, not eligible
   1 = Not received, should consider application
   2 = Received

In general, disabled (elderly) people may be eligible for:

- ___ Income support
- ___ Social Fund Community Care grant
- ___ Independent Living Fund grant
- ___ Housing Benefit
- ___ Community Charge benefit
- ___ Community Charge exemption if severely mentally impaired (*)
- ___ Attendance Allowance (two rates) (*)
- ___ Invalid Care allowance (*)
- ___ Mobility allowance (if aged <65 years)(*)

Reference   Not previously published.

Comment
This checklist was devised for use in the UK to help identify potential areas where environmental changes might reduce handicap.

Scored as:
 0 = Not got *and* not needed (use judgement)
 1 = Not got, *but* might be needed
 2 = Has got, *not* used
 3 = Has got, is used, needs check (or instructions)
 4 = Has got, is used, satisfactory

 __ For getting out of bed
 __ For incontinence
 __ For toileting
 __ For bathing/showering
 __ For cooking
 __ For getting about in house (exclude walking stick)
 __ For getting about outside house

Finance
The financial support available varies continuously, and up-to-date leaflets should always be used. Some indicated (*) are *not* means tested. Responses to be used are:
 0 = Not received, not eligible
 1 = Not received, should consider application
 2 = Received

In general, disabled (elderly) people may be eligible for:
 __ Income support
 __ Social Fund Community Care grant
 __ Independent Living Fund grant
 __ Housing Benefit
 __ Community Charge benefit
 __ Community Charge exemption if severely mentally impaired (*)
 __ Attendance Allowance (two rates) (*)
 __ Invalid Care allowance (*)
 __ Mobility allowance (if aged <65 years)(*)

Reference   Not previously published.

Comment
This checklist was devised for use in the UK to help identify potential areas where environmental changes might reduce handicap.

19   Measures of emotion and social interaction

Summary

1. Recovery Locus of Control
2. Hospital Anxiety and Depression Scale
3. Wakefield Self-assessment Depression Inventory
4. Beck Questionnaire
5. Hamilton Rating Scale for Depression
6. Zung Self-rating Depression Scale
7. General Health Questionnaire
8. Modified self-report measure of social adjustment
9. General Well-being Schedule
10. Agitated Behaviour Scale
11. Social Behaviour Schedule

Introduction

The measures in this chapter relate primarily to the impairments seen in psychiatric conditions, and to social interaction disabilities. For extensive discussion of scales measuring emotional states, refer to Thompson (1989). The intention of reproducing the scales here is to illustrate what is available and used. Many of these scales have been used extensively, but usually in patients with primary psychiatric illness. The use of such scales in disabling physical illness, especially that due to brain damage, has not been properly investigated.

The General Health Questionnaire (GHQ) is probably the most widely used measure, but the Hospital Anxiety and Depression Scale (HADS) is gaining popularity. The Recovery Locus of Control test needs further evaluation; if initial results are confirmed it would be a useful measure. The Agitated Behaviour Scale might be useful, but also requires further evaluation.

Recovery Locus of Control

For each statement, ask the patient whether he or she:

		Score	
		Internal	External
Type			
Question numbers		1–5	6–9
A	strongly agree	4	0
B	agree	3	1
C	do not know	2	2
D	disagree	1	3
E	strongly disagree	0	4

Please read each statement and tick response closest to your own opinion:

---

1. How I manage in the future depends upon me, not on what other people do for me.

   Strongly agree__   Agree__   Do not know__   Disagree__   Strongly disagree__

2. It's what I do to help myself that's really going to make all the difference.

   Strongly agree__   Agree__   Do not know__   Disagree__   Strongly disagree__

3. It's up to me to make sure I make the best recovery possible under the circumstances.

   Strongly agree__   Agree__   Do not know__   Disagree__   Strongly disagree__

4. Getting better now is a matter of my own determination rather than anything else.

   Strongly agree__   Agree__   Do not know__   Disagree__   Strongly disagree__

5. It doesn't matter how much help you get—in the end it's your own efforts that count.

   Strongly agree__   Agree__   Do not know__   Disagree__   Strongly disagree__

6. It's often best to just wait and see what happens.

   Strongly agree__   Agree__   Do not know__   Disagree__   Strongly disagree__

7. My own efforts are not very important, my recovery really depends on others.

   Strongly agree__   Agree__   Do not know__   Disagree__   Strongly disagree__

8. My own contribution to my recovery doesn't amount to much.

   Strongly agree__   Agree__   Do not know__   Disagree__   Strongly disagree__

9. I have little or no control over my progress from now on.

   Strongly agree__   Agree__   Do not know__   Disagree__   Strongly disagree__

Reference   Partridge and Johnston (1989)

Comment

This is supposed to be a measure of motivation—the extent to which a subject feels that he or she can influence his or her future state. Only used in one study on recovery after stroke. Studies on validity (as measure of motivation) and reliability have yet to be performed. Score ranges from 0 (very 'external' or passive) to 36 (very 'internal' or selfmotivated). The initial study suggested a positive relationship between a high score and a good recovery.

Hospital Anxiety and Depression Scale

Patients are asked to chose one response from the four given for each question. They should give an immediate response and be dissuaded from thinking too long about their answers. The questions relating to anxiety are marked 'A', and to depression 'D'. The score for each answer is given in brackets before the answer.

A I feel tense or 'wound up':
  (3) Most of the time
  (2) A lot of the time
  (1) From time to time, occasionally
  (0) Not at all

D I still enjoy the things I used to enjoy:
  (0) Definitely as much
  (1) Not quite so much
  (2) Only a little
  (3) Hardly at all

A I get a sort of frightened feeling as if something awful is about to happen:
  (3) Very definitely and quite badly
  (2) Yes, but not too badly
  (1) A little, but it doesn't worry me
  (0) Not at all

D I can laugh and see the funny side of things:
  (0) As much as I always could
  (1) Not quite so much now
  (2) Definitely not so much now
  (3) Not at all

A Worrying thoughts go through my mind:
  (3) A great deal of the time
  (2) A lot of the time
  (1) From time to time, but not too often
  (0) Only occasionally

D I feel cheerful:
   (3) Not at all
   (2) Not often
   (1) Sometimes
   (0) Most of the time

A I can sit at ease and feel relaxed:
   (0) Definitely
   (1) Usually
   (2) Not often
   (3) Not at all

D I feel as if I am slowed down:
   (3) Nearly all the time
   (2) Very often
   (1) Sometimes
   (0) Not at all

A I get a sort of frightened feeling like 'butterflies' in the stomach:
   (0) Not at all
   (1) Occasionally
   (2) Quite often
   (3) Very often

D I have lost interest in my appearance:
   (3) Definitely
   (2) I don't take as much care as I should
   (1) I may not take quite as much care
   (0) I take just as much care as ever

A I feel restless as if I have to be on the move:
   (3) Very much indeed
   (2) Quite a lot
   (1) Not very much
   (0) Not at all

D I look forward with enjoyment to things:
   (0) As much as I ever did
   (1) Rather less than I used to
   (2) Definitely less than I used to
   (3) Hardly at all

A I get sudden feelings of panic:
   (3) Very often indeed
   (2) Quite often
   (1) Not very often
   (0) Not at all

D I can enjoy a good book or radio or TV programme:
- (0) Often
- (1) Sometimes
- (2) Not often
- (3) Very seldom

Scoring (depression [D] and anxiety [A] separately):
- 0–7 = Normal
- 8–10 = Borderline abnormal
- 11–21 = Abnormal

Reference Zigmond and Snaith (1983)

Comment

Specifically designed for use with hospitalized, medically ill patients, this scale attempts to overcome bias caused by somatic complaints which feature in most other inventories. Also, it covers both depression (misery) and anxiety. Easy to use and score, but more work needed on validity and reliability in the context of brain damaged patients.

Wakefield Self-assessment Depression Inventory

Read each statement, and then choose one of the following four answers to indicate your response:

- a = Yes, definitely
- b = Yes, sometimes
- c = No, not much
- d = No, not at all

Response		Statement
—	1.	I feel miserable and sad.
—	2.	I find it easy to do the things I used to do.
—	3.	I get very frightened, or panic feelings, for no apparent reason at all.
—	4.	I have weeping spells, or feel like it.
—	5.	I still enjoy the things I used to.
—	6.	I am restless and can't keep still.
—	7.	I get off to sleep easily without sleeping tablets.
—	8.	I feel anxious when I go out of the house on my own.
—	9.	I have lost interest in things.
—	10.	I get tired for no reason.
—	11.	I am more irritable than usual.
—	12.	I wake up early, then sleep badly for the rest of the night.

Scoring

	Qs 2, 5, 7	Qs 1, 3, 4, 6, 8–12
a =	0	3
b =	1	2
c =	2	1
d =	3	0

Score range = 0–36.   Score of 15–36 indicates a high likelihood of depression.

References Snaith *et al.* (1971); Wade *et al.* (1987*b*)

Comment
Primarily designed for use with physically healthy young people, this scale has been used in several studies of stroke. Its validity as a diagnostic instrument in older people with physical disabilities has never been established. It is short and easy to use, and probably quantifies misery but not depression, the clinical illness.

Beck Questionnaire

In this questionnaire are groups of statements. Please read each group carefully. Then pick the one statement in each group which best describes the way you have been feeling during the *past week, including today*. Circle the number beside the statement you picked. If several statements in the group seem to apply equally well, circle each one. Be sure to read all statements in each group before making your choice.

---

1. 0 I do not feel sad.
    1 I feel sad.
    2 I am sad all the time and can't snap out of it.
    3 I am so sad or unhappy that I can't stand it.

2. 0 I am not particularly discouraged about the future.
    1 I feel discouraged about the future.
    2 I feel I have nothing to look forward to.
    3 I feel that the future is hopeless and that things cannot improve.

3. 0 I do not feel like a failure.
    1 I feel that I have failed more than the average person.
    2 As I look back on my life, all I can see is a lot of failures.
    3 I feel that I am a complete failure as a person.

4. 0 I get as much satisfaction out of things as I used to.
   1 I don't enjoy things the way I used to.
   2 I don't get real satisfaction out of anything anymore.
   3 I am dissatisfied or bored with everything.

5. 0 I don't feel particularly guilty.
   1 I feel guilty a good part of the time.
   2 I feel quite guilty most of the time.
   3 I feel guilty all of the time.

6. 0 I don't feel I am being punished.
   1 I feel I may be punished.
   2 I expect to be punished.
   3 I feel I am being punished.

7. 0 I don't feel disappointed in myself.
   1 I am disappointed in myself.
   2 I am disgusted with myself.
   3 I hate myself.

8. 0 I don't feel I am any worse than anybody else.
   1 I am critical of myself for my weaknesses or mistakes.
   2 I blame myself all the time for my faults.
   3 I blame myself for everything bad that happens.

9. 0 I don't have any thoughts of killing myself.
   1 I have thoughts of killing myself, but I would not carry them out.
   2 I would like to kill myself.
   3 I would kill myself if I had the chance.

10. 0 I don't cry any more than usual.
   1 I cry now more than I used to.
   2 I cry all the time now.
   3 I used to be able to cry, but now I can't cry even though I want to.

11. 0 I am no more irritated now than I ever am.
   1 I get annoyed or irritated more easily than I used to.
   2 I feel irritated all the time now.
   3 I don't get irritated at all by the things that used to irritate me.

12. 0 I have not lost interest in other people.
   1 I am less interested in other people than I used to be.
   2 I have lost most of my interest in other people.
   3 I have lost all my interest in other people.

13.　0　I make decisions about as well as I ever could.
　　　1　I put off making decisions more than I used to.
　　　2　I have greater difficulty in making decisions than before.
　　　3　I can't make decisions at all anymore.

14.　0　I don't feel I look any worse than I used to.
　　　1　I am worried that I am looking old or unattractive.
　　　2　I feel that there are permanent changes in my appearance that make me
　　　　look unattractive.
　　　3　I believe that I look ugly.

15.　0　I can work about as well as before.
　　　1　It takes an extra effort to get started at doing something.
　　　2　I have to push myself very hard to do anything.
　　　3　I can't do any work at all.

16.　0　I can sleep as well as usual.
　　　1　I don't sleep as well as I used to.
　　　2　I wake up 1–2 hours earlier than usual and find it hard to get back to sleep.
　　　3　I wake up several hours earlier than I used to and cannot get back to sleep.

17.　0　I don't get more tired than usual.
　　　1　I get tired more easily than I used to.
　　　2　I get tired from doing almost anything.
　　　3　I am too tired to do anything.

18.　0　My appetite is no worse than usual.
　　　1　My appetite is not as good as it used to be.
　　　2　My appetite is much worse now.
　　　3　I have no appetite at all any more.

19.　0　I haven't lost much weight, if any, lately.
　　　1　I have lost more than 5 lbs (2 kg).
　　　2　I have lost more than 10 lbs (5 kg).
　　　3　I have lost more than 15 lbs (7 kg).
　　　(I am purposefully trying to lose weight by eating less. Yes/no)

20.　0　I am no more worried about my health than usual.
　　　1　I am worried about physical problems such as aches and pains; or upset
　　　　stomach; or constipation.
　　　2　I am very worried about physical problems and it's hard to think of much
　　　　else.
　　　3　I am so worried about my physical problems that I cannot think about
　　　　anything else.

21. 0 I have not noticed any recent change in my interest in sex.
     1 I am less interested in sex than I used to be.
     2 I am much less interested in sex now.
     3 I have lost interest in sex completely.

References Beck *et al.* (1961); Salkind (1969); Steer *et al.* (1986); House *et al.* (1989)

Comment

Widely used, and often outside primarily psychiatric or hospital settings. Validity, reliability, and sensitivity, to effects of antidepressant medication all well-proven for physically healthy, psychiatrically ill patients. Although used in neurological disease; for example, with stroke, its validity as a *diagnostic* measure of depression with physically disabling disease has not been established. It probably measures distress, not depression, in disabled people.

Suggested cut-off values are:
   0–10 = No depression
   11–17 = Mild depression
   18–23 = Moderate depression
   24 + = Severe depression

Hamilton Rating Scale for Depression

1. *Depressed mood*
   Sad, hopeless, helpless, worthless
   0 Absent
   1 Gloomy attitude, pessimism, hopelessness
   2 Occasional weeping
   3 Frequent weeping
   4 Patient reports highlight these feeling states in his/her spontaneous verbal and non-verbal communication.

2. *Feelings of guilt*
   0 Absent
   1 Self-reproach, feels he/she has let people down
   2 Ideas of guilt or rumination over past errors or sinful deeds
   3 Present illness is punishment
   4 Hears accusatory or denunciatory voices and/or experiences threatening visual hallucinations. Delusions of guilt

3. *Suicide*
   0 Absent
   1 Feels life is not worth living
   2 Wishes he/she were dead, or any thoughts of possible death to self
   3 Suicide, ideas or half-hearted attempt
   4 Attempts at suicide (any serious attempt rates 4)

4. *Insomnia, early*
   0 No difficulty falling asleep
   1 Complaints of occasional difficulty in falling asleep i.e. more than half-hour
   2 Complaints of nightly difficulty in falling asleep

5. *Insomnia, middle*
   0 No difficulty
   1 Patient complains of being restless and disturbed during the night
   2 Waking during the night—any getting out of bed rates 2 (except voiding bladder)

6. *Insomnia, late*
   0 No difficulty
   1 Waking in the early hours of the morning but goes back to sleep
   2 Unable to fall asleep again if he/she gets out of bed

7. *Work and activities*
   0 No difficulty
   1 Thoughts and feelings of incapacity related to activities: work or hobbies
   2 Loss of interest in activity—hobbies or work—either directly reported by patient or indirectly seen in listlessness, in decisions and vacillation (feels he/she has to push self to work or activities)
   3 Decrease in actual time spent in activities or decrease in productivity. In hospital, rate 3 if patient does not spend at least three hours a day in activities
   4 Stopped working because of present illness. In hospital rate 4 if patient engages in no activities except supervised ward chores

8. *Retardation*
   Slowness of thought and speech; impaired ability to concentrate; decreased motor activity.
   0 Normal speech and thought
   1 Slight retardation at interview
   2 Obvious retardation at interview
   3 Interview difficult
   4 Interview impossible

9. *Agitation*
   0 None
   1 Fidgetiness
   2 Playing with hands, hair, obvious restlessness
   3 Moving about; can't sit sill
   4 Hand wringing, nail biting, hair pulling, biting of lips, patient is on the run

10. *Anxiety, psychic*
    Demonstrated by:
    • subjective tension and irritability, loss of concentration
    • worrying about minor matters
    • apprehension
    • fears expressed without questioning
    • feelings of panic
    • feeling jumpy

    0 Absent
    1 Mild
    2 Moderate
    3 Severe
    4 Incapacitating

11. *Anxiety, somatic*
    Physiological concomitants of anxiety such as:
    • gastrointestinal: dry mouth, wind, indigestion, diarrhoea, cramps, belching
    • cardiovascular: palpitations, headaches
    • respiratory: hyperventilation, sighing
    • urinary frequency
    • sweating
    • giddiness, blurred vision
    • tinnitus

    0 Absent
    1 Mild
    2 Moderate
    3 Severe
    4 Incapacitating

12. *Somatic symptoms: gastrointestinal*
    0 None
    1 Loss of appetite but eating without encouragement
    2 Difficulty eating without urging. Requests or requires laxatives or medication
      for GI symptoms

13. *Somatic symptoms: general*
    0 None
    1 Heaviness in limbs, back or head; backaches, headaches, muscle aches, loss of
      energy, fatiguability
    2 Any clear-cut symptom rates 2

14. *Genital symptoms*
Symptoms such as: loss of libido, menstrual disturbances:
0 Absent
1 Mild
2 Severe

15. *Hypochondriasis*
0 Not present
1 Self-absorption (bodily)
2 Preoccupation with health
3 Strong conviction of some bodily illness
4 Hypochondriacal delusions

16. *Loss of weight*
Rate either 'A' or 'B':

A   When rating by history:
0 No weight loss
1 Probable weight loss associated with present illness
2 Definite (according to patient) weight loss

B   Actual weight changes (weekly):
0 Less than 1 lb (0.5 kg) weight loss in one week
1 1–2 lb (0.5–1.0 kg) weight loss in week
2 Greater than 2 lb (1 kg) weight loss in week
3 Not assessed

17. *Insight*
0 Acknowledges being depressed and ill
1 Acknowledges illness but attributes cause to bad food, overwork, virus, need for rest, etc.
2 Denies being ill at all

Reference   Hamilton (1967)

Comment
This scale was designed to help clinicians assess the severity of depression, not to diagnose it. It requires a psychiatrically trained observer, and simply standardizes clinical judgements.

Zung Self-rating Depression Scale

Indicate which of the four responses applies for each statement given below.

Responses
   1 = None, *or* a little of the time
   2 = Some of the time
   3 = Good part of the time
   4 = Most *or* all of the time

No.	Answer	Statement
1.	____	I feel down-hearted, blue, and sad.
2.	____	Morning is when I feel the best.
3.	____	I have crying spells or feel like it.
4.	____	I have trouble sleeping through the night.
5.	____	I eat as much as I used to.
6.	____	I enjoy looking at, talking to, and being with attractive men/women.
7.	____	I notice that I am losing weight.
8.	____	I have trouble with constipation.
9.	____	My heart beats faster than usual.
10.	____	I get tired for no reason.
11.	____	My mind is as clear as it used to be.
12.	____	I find it easy to do the things I used to.
13.	____	I am restless and can't keep still.
14.	____	I feel hopeless about the future.
15.	____	I am more irritable than usual.
16.	____	I find it easy to make decisions.
17.	____	I feel that I am useful and needed.
18.	____	My life is pretty full.
19.	____	I feel that others would be better off if I were dead.
20.	____	I still enjoy the things I used to.

Scoring

A Reverse scores on questions 2, 5, 6, 11, 12, 14, 16, 17, 18, 20

B SDS index = Total score/80(= maximum score)* 100

C Interpretation:
   25–50 per cent = within normal range

Reference　Zung (1965)

Comment

This is another self-rating scale to detect and measure depression in a population without associated illness. It was the progenitor of other scales and it has been used in stroke research. Its validity as a measure of depression in patients disabled by neurological disease has not been established.

General Health Questionnaire*

We should like to know if you have had any medical complaints and how your health has been, over the past few weeks. Please answer *all* the questions on the following pages simply by marking the answer which you think most nearly applies to you. Remember that we want to know about present and recent complaints, not about those you have had in the past.

Somatic symptoms
Have you recently:

Been feeling perfectly well and in good health?	Better than usual	Same as usual	Worse than usual	Much worse than usual
Been feeling in need of a good tonic?	Not at all	No more than usual	Rather more than usual	Much more than usual
Been feeling run down and out of sorts?	Not at all	No more than usual	Rather more than usual	Much more than usual
Felt that you are ill?	Not at all	No more than usual	Rather more than usual	Much more than usual
Been getting any pains in your head?	Not at all	No more than usual	Rather more than usual	Much more than usual

Been getting a feeling of tightness or pressure in your head?	Not at all	No more than usual	Rather more than usual	Much more than usual
Been having hot or cold spells?	Not at all	No more than usual	Rather more than usual	Much more than usual

Anxiety and insomnia
Have you recently:

Lost much sleep over worry?	Not at all	No more than usual	Rather more than usual	Much more than usual
Had difficulty staying asleep once you were off?	Not at all	No more than usual	Rather more than usual	Much more than usual
Felt constantly under strain?	Not at all	No more than usual	Rather more than usual	Much more than usual
Been getting edgy and bad-tempered?	Not at all	No more than usual	Rather more than usual	Much more than usual
Been getting scared or panicky for no good reason?	Not at all	No more than usual	Rather more than usual	Much more than usual
Found everything getting on top of you?	Not at all	No more than usual	Rather more than usual	Much more than usual
Been feeling nervous and strung-up all the time?	Not at all	No more than usual	Rather more than usual	Much more than usual

Social dysfunction
Have you recently:

Been managing to keep yourself busy and occupied?	More so than usual	Same as usual	Rather less than usual	Much less than usual
Been taking longer over things you do?	Quicker than usual	Same as usual	Longer than usual	Much longer than usual
Felt on the whole you were doing things well?	Better than usual	About the same	Less well than usual	Much less well

Been satisfied with the way you've carried out your task?	More satisfied	About same as usual	Less satisfied than usual	Much less satisfied
Felt you are playing a useful part in things?	More so than usual	Same as usual	Less useful than usual	Much less useful
Felt capable of making decisions about things?	More so than usual	Same as usual	Less so than usual	Much less capable
Been able to enjoy your normal day-to-day activities?	More so than usual	Same as usual	Less so than usual	Much less than usual

Severe depression
Have you recently:

Been thinking of yourself as a worthless person?	Not at all	No more than usual	Rather more than usual	Much more than usual
Felt that life is entirely hopeless?	Not at all	No more than usual	Rather more than usual	Much more than usual
Felt that life isn't worth living?	Not at all	No more than usual	Rather more than usual	Much more than usual
Thought of the possibility that you might make away with yourself?	Definitely not	I don't think so	Has crossed my mind	Definitely have
Found at times you couldn't do anything because your nerves were too bad?	Not at all	No more than usual	Rather more than usual	Much more than usual
Found yourself wishing you were dead and away from it all?	Not at all	No more than usual	Rather more than usual	Much more than usual
Found that the idea of taking your own life kept coming into your mind?	Definitely not	I don't think so	Has crossed my mind	Definitely has

Scoring (A) (Likert)
'0' for left two columns, '1' for right two columns.

Scoring (B)
From '0' for leftmost column to '3' for rightmost column.

References Goldberg (1972); Goldberg and Hillier (1979); DePaulo *et al.* (1980); Wade *et al.* (1986*b*); Carnwath and Johnson (1987)
Copies and handbook with up-to-date information and references available from:
   NFER-Nelson Publishing Co. Ltd,
   Darville House, 2 Oxford Road East,
   Windsor SL4 1DF
by whose permission GHQ–28 is reproduced here for reference purposes only.

Comment
This is a widely used, well validated measure of good reliability. It is simple and quick to use. There are various versions derived from the original 60-question version, and the GHQ-28 shown here is probably comparable to the others. Using the Likert scoring method (i.e. 0, 0, 1, 1) a cut-off score of 4/5 is most efficient at separating cases from non-cases. It can be used to measure stress upon carers. As with all other measures of depression, its validity when used with neurologically disabled patients needs to be proved. The author's experience suggests that many patients cannot complete it, reducing its utility.

Modified self-report measure of social adjustment

For each question chose one of the following answers:

1. All the time
2. Most of the time
3. About half the time
4. Occasionally
5. Not at all

We are interested in how you have been in the past two weeks. We would like to ask you some questions about your work, spare time activities and your family life.

Work outside the home
The following questions are about how things have been in your job (full-time or part-time). If you do not have a job, go straight on to the next section.

Over the past two weeks have you:

__   1. Missed any time from work?
__   2. Been doing your job well?
__   3. Felt ashamed of how you have been doing your work?
__   4. Got angry with or argued with people at work?
__   5. Felt upset, worried or uncomfortable at work?
__   6. Been finding your work interesting?

Housework
The following questions are about how the housework has been.

Over the past two weeks have you:

__   7. Done the necessary housework each day?
__   8. Been doing the housework well?
__   9. Felt ashamed of how you have been doing the housework?
__ 10. Got angry with or argued with salespeople, tradesmen or neighbours?
__ 11. Felt upset, worried or uncomfortable while doing the housework?
__ 12. Found the housework boring, unpleasant or a drudge?

Social and leisure activities
The following questions are about your friends and what you have been doing in your spare time:

Over the past two weeks have you:

__ 13. Been in touch with any of your friends?
__ 14. Been able to talk about your feelings openly with your friends?
__ 15. Done things socially with your friends (for example, visiting, entertaining, going out together)?
__ 16. Spent your available time on hobbies or spare time interests?
__ 17. Got angry with or argued with your friends?
__ 18. Been offended or had your feelings hurt by your friends?
__ 19. Felt ill at ease, tense or shy when with people?
__ 20. Felt lonely and wished for companionship?
__ 21. Felt bored in your free time?

Extended family
The following questions are about your extended family, i.e. your parents, brothers, sisters, in-laws, and children not living at home. Please do *not* include your partner or children living at home.

Over the past two weeks have you:

__ 22. Got angry or argued with any of your relatives?
__ 23. Made an effort to keep in touch with your relatives?
__ 24. Been able to talk about your feelings openly with your relatives?
__ 25. Depended upon your relatives for help, advice or friendship?

___ 26. Worried more than necessary about things happening to your relatives?
___ 27. Been feeling that you have let your relatives down at any time?
___ 28. Been feeling that your relatives have let you down at any time?

Marital

The following questions are about how things have been between you and your partner. If you are *not* living with your partner or a person in a steady relationship, go straight on to the next section.

Over the past two weeks have you:

___ 29. Got angry with each other or argued with one another?
___ 30. Been able to talk about your feelings and problems with your partner?
___ 31. Been making most of the decisions at home yourself?
___ 32. Tended to give in to your partner and let him/her have his/her own way when there was disagreement?
___ 33. And your partner shared the responsibility for practical matters that have arisen?
___ 34. Had to depend on your partner to help you?
___ 35. Been feeling affectionate towards your partner?
___ 36. And your partner had sexual relationships? About how many times?
___ 37. Had any problems during sexual intercourse (for example, pain or difficulty in reaching climax)?
___ 38. Enjoyed your sexual relations with your partner?

Parental

The following questions about how things have been with your children. If you do *not* have any children living at home go straight on to the next section.

Over the past two weeks have you:

___ 39. Been interested in your children's activities; for example, school, friends, etc.?
___ 40. Been able to talk and listen to your children?
___ 41. Been shouting or arguing with your children?
___ 42. Been feeling affectionate towards your children?

Family unit

The following questions are about how you have been with your immediate family, that is your partner and children at home. If you do *not* have an immediate family, please ignore this section.

Over the past two weeks have you:

___ 43. Been worrying more than necessary about things happening to your family?
___ 44. Been feeling that you have let your immediate family down at any time?
___ 45. Been feeling that your immediate family has let you down at any time?

References   Weissman and Bothwell (1976); Cooper *et al.* (1982)

Comment
This scale is supposed to measure adjustment to a change in circumstances arising as a result of illness. The modified version shown here was evaluated in Britain, using an all female population with gynaecological problems. There was reasonable agreement between the modified self-report questionnaire and the interview full version. It is shown so that it can be considered for use with neurologically disabled patients.

General Well-being Schedule

These questions are about how you feel and how things have been going with you. Mark *one* answer for each question.

During the past month

A __ How have you been feeling in general?

    1 In excellent spirits
    2 In very good spirits
    3 In good spirits mostly
    4 I have been up and down in spirits a lot
    5 In low spirits mostly
    6 In very low spirits

B __ Have you been bothered by nervousness or your 'nerves'?

    1 Extremely so, to the point where I could not work or take care of things
    2 Very much so
    3 Quite a bit
    4 Some, enough to bother me
    5 A little
    6 Not at all

C __ Have you been in firm control of your behaviour, thoughts, emotions *or* feelings?

    1 Yes, definitely so
    2 Yes, for the most part
    3 Generally so
    4 Not too well
    5 No and I am somewhat disturbed
    6 No and I am very disturbed

D __   Have you felt so sad, discouraged, hopeless, or had so many problems that
you wondered if anything was worthwhile?

1 Extremely so, to the point I have just about given up
2 Very much so
3 Quite a bit
4 Some, enough to bother me
5 A little bit
6 Not at all

E __   Have you been under or felt you were under any strain, stress or pressure?

1 Yes, almost more than I could bear or stand
2 Yes, quite a bit of pressure
3 Yes, some—more than usual
4 Yes, some—but about usual
5 Yes, a little
6 Not at all

F __   How happy, satisfied, or pleased have you been with your personal life?

1 Extremely happy, could not have been more satisfied or pleased
2 Very happy
3 Fairly happy
4 Satisfied, pleased
5 Somewhat dissatisfied
6 Very dissatisfied

G __   Have you had any reason to wonder if you were losing your mind, or losing
control over the way you act, talk, think, feel or of your memory?

1 Not at all
2 Only a little
3 Some, but not enough to be concerned or worried about
4 Some, and I have been a little concerned
5 Some and I am quite concerned
6 Yes, very much so and I am very concerned

H __   Have you been anxious, worried or upset?

1 Extremely so, to the point of being sick or almost sick
2 Very much so
3 Quite a bit
4 Some, enough to bother me
5 A little bit
6 Not at all

I __ Have you been waking up fresh and rested?

1 Every day
2 Most every day
3 Fairly often
4 Less than half the time
5 Rarely
6 None of the time

J __ Have you been bothered by any illness, bodily disorder, pains or fears about your health?

1 All the time
2 Most of the time
3 A good bit of the time
4 Some of the time
5 A little of the time
6 None of the time

K __ Has your daily life been full of things that were interesting to you?

1 All the time
2 Most of the time
3 A good bit of the time
4 Some of the time
5 A little of the time
6 None of the time

L __ Have you felt down-hearted and blue?

1 All the time
2 Most of the time
3 A good bit of the time
4 Some of the time
5 A little of the time
6 None of the time

M __ Have you been feeling emotionally stable and sure of yourself?

1 All the time
2 Most of the time
3 A good bit of the time
4 Some of the time
5 A little of the time
6 None of the time

N __ Have you felt tired, worn out, used-up, or exhausted?

    1 All the time
    2 Most of the time
    3 A good bit of the time
    4 Some of the time
    5 A little of the time
    6 None of the time

For each of the four scales below, note that the words at each end of the 0 to 10 scale describe opposite feelings. Circle any number along the bar which seems closest to how you have generally felt during the past month.

O   How concerned or worried about your *health* have you been?

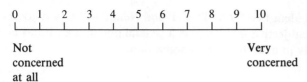

Not
concerned
at all

Very
concerned

P   How *relaxed* or *tense* have you been?

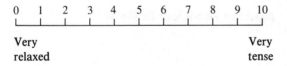

Very
relaxed

Very
tense

Q   How much *energy, pep, vitality* have you felt?

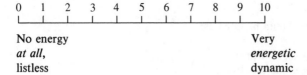

No energy
at all,
listless

Very
energetic
dynamic

R   How *depressed* or *cheerful* have you been?

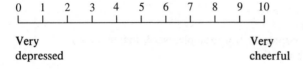

Very
depressed

Very
cheerful

The questions related to six topics:

Topic	Questions
Anxiety	B, E, H. P
Depression	D, L, R
Positive well-being	A, F, K
Self-control	C, G, M
Vitality	I, N, Q
General health	J, O

References Fazio (1977); McDowell and Newell (1989)

Comment
This index was identified by McDowell and Newell as being a good choice for measuring subjective well-being in a general population. It has been not used specifically in neurological rehabilitation.

Agitated Behaviour Scale (ABS)

Observation period
Choose a period of 30–60 min. Note times, and keep to same times (both duration and time of day) if observations are repeated.

Rating behaviour
  Each behaviour should be rated as:
  0 = absent
  1 = present to a slight degree
  2 = present to a moderate degree
  3 = present to an extreme degree
  The rating can be based on *frequency* or *severity*.

Other information to record
  (a) Observer(s)
  (b) Patient's environment (for example, ward, therapy, etc.)
  (c) Times of observation

Behaviours to observe

Score	Behaviour
__	1. Short attention span, easy distractibility, inability to concentrate.
__	2. Impulsive, impatient, low tolerance for pain or frustration.
__	3. Uncooperative, resistant to care, demanding.
__	4. Violent and/or threatening violence towards people or property.
__	5. Explosive and/or unpredictable anger.
__	6. Rocking, rubbing, moaning, or other self-stimulating behaviour.
__	7. Pulling at tubes, restraints, etc.
__	8. Wandering from treatment areas.
__	9. Restlessness, pacing, excessive movement.
__	10. Repetitive behaviours, motor and/or verbal.
__	11. Rapid, loud or excessive talking.
__	12. Sudden changes of mood.
__	13. Easily initiated or excessive crying or laughter.
__	14. Self-abusiveness, physical and/or verbal.
__	*Total score* (0–42)

Reference   Corrigan (1989)

Comment
A recently published scale for use with brain damaged patients who are aggressive, primarily in the context of post-injury confusion. It needs further evaluation.

Social Behaviour Schedule

Instructions
This schedule is administered to an informant about the patient's behaviour *over the preceding month*. The informant should consider both *severity* and *frequency* of abnormal behaviour, giving more weight to frequency if in doubt. For each behaviour the administrator and informant need to give a rating between 0 (normal) and 4 (most severe disturbance), with 3–4 being 'severe' and 2 'mild'.

Detailed guide-lines are available in original reference. The 23 areas are given here:

---

1. Communication: taking the initiative
2. Communication: incoherence
3. Conversation: oddity/inappropriateness
4. Social mixing: ability to make social contacts in an appropriate way
5. Social mixing: proportion of social contacts which are hostile in nature
6. Social mixing: attention-seeking behaviour
7. Suicidal and self-harming ideas and behaviour
8. Panic attacks and phobias
9. Overactivity and restlessness
10. Laughing and talking to self
11. Acting out of bizarre ideas (*only 0–2*)
12. Posturing and mannerisms
13. Socially unacceptable habits or manners
14. Destructive behaviour (*to property*)
15. Depression (*only 0–3*)
16. Inappropriate sexual behaviour
17. Personal appearance and hygiene
18. Slowness
19. Underactivity
20. Concentration (*only 0–2*)
21. Behaviours, not otherwise specified, that impede progress
22. Type of weekday occupation (*scored 0–5*)
23. Leisure: activities

References Wykes and Sturt (1986); Creed *et al.* (1990)

Comment

This schedule was designed to measure problem behaviours in chronic institutionalized patients. It has been used in a randomized trial of acute psychiatric treatment (day hospital vs. in-patient care). It is included here (in outline) to indicate (a) the range of behaviours it includes, and (b) a classification scheme. The original reference (Wykes and Sturt 1986) gives detailed guide-lines for assessing each behaviour. The schedule is reliable and it is an example of a psychiatric scale concentrating upon disability whereas most of the others concentrate upon impairment.

20   Multiple sclerosis

Summary

1. Kurtzke Multiple Sclerosis Rating Scales
     Functional Systems Scales
     Expanded Disability Status Scales
2. An illness-severity score for multiple sclerosis

Introduction

This chapter shows the Kurtzke Scales which are the only widely used and recognized instruments in multiple sclerosis research. They are impractical in clinical practice, and very insensitive to changes in disability. Their continued use cannot be recommended given the much better measures of disability now available.

Kurtzke Multiple Sclerosis Rating Scales

Functional Systems

A. *Pyramidal functions*
   - 0 = Normal
   - 1 = Abnormal signs without disability
   - 2 = Minimal disability
   - 3 = Mild or moderate paraparesis or hemiparesis, severe monoparesis
   - 4 = Marked paraparesis or hemiparesis; moderate quadraparesis; or monoplegia
   - 5 = Paraplegia, hemiplegia, or marked quadriparesis
   - 6 = Quadriplegia
   - V = Unknown

B. *Cerebellar functions*
   - 0 = Normal
   - 1 = Abnormal signs without disability
   - 2 = Mild ataxia
   - 3 = Moderate truncal or limb ataxia
   - 4 = Severe ataxia, all limbs
   - 5 = Unable to perform co-ordinated movements due to ataxia
   - V = Unknown
   - X = Used throughout after each number when weakness (Grade 3 or more on pyramidal) interferes with testing

C. *Brain-stem functions*
   0 = Normal
   1 = Signs only
   2 = Moderate nystagmus or other mild disability
   3 = Severe nystagmus, marked extraocular weakness or moderate disability of
        other cranial nerves
   4 = Marked dysarthria or other marked disability
   5 = Inability to swallow or speak
   V = Unknown

D. *Sensory functions* (1982 revision)
   0 = Normal
   1 = Vibration or figure-writing decrease only, in one or two limbs
   2 = Mild decrease in touch or pain or position sense, and/or moderate decrease
        in vibration in one or two limbs; or vibratory (c/s figure-writing) decrease
        alone in three or four limbs
   3 = Moderate decrease in touch or pain or position sense, and/or essentially lost
        vibration in one or two limbs; or mild decrease in touch or pain and/or
        moderate decrease in all proprioceptive tests in three or four limbs
   4 = Marked decrease in touch or pain or loss of proprioception, alone or
        combined, in one or two limbs; or moderate decrease in touch or pain
        and/or severe proprioceptive decrease in more than two limbs
   5 = Loss (essentially) of sensation in one or two limbs; or moderate decrease in
        touch or pain and/or loss of proprioception for most of body below the
        head
   6 = Sensation essentially lost below the head
   V = Unknown

E. *Bowel and bladder function* (1982 revision)
   0 = Normal
   1 = Mild urinary hesitancy, urgency, or retention
   2 = Moderate hesitancy, urgency, retention of bowel or bladder, or rare urinary
        incontinence
   3 = Frequent urinary incontinence
   4 = In need of almost constant catheterization
   5 = Loss of bladder function
   6 = Loss of bowel and bladder function
   V = Unknown

F. *Visual (or optic) functions*
   0 = Normal
   1 = Scotoma with visual acuity (corrected) better than 20/30
   2 = Worse eye with scotoma with maximal visual acuity (corrected) of 20/30
        to 20/59
   3 = Worse eye with large scotoma, or moderate decrease in fields, but with
        maximal visual acuity (corrected) of 20/60 to 20/99

4 = Worse eye with marked decrease of fields and maximal visual acuity (corrected) of 20/100 to 20/200; grade 3 plus maximal acuity of better eye of 20/60 or less

5 = Worse eye with maximal visual acuity (corrected) less than 20/200; grade 4 plus maximal acuity of better eye of 20/60 or less

6 = Grade 5 plus maximal visual acuity of better eye of 20/60 or less

V = Unknown

X = Added to grades 0–6 for presence of temporal pallor

G. *Cerebral (or mental) functions*

   0 = Normal

   1 = Mood alteration only (does not affect DSS score)

   2 = Mild decrease in mentation

   3 = Moderate decrease in mentation

   4 = Marked decrease in mentation (chronic brain syndrome moderate)

   5 = Dementia or chronic brain syndrome—severe or incompetent

   V = Unknown

Other functions

   0 = None

   1 = Any other neurologic finding attributed to MS (specify)

   V = Unknown

Kurtzke Multiple Sclerosis Scales

Expanded Disability Status Scale (EDSS)

---

0   Normal neurologic exam (all grade 0 in functional systems [FS]; Cerebral grade 1 acceptable).

1.0 No disability, minimal signs in one FS (i.e. grade 1 excluding Cerebral grade 1).

1.5 No disability, minimal signs in more than one FS (more than one grade 1 excluding Cerebral grade 1).

2.0 Minimal disability in one FS (one FS grade 2, others 0 or 1).

2.5 Minimal disability in two FS (two FS grade 2, others 0 or 1).

3.0 Moderate disability in one FS (one FS grade 3, others 0 or 1), or mild disability in three or four FS (three/four FS grade 2, others 0 or 1) though fully ambulatory.

3.5 Fully ambulatory but with moderate disability in one FS (one grade 3) and one or two FS grade 2; or two FS grade 3; or five FS grade 2 (others 0 or 1).

4.0 Fully ambulatory without aid, self sufficient, up and about some 12 hours a day despite relatively severe disability consisting of one FS grade 4 (others 0 or 1), or combinations of lesser grade exceeding limits of previous steps. Able to walk without aid or rest some 500 m.

4.5   Fully ambulatory without aid, up and about much of the day, able to work a full day, may otherwise have some limitation of full activity or require minimal assistance; characterized by relatively severe disability, usually consisting of one FS grade 4 (others 0 or 1) or combinations of lesser grades exceeding limits of previous steps. Able to walk without aid or rest for some 300 m.

5.0   Ambulatory without aid or rest for about 200 m; disability severe enough to impair full daily activities (for example, to work a full day without special provisions). (Usual FS equivalents are one grade 5 alone, others 0 or 1; or combinations of lesser grades usually exceeding specifications for step 4.0.)

5.5   Ambulatory without aid or rest for about 100 m; disability severe enough to preclude full daily activities. (Usual FS equivalents are one grade 5 alone, others 0 or 1; or combinations of lesser grades usually exceeding specifications for step 4.0.)

6.0   Intermittent or unilateral constant assistance (cane, crutch or brace) required to walk about 100 m with or without resting. (Usual FS equivalents are combinations with more than two FS grade 3 + .)

6.5   Constant bilateral assistance (canes, crutches or braces) required to walk about 20 m without resting. (Usual FS equivalents are combinations with more than two FS grade 3 + .)

7.0   Unable to walk beyond about 5 m even with aid, essentially restricted to wheelchair; wheels self in standard wheelchair and transfers alone; up and about in wheelchair some 12 hours a day. (Usual FS equivalents are combinations with more than one FS grade 4 + ; very rarely Pyramidal grade 5 alone.)

7.5   Unable to take more than a few steps; restricted to wheelchair; may need aid in transfer; wheels self but cannot carry on in a standard wheelchair for a full day; may require a motorized wheelchair. (Usual FS equivalents are combinations with more than one FS grade 4 + .)

8.0   Essentially restricted to bed or chair or perambulated in wheelchair but may be out of bed itself for much of the day; retains many self-care functions; generally has effective use of arms. (Usual FS equivalents are combinations, generally grade 4 + in several systems.)

8.5   Essentially restricted to bed much of the day; has some effective use of arm(s); retains some self-care functions. (Usual FS equivalents are combinations, generally 4 + in several systems.)

9.0   Helpless bed patient; can communicate and eat. (Usual FS equivalents are combinations, mostly grade 4 + .)

9.5   Totally helpless bed patient; unable to communicate effectively or eat/swallow. (Usual FS equivalents are combinations, almost all grade 4 + .)

10   Death due to MS.

References   Kurtzke (1955, 1965, 1981, 1983, 1989); Milligan *et al.* (1987); Willoughby and Paty (1988); Goodkin *et al.* (1988); Noseworthy *et al.* (1990)

Comment

Although of great historical importance, these two scales have little to commend their continued use. The Functional Systems concentrates upon impairments but includes reference to disability. The EDSS is a combination of a complicated way of converting a mixture of possible signs (the FS grades) into single numbers (the EDSS grades), together with a mobility scale. They cannot detect minor changes and it is almost certainly better to measure disability in trials of treatment (for example, Hauser *et al.* 1983) and to measure individual impairments as thought necessary. Reliability has been assessed recently (Noseworthy *et al.* 1990) and found to be reasonable —a two-step difference probably reflects a real difference.

An illness-severity score for multiple sclerosis

Mickey *et al.* (1984) devised a system of weights in order to derive an overall score for each patient, using the Kurtzke Functional Systems (KFS) and the Disability Status Scale (DSS) with additional information on activity and course.

(a) Activity is rated:
   1 = inactive; no increase in neurologic signs in preceding six months
   2 = active

(b) Course is rated:
   1 = relapsing type
   2 = relapsing and progressive
   3 = progressive only

Assigned rating	0	1	2	3	4	5	6	7	8	9
Activity (a)	0.0	1.4	2.4							
Course (b)	0.0	0.4	0.7	1.0						
KFS–A	0.0	1.1	1.8	2.6	3.4	4.2	5.4			
KFS–B	0.0	1.6	3.0	4.6	6.6	8.3				
KFS–C	0.0	0.9	1.5	2.0	2.8	3.6				
KFS–D	0.0	0.3	0.5	0.7	1.0	1.3				
KFS–E	0.0	0.2	0.4	0.5	0.6	0.8				
KFS–F	0.0	0.2	0.3	0.4	0.4	0.5	0.6			
KFS–G	0.0	0.2	0.4	0.6	0.7	0.8				
DSS	0.0	6.3	9.9	13.1	15.3	16.6	19.8	24.5	29.4	35.2

ISS score = 19.8 + sum of all weights

Reference   Mickey *et al.* (1984)

Comment

This scale demonstrates the relative unimportance of most of the Kurtzke scales, as only the motor sections (and disability scale) contribute significant weights. The scale is constructed to give a mean of 50 and a standard deviation of 10 with reference to the original population of 87 patients. Validity and reliability was investigated and found to be acceptable—the unreliability in rating the Kurtzke scales was probably lost given the low weight attached to most items.

21   Stroke scales

Summary

1. Mathew Stroke Scale
2. The National Institute of Health (NIH) Stroke Scale
3. Canadian Neurological Scale
4. Orgogozo Score
5. Hemispheric Stroke Scale
6. Clinical Classification of Stroke (Bamford)
7. Allen Score for prognosis after stroke
8. Guy's Hospital Score for haemorrhage

Introduction

This chapter shows eight measures which have been developed specifically for use with stroke patients. All concentrate upon impairment, and all (except the last) almost certainly 'measure' the severity of the stroke.

Two indices use clinical features to make a more detailed pathological diagnosis either of stroke site (Clinical Classification) or of stroke type (Guy's Hospital Score). The clinical classification is probably useful and relates to prognosis.

In practice, it is rarely necessary to use these measures because other data will give equivalent information more efficiently. A CT scan will diagnose stroke type more accurately. Single items such as urinary incontinence, severity of motor loss and level of consciousness may be sufficiently accurate in many circumstances.

If a scale is required, the NIH scale, the Canadian Neurological Scale, or the Hemispheric Stroke Scale should be used. The Mathew Scale has little to recommend it despite its frequent and continuing use, and indeed it should be avoided given the much better measures now available.

Mathew Stroke Scale

Mentation

___ Level of consciousness
    8 = Fully conscious
    6 = Lethargic but mentally intact
    4 = Obtunded
    2 = Stuperous
    0 = Comatose

___ Orientation (time, place, person)
    6 = Oriented × 3
    4 = Oriented × 2
    2 = Oriented × 1
    0 = Disoriented

Speech

___ 0–23, according to Reitan test

Cranial nerves

___ Homonymous hemianopsia
    3 = Intact
    2 = Mild
    1 = Moderate
    0 = Severe

___ Conjugate deviation of eyes
    3 = Intact
    2 = Mild
    1 = Moderate
    0 = Severe

___ Facial weakness
    3 = Intact
    2 = Mild
    1 = Moderate
    0 = Severe

Motor power

___ Right arm

___ Right leg

___ Left arm

___ Left leg
    5 = Normal strength
    4 = Contracts against resistance
    3 = Elevates against gravity

2 = Gravity eliminated
1 = Flicker
0 = No movements

Performance, or disability status scale

__ Score
28 = Normal
21 = Mild impairment
14 = Moderate impairment
 7 = Severe impairment
 0 = Death

Reflexes

__ Score
3 = Normal
2 = Asymmetrical or pathological reflexes
1 = Clonus
0 = No reflexes elicited

Sensation

__ Score
3 = Normal
2 = Mild sensory abnormality
1 = Severe sensory abnormality
0 = No response to pain

Reference   Mathew *et al.* (1972)

Comment
A widely used scale in stroke treatment studies, but it has nothing to commend it, and should be abandoned. It is invalid, combining many impairments and disabilities; reliability has never been demonstrated; the weighting is not logical and is dominated by level of consciousness (see Capildeo and Rose 1979). Much better measures now exist.

The National Institute of Health (NIH) Stroke Scale (Brott *et al.* 1989)

__ *Level of consciousness*
0 = Alert, keenly responsive
1 = Drowsy, but rousable by minor stimulation to obey, answer, or respond
2 = Stuporous, requires repeated stimulation to attend, or lethargic or obtunded, requiring strong or painful stimulation to make movements
3 = Coma, responds only with reflex motor or autonomic effects, or unresponsive

___ *Level of consciousness—questions*
Ask patient the month and his/her age. Score first answer.
    0 = Answers both correctly
    1 = Answers one correctly
    2 = Incorrect

___ *Level of consciousness—commands*
Ask patient to open/close hand and eyes. Score if he or she makes unequivocal attempt.
    0 = Obeys both correctly
    1 = Obeys one correctly
    2 = Incorrect

___ *Pupillary response*
    0 = Both reactive
    1 = One reactive
    2 = Neither reactive

___ *Best gaze*
    0 = Normal
    1 = Partial gaze palsy; abnormal but not forced deviation
    2 = Forced deviation/total gaze paresis

___ *Best visual*
Confrontation testing using finger movements, including double simultaneous stimulation. Use visual threat if consciousness or comprehension limit testing, scoring '1' for any asymmetry demonstrated.
    0 = No visual loss
    1 = Partial hemianopia
    2 = Complete hemianopia, to within 5 degrees of fixation

___ *Facial palsy*
    0 = Normal
    1 = Minor
    2 = Partial
    3 = Complete

___ *Best motor—arm*
Arms held for 10 sec at 90 degrees if sitting, 45 degrees if lying. Grade weaker arm. Place arms in position if comprehension reduced.
    0 = No drift in 10 sec
    1 = Drift, after brief hold
    2 = Cannot resist gravity, falling immediately but some effort made
    3 = No effort against gravity

__ *Best motor—leg*
While lying, patient to hold weaker leg raised 30 degrees for 5 sec. Place leg if comprehension reduced.
   0 = No drift in 5 sec
   1 = Drift, lowering within 5 sec
   2 = Cannot resist gravity, falling to bed but some effort made
   3 = No effort against gravity

__ *Plantar reflex*
   0 = Normal
   1 = Equivocal
   2 = One extensor
   3 = Bilateral extensor

__ *Limb ataxia*
Finger-nose and heel-to-shin tests performed; ataxia is scored only if out of proportion to weakness. If total paralysis, score as absent.
   0 = Absent
   1 = Present in arm or leg
   2 = Present in arm and leg

__ *Sensory*
Tested with pin; only hemisensory loss scored. If comprehension or consciousness reduced, only score if obvious evidence.
   0 = Normal
   1 = Partial loss, subjectively different but still felt
   2 = Dense loss, unaware of being touched

__ *Neglect*
   0 = No neglect
   1 = Partial neglect, visual, tactile or auditory
   2 = Complete neglect, affecting more than one modality

__ *Dysarthria*
   0 = Normal articulation
   1 = Mild to moderate dysarthria, slurring some words
   2 = Near unintelligible or worse

__ *Best language*
Assessed from responses during evaluation.
   0 = No aphasia
   1 = Mild to moderate aphasia; naming errors, paraphrasias, etc.
   2 = Severe aphasia
   3 = Mute

References   Brott *et al.* (1989); Goldstein *et al.* (1989)

Comment
Validity and reliability have been studied but this scale suffers from the
disadvantage of trying to summarise all impairments of stroke into one
scale. It is simple and short, taking from five to eight minutes to complete.

Canadian Neurological Scale

Mentation

— Level of consciousness
3.0 Alert
1.5 Drowsy

— Orientation
1.0 Oriented
0.0 Disoriented, or not applicable

— Speech
1.0 Normal
0.5 Expressive deficit
0.0 Receptive deficit

Motor function: weakness (no comprehension deficit)

— Face
0.5 None
0.0 Present

— Arm, proximal
1.5 None
1.0 Mild
0.5 Significant
0.0 Total

— Arm, distal
1.5 None
1.0 Mild
0.5 Significant
0.0 Total

— Leg, proximal
1.5 None
1.0 Mild
0.5 Significant
0.0 Total

— Leg, distal
1.5 None
1.0 Mild
0.5 Significant
0.0 Total

Motor response (comprehension deficit)

— Face
0.5 Symmetrical
0.0 Asymmetrical

— Arms
1.5 Equal
0.0 Unequal

— Legs
1.5 Equal
0.0 Unequal

References Cote *et al.* (1988, 1989)

Comment
A valid, reliable, quick (five minute) assessment which can be used by doctors, nurses or therapists. It mainly measures cognition and motor response. It should be compared with the Glasgow Coma Scale and the Motricity Index.

Orgogozo Score

— Consciousness
15 = Normal; awake and responsive to stimuli
10 = Drowsiness; can be woken to remain awake through examination
5 = Stupor; localizes and responds to painful stimuli
0 = Coma; non-purposeful response to painful stimuli

— Verbal communication
10 = Normal/not restricted; can sustain informative conversation
5 = Difficult; limited to essential ideas, dysarthria included
0 = Extremely difficult/impossible; for any reason

— Eyes and headshift
10 = Normal symmetrical horizontal eye movements
5 = Gaze failure/unilateral neglect; gaze restricted on one side
0 = Forced/tonic deviation; unable to gaze beyond midline

— Facial movements
5 = Normal/slight weakness; only minimal asymmetry at most
0 = Paralysis, or marked paresis

— Arm raising

    10 = Possible; can raise above horizontal against some resistance

    5 = Incomplete; only against gravity, not horizontally

    0 = Impossible; arm abduction impossible

— Hand movements

    15 = Normal; no disability

    10 = Skilled; restriction of fine movements, slow/clumsy use

    5 = Useful; gross movements possible, can hold a walking stick

    0 = Useless; cannot hold or carry objects even if moves

— Arm tone

    5 = Normal/near normal

    0 = Overt spasticity or flaccidity

— Leg raising

    15 = Normal; can be elevated from bed almost as other side

    10 = Possible against resistance; can be elevated, but weak

    5 = Possible against gravity; not against resistance

    0 = Impossible; cannot be lifted off bed

— Foot dorsiflexion

    10 = Possible against resistance; even if weaker than normal

    5 = Possible against gravity; can raise tip of foot off floor

    0 = Foot drop; active dorsiflexion impossible

— Leg tone

    5 = Normal/near normal

    0 = Overt spasticity or flaccidity

— *Total* (out of 100)

Reference   Orgogozo (1989)

Comment

One of many stroke scales concentrating upon impairment. Validity not formally established but contains the same items as other (valid) scales. Reliability has been tested and it is simple, with a score which is easily understood. Some items (for example, verbal communication) measure function (i.e. ability to communicate).

Hemispheric Stroke Scale

Scored to give 0 (= good) to 100 (= bad).

Level of consciousness
___   15 – Glasgow Coma Scale score

Language
___   Comprehension

Give three commands:
'Stick out your tongue' *or* 'Close your eyes'
'Point to the door'
'Place left/right hand on left/right ear and then on left/right knee' (using unaffected side)

Score on number correctly followed:
0 = 5
1 = 4
2 = 2
3 = 0

___   Naming

Ask patient to name the following items:
Watch *or* Belt
Watch strap *or* Belt buckle
Index finger *or* Ring finger

Score on number correctly named:
0 = 5
1 = 4
2 = 3
3 = 0

___   Repetition

Ask the patient to repeat the following:
A single word, such as 'dog' or 'cat'
'The president lives in Washington'
'No ifs, ands, or buts'

Score on number repeated:
0 = 5
1 = 4
2 = 2
3 = 0

___ Fluency

Score according to patient's spontaneous speech fluency, *or*
Ask patient to name as many words as he can within one minute beginning with the letter 'A' (excluding proper names).

Score as:
5 = Essentially no verbal output
3 = Moderately severe decrease in fluency (*or* 1–4 words)
1 = Mild decrease in fluency (*or* 5–10 words)
0 = Normal fluency (*or* 11 + words)

Other cortical functions, and cranial nerves

___ Visual fields

Test clinically and score hemi-field loss as:
3 = Severe loss: inability to recognize moving hand, no response to threat
2 = Moderate loss: inability to recognize stationary finger, sees moving finger
1 = Mild loss: defect to double simultaneous stimulation
0 = Normal

___ Gaze

Score eye movements:
2 = Gaze palsy, or persistent deviation
1 = Gaze preference, or difficulty with far lateral gaze
0 = Normal

___ Facial expression

Score movement:
3 = Severe weakness; drooling
2 = Moderate loss; asymmetry at rest
1 = Mild weakness; asymmetry on smiling
0 = Normal

___ Dysarthria

Score talking:
2 = Severe dysarthria
1 = Moderate dysarthria
0 = Normal

___ Dysphagia

Score swallow of glass water:
2 = Severe dysphagia
1 = Moderate dysphagia
0 = Normal

— Neglect syndrome

Ask about weak limbs, *and* ask to bisect a line 7 inches (20 cm) long on piece of paper in visual midline. Score:
   2 = Anosagnosia, or denial of body part
   1 = Consistently bisects line towards 'good' side of body
   0 = Bisects line in middle

— Visual construction

Ask patient to copy three figures given, and score:
   3 = Unable to copy any figure
   2 = Can copy a square
   1 = Can copy a 'Greek Cross' ('Cross of St. George')
   0 = Can copy 3D drawing of a cube

Motor function

— Arm, proximal

— Arm, distal

— Leg, proximal

— Leg, distal

All scored 0–7 as:
   7 = No movement (MRC 0)
   6 = Trace movement only (MRC 1)
   5 = Motion without gravity only (MRC 2)
   4 = Moves against gravity but not against resistance (MRC 3)
   3 = Moderate weakness (MRC 4 −)
   2 = Mild weakness (MRC 4)
   1 = Positive drift of arm/leg (MRC 4 +)
   0 = Normal (MRC 5)

— Deep tendon reflexes:

   2 = Hypoactive *or* hyperactive
   0 = Normal

— Pathologic reflexes

   2 = Babinski (plantar) *and* another abnormal
   1 = Babinski (plantar) *or* another abnormal
   0 = Normal

— Muscle tone

   2 = Increased *or* decreased
   0 = Normal

— Gait

Test ability to stand and walk, and score:
  6 = Unable to stand unsupported *or* cannot evaluate
  5 = Can stand with support but cannot walk
  4 = Severely abnormal; walking distance limited even with support (from aid or person)
  3 = Moderately abnormal; no assistance required (apart from a stick/cane), but distance limited
  2 = Mildly abnormal (weak, uncoordinated); can walk independently but slowly
  1 = Minimally abnormal, no reduction in speed or distance
  0 = Normal

Sensory

— Primary modalities (of affected side only), arm

— Primary modalities (of affected side only), leg

Test touch, pain and score as:
  4 = Anaesthesia
  3 = Severe hypaesthesia
  2 = Moderate hypaesthesia or deficit only; *or* extinction to double simultaneous stimulation
  1 = Mild hypaesthesia or dysaesthesia
  0 = Normal

— Stereoagnosis

Test ability to distinguish two coins and a key, and score:
  3 = Unable to achieve any distinctions
  2 = Can distinguish a coin from a key
  1 = Can distinguish between two very different sized coins (penny and ten-pence piece, penny and quarter)
  0 = Can distinguish between two similar sized coins (penny and nickel, or two-pence piece and ten-pence piece)

Reference Adams *et al.* (1987)

Comment

Another stroke scale, mixing many impairments with a few disabilities. Its validity has been tested against the Barthel Index and its reliability has been tested but it has no specific virtues.

Clinical Classification of Stroke (Bamford)

Total Anterior Circulation Syndrome (TACS)
Features:
• Unilateral motor deficit of face, arm and leg
• Homonymous hemianopia
• Higher cerebral dysfunction (for example, aphasia, neglect)

Partial Anterior Circulation Syndrome (PACS)
Features:
any *two* of:
• Unilateral motor and/or sensory deficit
• Ipsilateral hemianopia, *or* higher cerebral dysfunction
• Higher cerebral dysfunction alone, *or* isolated motor and/or sensory deficit restricted to one limb or the face

Posterior Circulation Syndromes (POCS)
Features:
One or more of:
• Bilateral motor or sensory signs not secondary to brain-stem compression by a large supra-tentorial lesion
• Cerebellar signs, unless accompanied by ipsilateral motor deficit (see ataxic hemiparesis)
• Unequivocal diplopia with or without external ocular muscle palsy.
• Crossed signs, for example, left facial and right limb weakness
• Hemianopia, alone or with any of four items above.

Lacunar Syndromes (LACS)

Pure Motor Stroke (PMS)
  • Unilateral, pure motor deficit
  • Clearly involving two of three areas (face, arm, leg)
  • With the whole of any limb being involved

Pure Sensory Stroke (PSS)
  • Unilateral purely sensory symptoms (+ / − signs)
  • Involving at least two of three areas (face, arm, leg)
  • With the whole of any limb being involved

Ataxic Hemiparesis (AH)
  • Ipsilateral cerebellar and cortico-spinal tract signs
  • With or without dysarthria
  • In the absence of higher cerebral dysfunction or a visual field defect

Sensory-motor Stroke (SMS)
  • PMS and PSS combined (i.e. unilateral motor and sensory signs and symptoms)
  • In the absence of higher cerebral dysfunction or a visual field defect

---

Reference   Bamford (1988)

Comment

A reliable clinical classification, validated against CTscan and also of considerable prognostic value, both in terms of morbidity and mortality.

Allen Score for prognosis after stroke

Features to be recorded
- Age in years
- Loss of consciousness at onset of stroke
- Drowsy or comatose 24 hours after onset (or later)
- Complete limb paralysis
  No movement better than palpable contraction (MRC 1)
- Higher Cerebral Dysfunction (HCD)
  Aphasia, and/or
  Parietal deficit:
  - sensory or visual inattention, *or*
  - visuospatial neglect *or*
  - loss of joint position sense
- Homonymous visual field deficit to confrontation (HHA)

Calculating score

Constant	$+40$
Complete limb paralysis	-12
HCD with HHA and hemiplegia	-11
Drowsy/comatose at 24 hours	-10
Age in years * 0.4	$-(\text{age} \times 0.4)$
Initial loss of consciousness	-9
Uncomplicated hemiparesis	$+8$
Total	_____

Interpretation of score
  Score <0 means: likely to die, or be left severely disabled
  Score >0 means: likely to survive and walk

Reference   Allen (1984)

Comment

The features essentially correlate with the volume of brain lost, as can be seen through their similarity to the features which distinguish total from partial anterior cerebral circulation infarcts.

Guy's Hospital Score for haemorrhage

Variable	Clinical feature		Score
Apoplectic onset • Loss of consciousness	One or none of these	=	0
• Headache within 2 hours • Vomiting • Neck stiffness	Two or more	=	+ 21.9
Level of consciousness (24 hours after onset)	Alert	=	0
	Drowsy	=	+ 7.3
	Unconscious	=	+ 14.6
Plantar responses	Both flexor/single extensor	=	0
	Both extensor	=	+ 7.1
Diastolic blood pressure (24 hours post-onset)	BP in mm of mercury	=	+ (BP*0.17)
Atheroma markers	None	=	0
• angina, claudication, history of diabetes	One or more	=	− 3.7
History of hypertension	Not present	=	0
	Present	=	− 4.1
Previous event (stroke or TIA)	None	=	0
	Any number	=	− 6.7
Heart disease	None	=	0
	Aortic/mitral murmur	=	− 4.4
	Cardiac failure	=	− 4.3
	Cardiomyopathy	=	− 4.3
	Atrial fibrillation	=	− 4.3
	Cardiomegaly (chest X-ray)	=	− 4.3
	Myocardial infarct within 6 months	=	− 4.3
	Constant	=	−12.6
	Total	=	_____

Interpretation of score:
−30 to 0 = 95 per cent probability of being infarct
25 to 50 = 95 per cent probability of being haemorrhage
See original paper for a more accurate graph

References   Allen (1983); Sandercock *et al.* (1985)

Comment
This clinical score was developed on one population and has been tested on a second sample. The clinical distinction, though reasonably accurate, is insufficiently reliable for making clinical decisions, for example about anticoagulation. (The most accurate method is to assume that every stroke is an infarct—this will be correct for 89 cases in every hundred.)

22 Head injury

Summary

1. Galveston Orientation and Amnesia Test (GOAT)
2. Rappaport Disability Rating Scale
3. Glasgow Assessment Schedule
4. Neurobehavioural Rating Scale

Introduction

This chapter shows four measures specifically related to head injury but other measures shown elsewhere, particularly the Glasgow Coma Scale and the Glasgow Outcome Scale are also important in head injury research. The GOAT is designed to assess when post-traumatic amnesia ends, whereas the other three are measures of disability and perhaps handicap.

The Galveston Orientation and Amnesia Test

Instructions
Can be administered daily. Score of 78 or more on three consecutive occasions is considered to indicate that patient is out of post-traumatic amnesia (PTA).

Question	Error score	Notes
What is your name?	−2 __	Must give both first name and surname
When were you born?	−4 __	Must give day, month, and year
Where do you live?	−4 __	Town sufficient
Where are you now?		
(a) City	−5 __	Must give actual town
(b) Building	−5 __	Usually in hospital or rehabilitation centre. Actual name unnecessary
When were you admitted to this hospital?	−5 __	Date
How did you get here?	−5 __	Mode of transport

Question	Error score	Notes
What is the first event you can remember after the injury?	−5 __	Any plausible event is sufficient (record answer)
Can you give some detail?	−5 __	Must give relevant detail
Can you describe the last event you can recall before the accident?	−5 __	Any plausible event is sufficient (record answer)
Can you give some detail?	−5 __	Any relevant detail
What time is it now?	−5 __	−1 for each half-hour error
What day of the week is it?	−3 __	−1 for each day error
What day of the month is it? (i.e. the date)	−5 __	−1 for each day error
What is the month?	−15 __	−5 for each month error
What is the year?	−3 __	−10 for each year error

Total error = __

Total actual score = 100 − total error = 100 − __ = __

Reference   Levin *et al.* (1979)

Comment

Designed to determine when head injured patients emerge from PTA: a score of 78 or more for three consecutive days signals the end of PTA. It has been validated against the Glasgow Coma Scale, CT-brain scans, and the Glasgow Outcome Scale. Reliability has also been established but it is too long for routine use in British hospital wards and it is impractical when PTA extends for many months.

Rappaport Disability Rating Scale

Score	Item	Categories
		Arousability/awareness/responsivity
____	*Eye opening*	0 = Spontaneous 1 = To speech 2 = To pain 3 = None

	Best verbal response	0 = Oriented
		1 = Confused
		2 = Inappropriate
		3 = Incomprehensible
		4 = None

	Best motor response	0 = Obeying commands
		1 = Localizes pain
		2 = Withdraws from pain
		3 = Flexes to pain
		4 = Extends to pain
		5 = None

Cognitive ability to undertake following activities
(Note: physical ability is not required/tested)

	Feeding	0 = Completely knows how to and when
	Toileting	1 = Partially knows how to and when
	Grooming	2 = Minimally knows how to and when
		3 = No cognitive ability to achieve tasks

Dependence upon others
(Note: this does take account of need for physical help)

	Level of functioning	0 = Completely independent
		1 = Independent in special environment
		2 = Mildly dependent
		3 = Moderately dependent
		4 = Markedly dependent
		5 = Totally dependent

Psycho-social adaptability

	'Employability'	0 = Not restricted
		1 = Selected jobs; competitive
		2 = Sheltered workshop; non-competitive
		3 = Not employable

	Total (out of 30)	

Rappaport: guidelines

Cognitive ability
Needs to show awareness of where and how to perform activity, ignoring motor impairments.

Complete. Patient shows continuous awareness that he knows how to feed, toilet or groom him or herself and can convey unambiguous information that he or she knows when this activity should occur.

Partial. Patient intermittently shows awareness and intermittently conveys reasonable clear information that he or she knows when the activity should occur.

Minimal. Patient shows questionable or infrequent awareness that he or she knows in a primitive way how to do the activity and shows infrequently by certain signs, sounds or activities that he or she is vaguely aware when the activity should occur.

Level of functioning

Completely independent. Patient is able to live as he or she wishes with no restrictions.

Independent in special environment. Patient can function independently when needed requirements (mechanical aids) are met.

Mildly dependent. Needs limited assistance; non-resident helper.

Moderately dependent. Needs moderate assistance; person in home.

Markedly dependent. Needs assistance with all major activities at all times.

Totally dependent. Requires 24-hour nursing care.

Employability
This considers overall cognitive and physical ability to be an employee, homemaker or student. The determination considers the patient's ability:
• to understand, remember and follow instructions
• to plan and carry out simple tasks and assignments
• to remain oriented, relevant and appropriate in work situations
• to get to and from work and shopping effectively
• to deal with number concepts
• to handle simple money exchange problems
• to meet schedules and keep appointments

Selected jobs, competitive. Can compete in a limited job market for a relatively narrow range of jobs; can assume many but not all responsibilities associated with home-making; or can carry out many but not all school assignments.

Sheltered workshop, non-competitive. Cannot compete successfully in any job market because of moderate or severe cognitive and/or physical limitations and cannot do home-making or school work without major assistance.

References   Rappaport *et al*. (1982); Gouvier *et al*. (1987)

Comment
A valiant and possibly valid attempt to monitor patients with head injury from the incident to final status. Reliability has been established and the DRS has been compared with other scales. It mixes impairments and handicaps, which reduces validity, but might be useful in large, multicentre studies.

Glasgow Assessment Schedule

Area assessed Component item	Scoring system	Score
Personality change		
(Ask patient, obtain corroboration from relatives)		
Emotional lability	N, M, S	____
Irritability	N, M, S	____
Aggressiveness	N, M, S	____
Any other behavioural change	N, M, S	____
Subjective complaints		
(Ask patient, obtain corroboration from relatives)		
Sleep disturbance	N, M, S	____
Incontinence	N, M, S	____
Family stress	N, M, S	____
Financial problems	N, M, S	____
Sexual problems	N, M, S	____
Alcohol, excess drinking or poor tolerance	N, M, S	____
Reduced leisure and sporting activities	N, M, S	____
Headache	N, M, S	____
Dizziness, loss of balance	N, M, S	____
Paraesthesiae	N, M, S	____
Reduced sense of smell	N, M, S	____
Reduced hearing	N, M, S	____
Reduced vision	N, M, S	____
Occupational functioning		
At work—same job or similar job	0	
At work—less skilled job	1	
Not at work—employable	2	
Not at work—unemployable	3	____

Area assessed	Scoring	Score
Component item	system	

Cognitive functioning
Immediate recall:
  name, address, telephone number — N, M, S ——
Two-minute recall:
  name, address, telephone number — N, M, S ——
Attention and concentration:
  serial 7s subtracted from 100, *or*
  serial 3s subtracted from 20 — N, M, S ——
Orientation:
  time, place and person — N, M, S ——
Current intelligence status:
  simple arithmetic and general knowledge — N, M, S ——

Physical examination
Dysphasia (aphasia) — N, M, S ——
Dysarthria — N, M, S ——
Abnormal muscle tone:
  right leg — N, M, S ——
  left leg — N, M, S ——
  arms — N, M, S ——
Walking — N, M, S ——
Cranial nerve deficits — N, M, S ——
Seizures — N, M, S ——

Activities of daily living
Cooking — O, W, U ——
Other domestic tasks — O, W, U ——
Shopping — O, W, U ——
Travelling — O, W, U ——
Personal hygiene — O, W, U ——
Feeding — O, W, U ——
Dressing — O, W, U ——
Mobility — O, W, U ——

Scoring systems
All items are scored on a three-point scale:
  0 = Not present or only mildly present
  1 = Moderately severe
  2 = Severe

A. N, M, S =   B. O, W, U =
   Normal   On own
   Moderately severe   With help
   Severe   Unable to manage

Reference   Livingstone and Livingstone (1985)

Comment
Designed as a brief, disability problem orientated scale, this has been tested for reliability and also used in one published study. However, the component parts could be assessed using other scales, and it mixes impairments and disabilities.

Neurobehavioural Rating Scale

Item Description	Score
Inattention/reduced alertness Fails to sustain attention, easily distracted, fails to notice aspects of environment, difficulty directing attention, decreased alertness	____
Somatic concern Volunteers complaints or elaborates about somatic symptoms (for example, headache, dizziness, blurred vision), and about physical health in general	____
Disorientation Confusion, or lack of proper association for person, place or time	____
Anxiety Worry, fear, overconcern for present or future	____
Expressive deficit Word-finding disturbance, anomia, pauses in speech, effortful and agrammatic speech, circumlocution	____
Emotional withdrawal Lack of spontaneous interaction, isolation, deficiency in relating to others	____
Conceptual disorganization Thought processes confused, disconnected, disorganized, disrupted, tangential social communication, perseverative	____
Disinhibition Socially inappropriate comments and/or actions, including aggressive/sexual content, or inappropriate to the situation, outbursts of temper	____

Item Description	Score

Guilt feelings
Self-blame, shame, remorse for past behaviour   ——

Memory deficit
Difficulty learning new information, rapidly forgets recent events,
although immediate recall (forward digit span) may be intact   ——

Agitation
Motor manifestations of overactivation (for example, kicking, arm
flailing, picking, roaming, restlessness, talkativeness)   ——

Inaccurate insight and self-appraisal
Poor insight, exaggerated self-opinion, overrates level of ability and
underrates personality change in comparison with evaluation by
clinicians and family   ——

Depressive mood
Sorrow, sadness, despondency, pessimism   ——

Hostility/uncooperativeness
Animosity, irritability, belligerence, disdain for others, defiance of
authority   ——

Decreased initiative/motivation
Lacks normal initiative in work or leisure, fails to persist in tasks, is
reluctant to accept new challenges   ——

Suspiciousness
Mistrust, belief that others harbour malicious or discriminatory intent ——

Fatiguability
Rapidly fatigues on challenging cognitive tasks or complex activities,
lethargic   ——

Hallucinatory behaviour
Perceptions without normal external stimulus correspondence   ——

Motor retardation
Slowed movements or speech (excluding primary weakness)   ——

Unusual thought content
Unusual, odd, strange, bizarre thought content   ——

Blunted affect
Reduced emotional tone, reduction in normal intensity of feelings,
flatness   ——

Excitement
Heightened emotional tone, increased reactivity   ——

Poor planning ___
Unrealistic goals, poorly formulated plans for the future, disregards prerequisites (for example, training), fails to take disability into account

Lability of mood ___
Sudden change in mood which is disproportionate to the situation

Tension ___
Postural and facial expression of heightened tension, without the necessity of excessive activity involving the limbs or trunk

Comprehension deficit ___
Difficulty in understanding oral instructions on single or multistage commands

Speech articulation defect ___
Misarticulation, slurring or substitution of sounds which affect intelligibility (rating is independent of linguistic content)

Reference   Levin *et al.* (1987)

Comment
This scale assesses the behavioural consequences of cognitive impairments and impairment of social control mechanisms. It covers areas of importance in the long-term after head injury. Validity and reliability need to be established and clinical utility needs to be confirmed. Further work by other centres using this scale is needed. However, there is no real competition so this scale should be considered.

23 Parkinson's disease and other movement disorders

Summary

1. Columbian Rating Scale
2. Parkinson's disease: impairment index (McDowell *et al*.)
3. Parkinson's disease: disability index (McDowell *et al*.)
4. Parkinson's disease: Lieberman's index
5. Hoehn and Yahr Grades
6. Northwestern University Disability Scales
7. Self-assessment Parkinson's Disease Disability Scale
8. Webster Rating Scale
9. New York Rating Scale
10. Unified Parkinson's Disease Rating Scale (Version 3.0)
    I Mentation, behaviour, and mood
    II Activities of daily living
    III Motor examination
    IV Complications of therapy (in the past week):
        Dyskinesia
        Clinical fluctuations
        Other
    V Modified Hoehn and Yahr staging
    VI Schwab and England Activities of Daily Living Scale
11. Tourette's Syndrome Global Scale
12. Fahn–Marsden Scale for Primary Torsion Dystonias
13. Abnormal Involuntary Movement Scale (AIMS)

Introduction

There are many measures for use with patients with Parkinson's disease, perhaps because the evolution of specific treatments stimulated their development. Most of them cover the same impairments and disabilities. The Unified Parkinson's disease Rating Scale shown here is now probably the only scale to use in large research studies but it is far too long and complicated for routine use. It could be improved and shortened. More detailed information and reviews are available (Marsden and Schacheter 1981; Fahn 1989; Lang and Fahn 1989), and comparative studies have been carried out (Diamond and Markham 1983).

Measures have been devised for other movement disorders and a few are reproduced here. Not shown are measures for Huntington's chorea (Folstein *et al*. 1983) or measures dependent upon videotape for use with Gilles de la Tourette's syndrome (Goetz *et al*. 1987).

In routine clinical practice for all these conditions, simple measures are probably sufficient, such as the Barthel ADL Index, gait speed, and the Nine-hole Peg Test for physical disabilities and the Short Orientation-Memory-Concentration Test and an extended ADL test for the assessment of cognitive dysfunction. If any of these measures are used, the McDowell Impairment Index and the Self-assessment Disability Scale could both be useful.

Columbian Rating Scale

Tremor

Arm (score right and left)
  0 = Absent
  1 = Slight, and infrequently present
  2 = Moderate in amplitude, but only intermittently present
  3 = Moderate and present most of the time
  4 = Marked in amplitude and present most of the time

Head
  0 = Absent
  1 = Slight, and infrequently present
  2 = Moderate in amplitude, but only intermittently present
  3 = Moderate and present most of the time
  4 = Marked in amplitude and present most of the time

Leg (score right and left)
  0 = Absent
  1 = Slight, and infrequently present
  2 = Moderate in amplitude, but only intermittently present
  3 = Moderate and present most of the time
  4 = Marked in amplitude and present most of the time

_____ /20   Total tremor score

Rigidity
Judged on passive movement of major joints with patient relaxed in sitting position, cogwheeling to be ignored.

Arm (score right and left separately)
  0 = Absent
  1 = Slight or detectable only when activated by mirror or other movements
  2 = Mild to moderate
  3 = Marked, but full range of motion easily achieved
  4 = Severe, range of motion achieved with difficulty

Neck
   0 = Absent
   1 = Slight or detectable only when activated by minor or other movements
   2 = Mild to moderate
   3 = Marked, but full range of motion easily achieved
   4 = Severe, range of motion achieved with difficulty

Leg (score right and left separately)
   0 = Absent
   1 = Slight or detectable only when activated by minor or other movements
   2 = Mild to moderate
   3 = Marked, but full range of motion easily achieved
   4 = Severe, range of motion achieved with difficulty

____ /20   Total rigidity score

Bradykinesia
Five separate items, to be evaluated with the patient performing as naturally as possible without coaxing or special encouragement.

Bradykinesia
(combining both slowness and poverty of movement in general)
   0 = None
   1 = Minimal slowness giving movement a deliberate character, could be normal for some persons
   2 = Mild degree of slowness and poverty of movement which is definitely abnormal
   3 = Moderate slowness with occasional hesitation on initiating movement and arrests of ongoing movement
   4 = Marked slowness and poverty of movement, with frequent freezing and long delays in initiating movement

Gait disturbance
   0 = Freely ambulatory, good stepping, turns regularly
   1 = Walks slowly, may shuffle with short steps but no festination or propulsion
   2 = Walks with great difficulty, great festination, short steps, freezing and pulsion but requires little or no assistance
   3 = Severe disturbance of gait requiring frequent assistance
   4 = Cannot walk at all even with help

Posture
   0 = Normal erect
   1 = Not quite erect, slightly stooped posture, could be normal for older persons
   2 = Moderate simian posture, definitely abnormal
   3 = Marked simian posture with kyphosis
   4 = Severe flexion with extreme abnormality of posture

Postural stability
If Romberg Test is normal, judge response to posterior displacement produced by push on sternum

0 = Normal
1 = Retropulsion but recovers unaided
2 = Absence of postural response, would fall if not caught by examiner
3 = Very unstable, tends to fall spontaneously on the Romberg Test
4 = Unable to stand without assistance

Arising from chair (straightback wooden or metal chair)

0 = Normal
1 = Slow
2 = Pushes self up from arms of seat
3 = Tends to fall back and may have to try several times but can get up without help
4 = Unable to arise without help

_____ /20   Total bradykinesia score

Functional performance
Finger dexterity
Patient taps thumb with forefinger, then with each finger in rapid succession

0 = Normal
1 = Slightly slow
2 = Slow
3 = Markedly slow
4 = Unable

Succession movements
Patient taps knees alternately with palm and dorsum of hands

0 = Normal
1 = Slightly slow
2 = Slow
3 = Markedly slow
4 = Unable

Foot tapping
Putting heel at floor, patient taps floor with ball of foot as rapidly as possible

0 = Normal
1 = Slightly slow
2 = Slow
3 = Markedly slow
4 = Unable

Facial expression
 0 = Normal
 1 = Minimal hypomimia, could be normal 'poker face'
 2 = Slight but definitely abnormal diminution of facial expression
 3 = Moderate hypomimia
 4 = Masked or fixed facies with severe or complete loss of facial expression

Seborrhea
 0 = Normal
 1 = Greasy forehead, no dermatitis
 2 = Mild dermatitis, erythema, and scaling
 3 = Moderate dermatitis
 4 = Severe dermatitis

Sialorrhea
 0 = None
 1 = Slight but definite excess of saliva in pharynx, patient may be unaware thereof,
     no drooling
 2 = Moderately excessive saliva with minimal drooling if any
 3 = Marked excess of saliva with some drooling
 4 = Marked drooling, requires special measures

Speech disorder
 0 = None
 1 = Slight loss of expression, diction, and/or volume
 2 = Monotone, slurred but understandable
 3 = Marked impairment, difficult to understand
 4 = Unintelligible

____ /24   Functional performance score

References   Yahr *et al.* (1969); Lang and Fahn (1989)

Comment
One of several widely used scales for Parkinson's disease, it focuses mainly
on impairments (despite the title of the last section).

Parkinson's disease: impairment index (McDowell *et al.*)

Symptom/sign	Weight	×	Severity	Score
			0, 1, 2	
Akinesia	9	×	_____	_____
Dementia	8	×	_____	_____
Rigidity	7	×	_____	_____
Tremor	5	×	_____	_____
Depression	5	×	_____	_____
Postural abnormality	3	×	_____	_____
Seborrhea	2	×	_____	_____
Sialorrhea	2	×	_____	_____
Blepharospasm	2	×	_____	_____
Mask facies	1	×	_____	_____
Total				_____ /88

Reference   McDowell *et al.* (1970)

Comment

Basically a measure of impairments seen in Parkinson's disease although it includes some complications such as depression and dementia. There are no published guide-lines; it has not been used since first study; no explanation (justification) of weights used has been given; and the scoring system is counterintuitive (0 is best, 88 worst). None the less it does have face validity, its reliability is said to be 'acceptable' (but may vary by as much as 40 per cent between observers), and it is able to detect improvement brought about by L-dopa.

Parkinson's disease: disability index (McDowell *et al.*)

Activity	Weight	×	Severity 0, 1, 2	Score
Walking	10	×	____	____
Speech	10	×	____	____
Eating	7	×	____	____
Use of toilet	6	×	____	____
Bathing	6	×	____	____
Getting out of bed	6	×	____	____
Getting out of a chair	5	×	____	____
Handwriting	5	×	____	____
Dressing	5	×	____	____
Turning in bed	4	×	____	____
Climbing stairs	2	×	____	____
Total				____ /132

Reference   McDowell *et al.* (1970)

Comment

Designed to detect reduction in disability in a trial of L-dopa. There are no published guidelines; it has not been used since the first study; no explanation of weights used has been given; and the scoring system is counterintuitive (0 is best, 132 worst). However it does include some disabilities characteristic of Parkinson's disease (for example, turning in bed, getting up from chair) and so it has face validity. Reliability is said to be 'acceptable' but may vary by as much as 40 per cent between observers. Sensitivity is sufficient to detect improvement brought about by L-dopa.

Parkinson's disease: Lieberman's index

Rigidity
Evaluated at rest. Record most rigid limb (or neck), usually wrist:
  0 = Absent
  1 = Minimal
  2 = Moderate
  3 = Marked; full range easily achieved
  4 = Severe; full range achieved with difficulty

Tremor
Evaluated at rest, and using each limb separately. Record most tremor seen, usually hand:
  0 = Absent
  1 = Minimal amplitude
  2 = Moderate amplitude
  3 = Marked amplitude, but only intermittent
  4 = Severe; constant marked amplitude

Bradykinesia
Seated patient is asked to open and close hands while moving feet up and down as though walking. Slowest movement scored:
  0 = No bradykinesia
  1 = Minimal slowness; movement looks deliberate
  2 = Moderate slowness and poverty of movement
  3 = Marked slowness and poverty of movement with hesitancy and arrests of ongoing movement
  4 = Severe slowness; unable to perform simultaneous movement in four limbs

Gait qualitatively assessed
  0 = Normal; good stepping, turns readily
  1 = Minimal impairment; slow, may shuffle with short steps but no festination
  2 = Moderate impairment; has difficulty, short steps, freezing and festination, no assistance required
  3 = Marked impairment; has difficulty, frequent freezing and festination, requires assistance
  4 = Severe impairment; great difficulty, always needing assistance
  5 = Unable to walk even with assistance

Gait quantitatively assessed
Walking is timed, patient walking 10 metres away and then returning, using any aid he wishes.
   0 = Under 15 sec
   1 = 16–20 sec
   2 = 21–30 sec
   3 = 31–40 sec
   4 = 41 or more seconds
   5 = Unable to walk

Reference   Lieberman (1974)

Comment
The first three items are impairments, the fourth, a mixture of impairment and disability and the last, disability. The last item loses useful information: it would be better simply to record the time taken. The first three items have face validity but the scores of the last two should not be added on.

Hoehn and Yahr Grades

Stage I
   Unilateral involvement only, usually with minimal or no functional impairment.

Stage II
   Bilateral or midline involvement, without impairment of balance.

Stage III
   First sign of impaired righting reflexes. This is evident by unsteadiness as the patient turns, or is demonstrated when he is pushed from standing equilibrium with feet together and eyes closed. Functionally, the patient is somewhat restricted in his activities but may have some work potential, depending upon type of employment. Patients are physically capable of leading independent lives and their disability is mild to moderate.

Stage IV
   Fully developed, severely disabling disease; the patient is still able to walk and stand unassisted but is markedly incapacitated.

Stage V
   Confinement to bed or wheelchair unless aided.

Reference   Hoehn and Yahr (1967)

Comment

This 'scale' should no longer be used. It was a first attempt to classify the problems of Parkinson's disease, but now is only of historical importance because there are many more appropriate scales. This scale mixes presumed pathology (unilateral/bilateral) with impairments and disabilities (and even handicap; employment). There is no justification of the categories used. Reliability is untested.

Northwestern University Disability Scales

Walking

Never walks alone
   0 = Cannot walk at all with all help possible
   1 = Considerable help needed; cannot walk outdoors
   2 = Moderate help needed indoors; considerable help outdoors
   3 = Potential help needed indoors; active help outdoors

Sometimes walks alone
   4 = Room to room slowly, using an aid; never alone outside
   5 = Room to room with difficulty; occasionally walks alone outside
   6 = Short distances with ease; outdoors difficult but possible without help over short distance

Always walks alone
   7 = Extremely abnormal gait: slow, shuffling, posture grossly affected, may be propulsion
   8 = Poor, slow gait: posture moderately affected, mild propulsion possible, turning difficult
   9 = Gait mildly abnormal: normal posture, turning difficult
 10 = Normal

Dressing

Requires complete assistance
   0 = Patient is a hindrance, not a help
   1 = Patient neither hinders nor helps
   2 = Can give some help through bodily movements
   3 = Gives considerable help through body movements

Requires partial assistance
   4 = Only gross dressing unaided (for example, hat, coat)
   5 = Half dresses alone
   6 = Over half dressing alone, slowly and with effort
   7 = Only able to do fine activities (for example, buttons, zips)

No assistance required
   8 = Very slow, needs great effort
   9 = Slightly slow
   10 = Normal

Hygiene

Requires complete assistance
   0 = Unable to maintain even with full help
   1 = Reasonable hygiene but gives no help
   2 = Good hygiene, gives some help

Requires partial assistance
   3 = Performs a few tasks alone if unsupervised
   4 = Needs help for half of toilet needs
   5 = Needs help for some tasks
   6 = Manages most alone (may use aids)

Independent
   7 = Very slow, needs great effort, accidents occur, uses aids
   8 = Moderately slow, few accidents, no aids
   9 = Slightly slow
   10 = Normal

Eating and feeding (two scores added)

Eating
   0 = Hospital admission required for adequate nutrition
   1 = Only eats liquids and soft food, very slowly
   2 = Liquids/soft food easily eaten; hard food eaten rarely and slowly
   3 = Hard food eaten regularly, but slowly
   4 = Normal diet; chewing/swallowing are laboured
   5 = Normal

Feeding
   0 = Requires complete assistance
   1 = Few feeding tasks independently performed
   2 = Most feeding alone, but slowly with effort; needs help with some tasks (for example, cutting meat)
   3 = All feeding alone but slow; has accidents
   4 = Slow, but accidents are rare
   5 = Normal

Speech
   0 = No vocalization
   1 = Vocalizes but rarely communicates
   2 = Calls attention to self
   3 = Attempts to speak, but has difficulty in initiation and may stop midway through
   4 = Uses speech, articulation unintelligible, slight initiation difficulty, uses single words/short phrases
   5 = Articulation poor; usually uses complete sentences
   6 = Speech always understood if listener attends hard; defective voice and articulation
   7 = Communication easy, but speech detracts from content
   8 = Speech easily understood, but voice or speech rhythm abnormal
   9 = Speech adequate; minor voice disturbances
   10 = Normal

Reference   Canter *et al.* (1961)

Comment
Recommended by Marsden and Schachter (1981). To be used as a profile, giving each item's score separately. Has face/content validity for the areas assessed but not really specific to Parkinson's disease. It had good reliability in the original study but it's difficult to believe that it could be sustained.

Self-assessment Parkinson's Disease Disability Scale

Please read the questions below. For each item circle the number which describes best how easy or difficult it is for you to perform that activity. If you are more able at some times than others, indicate how you are *in general* at the times of day you would normally perform these activities. If you use a frame or walking stick or any special aids to help you, please answer according to how well you would manage *without* the aid.

   1 Able to do alone without difficulty
   2 Able to do alone with a little effort
   3 Able to do alone with a lot of effort or with a little help
   4 Able to do but only with a lot of help
   5 Unable to do at all

1.	Get out of bed	1 2 3 4 5
2.	Get up from an armchair	1 2 3 4 5
3.	Walk around the house/flat	1 2 3 4 5
4.	Walk outside, for example, to the local shops	1 2 3 4 5
5.	Travel by public transport	1 2 3 4 5
6.	Walk up stairs	1 2 3 4 5
7.	Walk down stairs	1 2 3 4 5
8.	Wash face and hands	1 2 3 4 5
9.	Get into a bath	1 2 3 4 5
10.	Get out of a bath	1 2 3 4 5
11.	Get dressed	1 2 3 4 5
12.	Get undressed	1 2 3 4 5
13.	Brush your teeth	1 2 3 4 5
14.	Open tins (not using an electric opener)	1 2 3 4 5
15.	Pour milk from a bottle or carton	1 2 3 4 5
16.	Make a cup of tea of coffee	1 2 3 4 5
17.	Hold a cup and saucer	1 2 3 4 5
18.	Wash and dry dishes	1 2 3 4 5
19.	Cut food with a knife and fork	1 2 3 4 5
20.	Pick up an object from the floor	1 2 3 4 5
21.	Insert and remove an electric plug	1 2 3 4 5
22.	Dial a telephone	1 2 3 4 5
23.	Hold and read a newspaper	1 2 3 4 5
24.	Write a letter	1 2 3 4 5
25.	Turn over in bed	1 2 3 4 5

Reference Brown *et al.* (1988, 1989)

Comment

This disability scale has eleven items relating to mobility (1–10, 25) and fourteen relating to manual dexterity. It has been tested and might be usefully given to out-patients who are waiting to be seen in the clinic (although they might need help marking the form!). Needs further evaluation.

Webster Rating Scale

__ *Bradykinesia* (of hands, including handwriting)

  0 No involvement

  1 Detectable slowing of the supination–pronation rate evidenced by beginning to have difficulty in handling tools, buttoning clothes and with handwriting

  2 Moderate slowing of supination–pronation rate, one or both sides, evidenced by moderate impairment of hand function. Handwriting is greatly impaired, micrographia present

3 Severe slowing of supination–pronation rate. Unable to write or button clothes. Marked difficulty in handling utensils

___ *Rigidity*

0 Non-detectable

1 Detectable rigidity in neck and shoulders. Activation phenomenon is present. One or both arms show mild, negative resting rigidity

2 Moderate rigidity in neck and shoulders. Resting rigidity is positive when patient not on medication

3 Severe rigidity in neck and shoulders. Resting rigidity cannot be reversed by medication.

___ *Posture*

0 Normal posture. Head flexed forward less than 4 inches (10 cm)

1 Beginning poker spine. Head flexed forward up to 5 inches (12 cm)

2 Beginning arm flexion. Head flexed forward up to 6 inches (15 cm). One or both arms raised but still below waist

3 Onset of simian posture. Head flexed forward more than 6 inches (15 cm). One or both hands elevated above the waist. Sharp flexion of hand, beginning interphalangeal extension. Beginning flexion of knees

___ *Upper extremity swing*

0 Swings both arms well

1 One arm definitely decreased in amount of swing

2 One arm fails to swing

3 Both arms fail to swing

___ *Gait*

0 Steps out well with 18- to 30-inch stride (45–75 cm). Turns about effortlessly

1 Gait shortened to 12- to 18-inch stride (30–45 cm). Beginning to strike one heel. Turn around time slowing. Requires several steps

2 Stride moderately shortened—now 6–12 inches (15–30 cm). Both heels beginning to strike floor forcefully

3 Onset of shuffling gait, steps less than 3 inches (8 cm). Occasional stuttering-type or blocking gait. Walks on toes—turns around very slowly

___ *Tremor*

0 No detectable tremor found

1 Less than 1 inch (2 cm) of peak-to-peak tremor movement observed in limbs or head at rest or in either hand while walking or during finger to nose testing.

2 Maximum tremor envelope fails to exceed 4 inches (10 cm). Tremor is severe but not constant and patient retains some control of hands

3 Tremor envelope exceeds 4 inches (10 cm). Tremor is constant and severe. Patient cannot get free of tremor while awake unless it is pure cerebellar type. Writing and feeding self are impossible

— *Facies*

0 Normal. Full animation. No stare

1 Detectable immobility. Mouth remains closed. Beginning to display features of anxiety or depression.

2 Moderate immobility. Emotion breaks through at markedly increased threshold. Lips parted some of the time. Moderate appearance of anxiety or depression. Drooling may be present

3 Frozen facies. Mouth open ¼ inch (60 mm) or more. Drooling may be severe.

— *Seborrhea*

0 None.

1 Increased perspiration, secretion remaining thin

2 Obvious oiliness present—secretion much thicker

3 Marked seborrhea, entire face and head covered by thick secretion

— *Speech*

0 Clear, resonant, easily understood

1 Beginning of hoarseness with loss of inflection and resonance. Good volume and still easily understood

2 Moderate hoarseness and weakness. Constant monotone, unvaried pitch Beginning of dysarthria, hesitancy, stuttering, difficult to understand

3 Marked harshness and weakness. Very difficult to hear and understand

— *Self-care*

0 No impairment

1 Still provides full self-care, but rate of dressing definitely impeded. Able to live alone and often still employable

2 Requires help in certain critical areas, such as turning in bed, rising from chairs etc. Very slow in performing most activities but manages by taking much time

3 Continuously disabled. Unable to dress, feed self, or walk alone

---

Reference   Webster (1968)

Comment

This measure has been widely used but there have not been any formal studies of reliability.

New York Rating Scale

Head
Ocular movements
Consider rapidity of conjugate gaze in all directions and the ability to open eyes after closure. Limitation of voluntary control is:

0 = None
1 = Mild
2 = Moderate
3 = Severe
4 = Complete

Blinking frequency
0 = Free
1 = 10–30 sec
2 = 30–60 sec
3 = 60+ sec
4 = inability to blink

Emotional facial control
Check degree of flattening of facial lines. Note facial expression with smiling. Score absence of control in upper face (forehead, eyes, nose) and lower face (mouth) separately:

0 = Normal
1 = Mild absence
2 = Moderate absence
3 = Severe absence
4 = Complete absence

Voluntary facial control
Ask patient to frown upward, inward; wrinkle his nose; close his eyes (all upper face) and to grimace and purse lips (lower face). Score absence of control in upper and lower face separately:

0 = Normal
1 = Mild absence
2 = Moderate absence
3 = Severe absence
4 = Complete absence

Swallowing
0 = Normal
1 = Drooling, occasional choking
2 = Slow
3 = Not voluntary, and chokes by reflex
4 = Unable to swallow

Motor speech
Degree to which speech is inaudible and unintelligible. Score as ability to talk:
 0 = Normal
 1 = Mildly abnormal
 2 = Moderately abnormal
 3 = Severely abnormal
 4 = Unable to talk

Tongue movement
 0 = Normal
 1 = Full movement but slowed
 2 = Can protrude tongue beyond lips, but not full forward or in other directions
 3 = Can protude tongue to lip margin
 4 = Unable to move tongue

Neck rotation (sitting)
Best rating taken. Rate 90 degrees as 100 per cent. Score both to left and to right separately.
 0 = 75–100%
 1 = 50–75%
 2 = 25–50%
 3 = 0–25%
 4 = unable to rotate

Shoulder elevation (sitting)
Best rating taken. Score both left and right separately.
 0 = 75–100%
 1 = 50–75%
 2 = 25–50%
 3 = 0–25%
 4 = unable to elevate

Lowering head to plinth (lying supine)
 0 = Normal
 1 = Can, moderate speed
 2 = Can, slowly
 3 = Can lower, but not as far as plinth
 4 = Unable to lower at all

Elevation of arms (sitting)
 0 = Full hyperabduction
 1 = Partial hyperabduction
 2 = Shoulder level
 3 = Below shoulder
 4 = Unable

Handwriting
  0 = Normal
  1 = Mild difficulty
  2 = Moderate difficulty
  3 = Severe difficulty, few words
  4 = Unable

Arising from standard chair with sidearms
  0 = Can arise with arms folded
  1 = Can arise with moderate arm support by self
  2 = Can arise with maximal arm support by self
  3 = Can arise with examiner's support
  4 = Unable

Walking
  0 = Can walk well
  1 = Can walk independently but slowly
  2 = Can walk with arm support by self
  3 = Can walk with observer's assistance
  4 = Cannot walk

Walking, on heels and toes
Score right and left side separately
  0 = able, without support
  1 = able, on heels *and* toes, with moderate support
  2 = able, on heels *or* toes, with moderate support
  3 = able, on heels *or* toes, with maximal support
  4 = unable

Climbing
Score right and left side separately
  0 = Can lift foot in walking, and climb 8 in (20 cm) step without support
  1 = Can lift foot in walking and climb with own support
  2 = Can lift foot in walking and climb with observer's support
  3 = Can lift foot in walking with observer's support but cannot climb
  4 = Cannot lift foot in walking and climbing

Trunk raising (supine position)
Lifting head and shoulders off table
  0 = Can arise to sitting position with arms on head
  1 = Off table with hands on head
  2 = Off table with hands on abdomen or chest
  3 = Off table with hands on side of plinth
  4 = Cannot lift head and shoulders off table

Trunk turning (supine position)
    0 = Can turn to both sides without using arms
    1 = Can turn to both sides using arms
    2 = Can turn to one side using arms, but not other
    3 = Can make some attempt to turn using arms
    4 = Cannot turn to right or left

Straight leg raising
Assess thigh flexion; score right and left leg separately
    0 = 60 degrees lifting, knee fully extended
    1 = 60 degrees lifting, knee partially extended
    2 = 30 degrees lifting, knee partially extended
    3 = Some lifting, heel remains on bed
    4 = Cannot flex thigh

Movement of ankles and toes
Score right and left sides separately
    0 = Free movement
    1 = Good, but slowed movement
    2 = Moderate movement
    3 = Slight movement
    4 = No spontaneous movement

General mobility
    0 = Freely mobile
    1 = Moderate mobility in trunk and extremities
    2 = Slight mobility in trunk and extremities
    3 = Mobility limited to head and neck
    4 = Complete immobility at rest

Abnormal tone (rigidity)
Score for following two midline and 12 bilateral areas: neck; back; shoulders; elbows; wrists and fingers; hips; knees; and ankles and toes.
    0 = Normal tone
    1 = Mild rigidity
    2 = Moderate rigidity
    3 = Severe rigidity
    4 = Complete rigidity

Contractures and deformities
Score for following two midline and 12 bilateral areas: neck; back; shoulders; elbows; wrists and fingers; hips; knees; and ankles and toes.
    0 = Normal range, no deformity
    1 = Mild restriction/deformity
    2 = Moderate restriction/deformity
    3 = Severe restriction/deformity
    4 = Complete restriction/deformity

Tremor
Score on amount of time tremor present in following nine areas: eyelids; face; jaw; tongue; neck; arms; legs.

  0 = Never
  1 = Occasional % time
  2 = Moderate % time
  3 = Considerable % time
  4 = Constant

Reference   Alba *et al.* (1968)

Comment
A massive amount of data, mixing impairments and disabilities. Many items are poorly defined. It is not recommended.

Unified Parkinson's Disease Rating Scale

(Version 3.0, February 1987)

I   *Mentation, behaviour, and mood*

— Intellectual impairment
  0 = None
  1 = Mild: consistent forgetfulness with partial recollection of events and no other difficulties
  2 = Moderate memory loss, with disorientation and moderate difficulty handling complex problems; mild but definite impairment of function at home, with need of occasional prompting
  3 = Severe memory loss with disorientation for time and often for place, severe impairment in handling problems
  4 = Severe memory loss with orientation preserved to person only; unable to make judgements or solve problems; requires much help with personal care; cannot be left alone at all

— Thought disorder (due to dementia or drug intoxication)
  0 = None
  1 = Vivid dreaming
  2 = 'Benign' hallucinations with insight retained
  3 = Occasional to frequent hallucination or delusions without insight; could interfere with daily activities
  4 = Persistent hallucinations, delusions, or florid psychosis; not able to care for self

— Depression
  0 = Not present
  1 = Periods of sadness or guilt greater than normal but never sustained for days or weeks
  2 = Sustained depression (1 week or more)
  3 = Sustained depression with vegetative symptoms (insomnia, anorexia, weight loss, loss of interest)
  4 = Sustained depression with vegetative symptom and suicidal thoughts or intent

— Motivation/initiative
  0 = Normal
  1 = Less assertive than usual; more passive
  2 = Loss of initiative or interest in elective (non-routine) activities
  3 = Loss of initiative or interest in day-to-day (routine) activities
  4 = Withdrawn, complete loss of motivation

II *Activities of daily living*

— Speech
  0 = Normal
  1 = Mildly affected, no difficulty in being understood
  2 = Moderately affected, sometimes asked to repeat statements
  3 = Severely affected, frequently asked to repeat statements
  4 = Unintelligible most of the time

— Salivation
  0 = Normal
  1 = Slight but definite excess of saliva in mouth; may have night-time drooling
  2 = Moderately excessive saliva; may have minimal drooling
  3 = Marked excess of saliva; some drooling
  4 = Marked drooling; requires constant use of tissue or handkerchief

— Swallowing
  0 = Normal
  1 = Rare choking
  2 = Occasional choking
  3 = Requires soft food
  4 = Requires nasogastric tube or gastrostomy feeding

— Handwriting
  0 = Normal
  1 = Slightly slow or small
  2 = Moderately slow or small; all words are legible
  3 = Severely affected; not all words are legible
  4 = The majority of words are not legible

__ Cutting food and handling utensils
0 = Normal
1 = Somewhat slow and clumsy, but no help needed
2 = Can cut most foods, although clumsy and slow; some help needed
3 = Food must be cut by someone but can still feed slowly
4 = Needs to be fed

__ Dressing
0 = Normal
1 = Somewhat slow, but no help needed
2 = Occasional assistance needed with buttoning, getting arms into sleeves
3 = Considerable help required, but can do some things alone
4 = Helpless

__ Hygiene
0 = Normal
1 = Somewhat slow but no help needed
2 = Needs help to shower or bathe; very slow in hygiene care
3 = Requires assistance for washing, brushing teeth, combing hair, going to bathroom (toilet)
4 = Needs Foley (bladder) catheter or other aids

__ Turning in bed and adjusting bedclothes
0 = Normal
1 = Somewhat slow and clumsy, but no help needed
2 = Can turn alone or adjust sheets, but with great difficulty
3 = Can initiate attempt but cannot turn or adjust sheets alone
4 = Helpless

__ Falling (unrelated to freezing)
0 = None
1 = Rare falling
2 = Occasional falls, less than once daily
3 = Falls an average of once daily
4 = Falls more than once daily

__ Freezing when walking
0 = None
1 = Rare freezing when walking; may have start hesitation
2 = Occasional freezing when walking
3 = Frequent freezing; occasionally falls because of freezing
4 = Frequently falls because of freezing

__ Walking
0 = Normal
1 = Mild difficulty; may not swing arms or may tend to drag leg
2 = Moderate difficulty, but requires little or no assistance
3 = Severe disturbance of walking; requires assistance
4 = Cannot walk at all, even with assistance

__ Tremor
   0 = Absent
   1 = Slight and infrequently present
   2 = Moderate; bothersome to patient
   3 = Severe; interferes with many activities
   4 = Marked; interferes with most activities

__ Sensory complaints related to Parkinsonism
   0 = None
   1 = Occasionally has numbness
   2 = Frequently has numbness, tingling, or aching; not distressing
   3 = Frequent painful sensations
   4 = Excruciating pain

III *Motor examination*

__ Speech
   0 = Normal
   1 = Slight loss of expression, diction and/or volume
   2 = Monotone, slurred but understandable; moderately impaired
   3 = Marked impairment, difficult to understand
   4 = Unintelligible

__ Facial expression
   0 = Normal
   1 = Minimal hypomimia; could be normal 'poker face'
   2 = Slight but definitely abnormal diminution of facial expression
   3 = Moderate hypomimia; lips parted some of the time
   4 = Masked or fixed facies, with severe or complete loss of facial expression; lips parted ¼ inch (6 mm) or more

__ Tremor at rest
   0 = Absent
   1 = Slight, and infrequently present
   2 = Mild in amplitude and persistent, or moderate in amplitude but only intermittently present
   3 = Moderate in amplitude and present most of the time
   4 = Marked in amplitude and present most of the time

__ Action or postural tremor of hands
   0 = Absent
   1 = Slight; present with action
   2 = Moderate in amplitude; present with action
   3 = Moderate in amplitude; present with posture-holding as well as with action
   4 = Marked in amplitude; interferes with feeding

— Rigidity

Judged on passive movement with patient relaxed in sitting position; 'cogwheeling' to be ignored

0 = Absent

1 = Slight or detectable only when activated by mirror or other movements

2 = Mild to moderate

3 = Marked, but full range of motion easily achieved

4 = Severe, range of motion achieved with difficulty

— Finger taps

Patient taps thumb with index finger in rapid succession with widest amplitude possible, each hand separately

0 = Normal

1 = Mild slowing and/or reduction in amplitude

2 = Moderately impaired; definite and early fatiguing; may have occasional arrests in movement

3 = Severely impaired; frequent hesitation in initiating movements or arrests in ongoing movement

4 = Can barely perform task

— Hand movements

Patient opens and closes hands in rapid succession with widest amplitude possible, each hand separately.

0 = Normal

1 = Mild slowing and/or reduction in movement

2 = Moderately impaired; definite and early fatiguing; may have occasional arrests in movement

3 = Severely impaired; frequent hesitation in initiating movements or arrests in ongoing movement

4 = Can barely perform task

— Rapid alternating movements of hand

Pronation–supination movements of hands, vertically or horizontally, with as large an amplitude as possible, both hands simultaneously.

0 = Normal

1 = Mild slowing and/or reduction in movement

2 = Moderately impaired; definite and early fatiguing; may have occasional arrests in movement

3 = Severely impaired; frequent hesitation in initiating movements or arrests in ongoing movement

4 = Can barely perform task

___ Leg agility
Patient taps heel on ground in rapid succession, picking up entire leg; amplitude
should be about 3 inches (75 mm).
0 = Normal
1 = Mild slowing and/or reduction in movement
2 = Moderately impaired; definite and early fatiguing; may have occasional
    arrests in movement
3 = Severely impaired; frequent hesitation in initiating movements or arrests in
    ongoing movement
4 = Can barely perform task

___ Arising from chair
Patient attempts to arise from a straight-backed wood or metal chair, with arms
folded across chest.
0 = Normal
1 = Slow, or may need more than one attempt
2 = Pushes self up from arms of seat
3 = Tends to fall back and may have to try several times but can get up without
    help
4 = Unable to arise without help

___ Posture
0 = Normal erect
1 = Not quite erect, slightly stooped posture; could be normal for older person
2 = Moderately stooped posture, definitely abnormal; can be slightly leaning to
    one side
3 = Severely stooped posture with kyphosis; can be moderately leaning to one
    side
4 = Marked flexion, with extreme abnormality of posture

___ Gait
0 = Normal
1 = Walks slowly, may shuffle with short steps but no festination or propulsion
2 = Walks with difficulty, but requires little or no assistance; may have some
    festination, short steps, or propulsion
3 = Severe disturbance of gait; requires assistance
4 = Cannot walk at all even with assistance

___ Postural stability
Response to sudden posterior displacement produced by a pull on shoulders
while patient is erect, with eyes open and feet slightly apart; patient *is* prepared.
0 = Normal
1 = Retropulsion but recovers unaided
2 = Absence of postural response, would fall if not caught by examiner
3 = Very unstable, tends to lose balance spontaneously
4 = Unable to stand without assistance

__ Body bradykinesia and hypokinesia
Combining slowness, hesitancy, decreased arm swing, small amplitude, and
poverty of movement in general.
0 = None
1 = Minimal slowness giving movement a deliberate character, could be normal
   for some persons; possibly reduced amplitude
2 = Mild degree of slowness and poverty of movement that is definitely abnormal; alternatively some reduced amplitude
3 = Moderate slowness; poverty or small amplitude of movement
4 = Marked slowness; poverty or small amplitude of movement

IV *Complications of therapy (in the past week): dyskinesia*

__ Duration
What proportion of the waking day are dyskinesias present? (Historical
information)
0 = None
1 = 1–25% of day
2 = 26–50% of day
3 = 51–75% of day
4 = 76–100% of day

__ Disability
How disabling are the dyskinesias? (Historical information, may be modified by
office examination)
0 = Not disabling
1 = Mildly disabling
2 = Moderately disabling
3 = Severely disabling
4 = Completely disabling

__ Painful dyskinesias
How painful are the dyskinesias?
0 = No painful dyskinesia
1 = Slightly
2 = Moderately
3 = Severely
4 = Markedly

__ Presence of early morning dystonia. (Historical information)
0 = No
1 = Yes

Complications of therapy (in the past week): clinical fluctuations

__ Are there any 'off' periods predictable as to timing after a dose of medication?
0 = No
1 = Yes

___ Are there any 'off' periods unpredictable as to timing after a dose of medication?
0 = No
1 = Yes

___ Do any 'off' periods come on suddenly (i.e. within a few seconds)?
0 = No
1 = Yes

___ What proportion of the waking day is the patient 'off' on average?
0 = None
1 = 1–25% of day
2 = 26–50% of day
3 = 51–75% of day
4 = 76–100% of day

Complications of therapy (in the past week): other

___ Does the patient have anorexia, nausea, or vomiting?
0 = No
1 = Yes

___ Does the patient have any sleep disturbances (for example, insomnia or hypersomnolence)?
0 = No
1 = Yes

___ Does the patient have symptomatic orthostasis?
0 = No
1 = Yes

V   *Modified Hoehn and Yahr staging*
0   = No signs of disease
1   = Unilateral disease
1.5 = Unilateral plus axial involvement
2   = Bilateral disease without impairment of balance
2.5 = Mild bilateral disease with recovery on pull test
3   = Mild to moderate bilateral disease; some postural instability; physically independent
4   = Severe disability; still able to walk or stand unassisted
5   = Wheelchair-bound or bedridden unless aided

VI   *Schwab and England Activities of Daily Living Scale*
Ask patient and relative to score patient's ability over the preceding week to the nearest 5 per cent using the following guide-lines.

100% = Completely independent; able to do all chores without slowness, difficulty, or impairment; essentially normal; unaware of any difficulty

90% = Completely independent; able to do all chores with some degree of slowness, difficulty, and impairment; may take twice as long as usual; beginning to be aware of difficulty

80% = Completely independent in most chores; takes twice as long as normal conscious of difficulty and slowness

70% = Not completely independent; more difficulty with some chores; takes three to four times as long as normal in some; must spend a large part of the day with some chores

60% = Some dependency; can do most chores, but exceedingly slowly and with considerable effort and errors; some chores impossible

50% = More dependent; needs help with half the chores, slower, etc.; difficulty with everything

40% = Very dependent; can assist with all chores but does few alone

30% = With effort, now and then does a few chores alone or begins alone; much help needed

20% = Does nothing alone; can be a slight help with some chores; severe invalid

10% = Totally dependent and helpless; complete invalid

0% = Vegetative functions such as swallowing, bladder and bowels are not functioning; bedridden

---

References   Lang and Fahn (1989); Schwab and England (1969); Hoehn and Yahr (1967)

Comment
Developed from parts of other scales and in five sections, most components of this index have been tested for reliability. It is probably now the preferred measure for large studies although the Hoehn and Yahr Grades and Schwab and England scale should be dropped—they add nothing. As stated in Chapter 11, the author's preference would be to use general measures of disability—they are shorter, simpler and probably as sensitive.

Tourette's Syndrome Global Scale

	Frequency	Disruption	Score (Code)
			(F × D)
MOTOR SYMPTOMS			
Simple motor Non-purposeful tics, jerks and/or movement	____	____	____ (SM)
Complex motor Purposeful, thoughtful actions (systematic actions), rituals, touching self, others or objects	____	____	____ (CM)
Simple phonic Non-purposeful noises, throat clearing, coughing	____	____	____ (SP)
Complex phonic Purposeful, insults, coprolalia words, distinguishable speech	____	____	____ (CP)
'SOCIAL FUNCTIONING'			
Behaviour (conduct)			____ (B)
Motor restlessness			____ (MR)
School and learning problems			____ (SL)
Work and occupation problems			____ (WO)

GLOBAL SCORE = [(SM + CM)/2] + [(SP + CP)/2] + [(B + MR + SL or WO) × 2/3]

Guidelines: general
The use of the TSGS requires the rater to have clinical experience with TS patients and knowledge of the range of TS symptomatology. Information for making a rating is based on a synthesis of the clinician's observation along with the patient, parent, school, and work reports for the past week. Whether or not the patient is on medication is not taken into account.

Guidelines: frequency codes
1. One or less in 5 min
2. One in 2–4.9 min
3. One to four in 1–1.9 min
4. Five or more in 1 min
5. Virtually uncountable

Guidelines: disruption

1. Camouflaged
   Some tics, but untrained person would not recognize (for example, tossing hair back).

2. Audible/visible, no problem
   Recognizable, but does not interfere (for example, picking at hair, throat clearing).

3. Some problem
   Significant problem but functioning continues (for example, interrupted speech, head-jerks, interruptions while reading).

4. Impaired function
   Symptom definitely a problem (for example, prolonged complex movements, series of non-stop tics).

5. Cannot function.
   Cannot do anything when symptom is present.

Simple motor tics
Rapid, darting, meaningless. Eye-blinking, grimacing, nose twitching, lip pouting, shoulder shrugs, arm jerks, head jerks, abdominal tensing, rapid kicks, finger movements, jaw snaps, tooth clicking, frowning, rapid jerking of any part of body.

Complex motor tics
Slower, 'purposeful': hopping, clapping, touching objects or others or self, throwing, arranging, gyrating and bending, 'dystonic' postures, biting mouth, lip, arm, headbanging, thrusting arms, striking out, picking scabs, writhing movements, rolling eyes to ceiling, holding funny expressions, sticking out tongue, kissing, pinching, writing over and over the same letter or word, pulling back on pencil while writing, tearing paper or books.

Simple phonic symptoms
Fast, 'meaningless' sounds: whistling, coughing, sniffling, spitting, screeching, barking, grunting, gurgling, clacking, hawking, hissing, sucking, 'uh-uh', 'eeee', 'ah-uh', 'ah' and innumerable other sounds.

Complex phonic symptoms
Language; words, phrases, statements: . . . 'shut up' . . . 'stop that' . . . 'OK' . . . 'I've got to' . . . 'I'm going to get better—right?' . . . 'Right.' . . . 'What makes me do this?' . . . 'How about it?' . . . 'Now you've seen it.' . . . 'all right.' . . . 'oh boy.' . . .
Also *rituals*: counting. Repeating a phrase until it is just right
Speech atypicalities: Unusual rhythms, tone, accents, intensity of speech
Coprolalia: obscene and aggressive words and statements

SOCIAL FUNCTIONING
Each area is given a score between 0 and 25. The guidelines below indicate some fixed points, and extrapolation between is allowed. (The original paper gives further examples.)

Behaviour
With three main areas of interaction: peers, school or authority figures and family relations. Provocative, argumentative, poor frustration tolerance, temper fits.
  0 = No problems, normal relationships
  5 = Subtle problems, no particular relationship threatened
  10 = Visible problem, at least one relationship impaired
  15 = Clear impairment in more than one area
  20 = Serious impairment affects all areas, occasional interactions
  25 = Unacceptable social behaviour, no attempt at good social interaction. Cannot be trusted, constant supervision

Motor restlessness
Increased motor activity, more than normal movement for task.
  0 = Normal movement for task—good concentration
  5 = Adventitial, occasional increased movement, mostly fine motor, visible but no problem
  10 = Increased motor restlessness, clearly visible (for example, shaking, fidgety, would be trouble at dinner table or movies), mild interference
  15 = Clear motor restlessness, fidgeting, hyperactive, some impairment (intervention)
  20 = Mostly in motion but occasionally stops, impaired direction, difficulty with structure, functioning greatly impaired
  25 = Non-stop motion, impaired concentration, unable to sit still, always in motion, clearly cannot function

School and learning problems
  0 = No problem, at grade level, doing at least average work
  5 = Low grades, not working up to potential
  10 = Should be, or is in special classes, special teacher, learning laboratory, tutor, or repeating grade (academic year)
  15 = All special classes, or repeated more than one grade (year)
  20 = Special school
  25 = Unable to remain in school, home bound, unable to learn

Work and occupational problems
  0 = Have job, no problems
  5 = Has held down job for at least six months, some problems doing work, getting along with co-workers, or taking orders
  10 = Poor functioning, changed jobs a few times in the past year. Serious problems (two or three jobs)
  15 = Cannot hold a job for long, lost lots of jobs
  20 = Almost never employed, sporadic employment, out of work 2–3 months
  25 = Unemployed—did not work for six or more months

Reference Harcherik *et al.* (1984)

Comment
Mixes impairments and disabilities. It is difficult to know how reliable this measure would be in routine practice. A shorter, simpler measure is needed separating the impairments from the disabilities.

Fahn-Marsden Scale for Primary Torsion Dystonias

Region	Provoking factor		Severity factor	Weight	Product (score)
Eyes	____	×	____	0.5	__ /8
Mouth	____	×	____	0.5	__ /8
Speech/swallowing	____	×	____	1.0	__ /16
Neck	____	×	____	0.5	__ /8
Right arm	____	×	____	1.0	__ /16
Left arm	____	×	____	1.0	__ /16
Trunk	____	×	____	1.0	__ /16
Right leg	____	×	____	1.0	__ /16
Left leg	____	×	____	1.0	__ /16
Total					__ /120

Provoking factor

General
   0 = No dystonia at rest or with action
   1 = Dystonia on particular occasion
   2 = Dystonia on many actions
   3 = Dystonia on action of distant part of body or intermittently at rest
   4 = Dystonia present at rest

Speech and swallowing
   1 = Occasional, either or both
   2 = Frequent either
   3 = Frequent one, and occasional other
   4 = Frequent both

Severity factors

Eyes
   0 = No dystonia present
   1 = Slight, occasional blinking
   2 = Mild. Frequent blinking without prolonged spasms of eye closure
   3 = Moderate. Prolonged spasm of eyelid closure but eyes open much of the time
   4 = Severe. Prolonged spasms of eyelid closure with eyes closed at least 30 per cent of the time

Mouth
0 = No dystonia present
1 = Slight. Occasional grimacing or other mouth movements (for example, jaw open or clenched; tongue movement)
2 = Mild. Movement present less than 50 per cent of the time
3 = Moderate dystonic movements or contractions present most of the time
4 = Severe dystonic movements or contractions present most of the time

Speech and swallowing
0 = No dystonia present
1 = Slightly involved; speech easily understood or occasional choking
2 = Some difficulty in understanding speech or frequent choking
3 = Marked difficulty in understanding speech or inability to swallow firm foods
4 = Complete or almost complete anarthria, or marked difficulty swallowing soft foods and liquids

Neck
0 = No dystonia present
1 = Slight. Occasional pulling
2 = Obvious torticollis, but mild
3 = Moderate pulling
4 = Extreme pulling

Arm
0 = No dystonia present
1 = Slight dystonia. Clinically insignificant
2 = Mild. Obvious dystonia, but not disabling
3 = Moderate. Able to grasp, with some manual function
4 = Severe. No useful grasp

Trunk
0 = No dystonia present
1 = Slight bending, clinically insignificant
2 = Definite bending, but not interfering with standing or walking
3 = Moderate bending; interfering with standing or walking
4 = Extreme bending of trunk preventing standing or walking

Leg
0 = No dystonia present
1 = Slight dystonia, but not causing impairment; clinically insignificant
2 = Mild dystonia—walks briskly and unaided
3 = Moderate dystonia—severely impairs walking or requires assistance
4 = Severe. Unable to stand or walk on involved leg

References   Burke *et al.* (1985); Fahn (1989)

Comment

The validity of this scale was tested by comparison with a disability scale but in fact the dystonia scale also includes disability, making the test of validity rather weak. Inter-observer and intra-observer reliability was good. A range of more detailed scales have been developed for blepharospasm, oromandibular dystonia, torticollis, arm dystonia, leg dystonia and trunk dystonia (see Fahn 1989) but these are so far untested for validity and reliability.

Abnormal Involuntary Movement Scale (AIMS)

Procedure
- Ensure patient is not chewing gum, etc.
- Ask patient if he/she notices any involuntary movements and, if so, do the movements bother or disable the patient?
- Observe patient sitting with hands on knees and then with arms hanging.
- Ask patient to open mouth (observe tongue) and protrude tongue. Repeat once.
- Ask patient to tap thumb with each finger as fast as possible for 10–15 seconds. Each hand separately.
- Ask patient to sit with arms outstretched, palms down.
- Ask patient to stand up, wait (observe), walk few paces, turn and sit down again.
- Test tone in each arm.

Then rate highest observed category on scale below (but one less if seen on activation), using coding:
   0 = None
   1 = Minimal, may be extreme normal
   2 = Mild
   3 = Moderate
   4 = Severe

__ Muscle of facial expression
   e.g. movements of forehead, eyebrows, periorbital area, cheeks including frowning, blinking, smiling, grimacing

__ Lips and perioral areas
   e.g. puckering, pouting, smacking

__ Jaw
   e.g. biting, clenching, chewing, mouth opening, lateral movement

__ Tongue
   Rate only increase in movement both in and out of mouth, *not* inability to sustain movement

__ Upper limb
   Include choreic movements (i.e. rapid, objectively purposeless, irregular, spontaneous) and athetoid movements (i.e. slow, irregular, complex, serpentine) Do *not* include tremor (i.e. repetitive, rhythmic, regular)

— Lower limb
  e.g. lateral knee movement, foot tapping, heel dropping, foot squirming, inversion and eversion of the foot
— Trunk: neck, shoulders, hips
  e.g. rocking, twisting, squirming, pelvic gyrations
— Global judgement: severity of abnormal movements
— Global judgement: incapacitation due to abnormal movements
— Patient's awareness of abnormal movements (self-report)
  0 = Unaware
  1 = Aware, no distress
  2 = Aware, mild distress
  3 = Aware, moderate distress
  4 = Aware, severe distress

Reference   Chien *et al.* (1980)

Comment
Its validity has been tested against counting movements, electronic measurement and three other rating scales. It had good validity and high inter-rater reliability ($r = 0.87$). The author does not know how widely this measure is used.

24   Miscellaneous measures

Summary

1. Behavioural Mapping
2. Engagement Levels
3. Spinal Injury: Frankel Scale
4. Spinal Cord Injury Motor Index and Sensory Indices
5. A Caregiver Strain Index
6. Rivermead Behavioural Memory Test
7. Rivermead Perceptual Assessment Battery
8. Wechsler Adult Intelligence Scales
9. Wechsler Memory Scale
10. Behavioural Inattention Test

Introduction

This chapter contains a variety of measures, including an outline of the components of some commonly used test batteries. The first two measures (Behavioural Mapping and Engagement Levels) enable measurement of the work undertaken within a rehabilitation unit. The next two are the only two the author has found relating to spinal injury. The Caregiver Strain Index is the only measure the author has found which explicitly measures stress on the carer; it needs to be compared with the General Health Questionnaire. The last five are test batteries and only the component items are shown.

Behavioural Mapping

Observers move through the unit at random intervals (1–2×/hour) and each location is visited by a predetermined route. Subjects can include all patients, staff and visitors present on the unit when observations are made. The behaviour, patterns of interaction and location of all subjects is appropriately recorded using the following categories:

Solitary behaviour
(a) *Isolated disengagement.* This is applied when little external activity occurs in physical isolation; for example, non-specific gaze while sitting or lying, or sleeping.

(b) *Inactive individual task*. Any activity carried out without interaction, not related to self-care but involving the same level of engagement with the environment: includes focused attention on objects, watching TV, listening to radio and observing others. (Excludes tasks involving gross physical movements.)

(c) *Active individual task*. Any activity carried out without interaction not related to self-care and excluding inactive tasks. Includes most solitary tasks involving gross physical movement, such as walking, using wheelchair, carrying equipment, doing physiotherapy exercises and using equipment.

(d) *Independent self-maintenance*. All activities associated with the following specific forms of self-care without assistance: eating, going to the toilet, bathing and dressing.

(e) *Deviant behaviour*. All excessive behaviour which is considered inappropriate by the observer.

Interactive behaviour

(f) *Individual interaction task*. All one-to-one communications associated with providing or receiving task type service facilities, or focused around task type activity. This includes taking temperatures and blood pressure readings, using physiotherapy and occupational therapy equipment, and catheterization help.

(g) *Individual interaction verbal*. All one-to-one communication during non-task activity or recreation with the focus on verbal aspects of communication. This involved informal discussion, giving advice, verbal instructions, conversation, counselling, and attentive listening.

(h) *Group interaction task*. As behavioural category (f) but involving more than two persons and excluding formal meetings.

(i) *Group interaction verbal*. As behavioural category (g) but involving more than two persons and excluding formal meetings.

(j) *Formal meetings*. All formal meetings involving staff, visitors or patients. This includes ward meetings, ward rounds, case conferences, unit meetings and meetings with visitors.

References   Kennedy *et al.* (1988); Tinson (1989); Lincoln *et al.* (1989)

Comment

This is a useful way of describing what actually happens in any unit managing patients with disability. With initial discussion between observers, rates of agreement usually approach 90 per cent. An objective measure like this would give managers much more information than the routine statistics of care given which are usually collected: the information would be relevant, reliable and probably cost less money if routine reports were abandoned.

Engagement Levels

Subjects are observed randomly by an observer. Each subject is observed once during each observation period, for five seconds. The observer records behaviour on three dimensions: his or her (body) position; his or her activity; and his or her location within the unit. The following categories can be used:

Position
  1a. Sitting, eyes closed
  1b. Sitting, eyes open
  2a. Laying down, eyes closed
  2b. Laying down, eyes open
  3a. Walking with assistance
  3b. Walking without assistance
  4. Standing
  5. Not visible

Activity
  10. No activity
  11. In conversation
  12. Watching TV or listening to radio
  13. In physiotherapy
  14. In occupational therapy
  15. Inappropriate behaviour (crying, screaming, shouting)
  16. Reading
  17. Playing cards or other games
  18. Being attended to by a nurse or physician
  19. Eating or drinking
  20. Other activity

Location
A coding suitable to the structure of the unit should be used.

Reference   Newton *et al.* (1989)

Comment
Another way of monitoring activity in a rehabilitation setting.

Spinal Injury: Frankel Scale

Score	Description
A	*Complete injury* No motor or sensory function below the level of injury.
B	*Sensation only* Some preserved sensation below the level of injury; this does not apply to a slight discrepancy between the motor and sensory level, but does apply to sacral sparing.
C	*Motor function useless* Some preserved motor function below the level of injury, but it is of no practical use to the patient.
D	*Motor function useful* Preserved useful motor function below the level of the injury; patients in this group can walk with or without aids.
E	*Recovery* Normal motor and sensory function; abnormal reflexes may be present.

References   Frankel *et al.* (1969); Piepmeier and Jenkins (1988)

Comment

A global scale, devised many years ago. Its validity and reliability are untested.

Spinal Cord Injury Motor Index and Sensory Indices

The following ten joint movements are assessed on both sides using the scoring system given.

Scoring system:
  0 = Absent, total paralysis
  1 = Trace; palpable or visible contraction
  2 = Poor; active movement through range of movement (RoM) with gravity eliminated
  3 = Fair; active movement through RoM against gravity
  4 = Good; active movement through RoM against resistance
  5 = Normal

Motor index

Level	Movement	Left	Right
C5	Shoulder abduction	__ /5	__ /5
C6/7	Wrist extension	__ /5	__ /5
C7/8	Elbow extension	__ /5	__ /5
C7/8	Grip	__ /5	__ /5
C8/T1	Finger abduction	__ /5	__ /5
L1–3	Hip flexion	__ /5	__ /5
L3/4	Knee extension	__ /5	__ /5
L4/5	Ankle dorsiflexion	__ /5	__ /5
L5	Great toe extension	__ /5	__ /5
S1/2	Ankle plantar flexion	__ /5	__ /5
Total		__ /50	__ /50

Sensory testing
Pinprick sensation is assessed for each dermatome level below level of injury. Scoring is:

1 = normal
0.5 = impaired
0 = absent

The total can be expressed as a percentage of the maximum possible from that level.

Joint position sense is assessed in both great toes, scored as:

1 = present
0 = absent

References   Lucas and Ducker (1979); Li *et al.* (1990)

Comment
Two ways of measuring impairment, designed for use in acute phase. Predictive validity has been established for high cervical lesions but otherwise it has been little tested.

A Caregiver Strain Index

Score: 'Yes' = 1
      'No' = 0

'I am going to read a list of things which other people have found to be difficult in helping with after someone comes home from the hospital.'

(*or*)

'I am going to read a list of things which other people have found to be difficult when helping someone who has an illness.'

'Would you please tell me whether any of these apply to you?' (*give examples*)

__ Sleep is disturbed (e.g. because ..... is in and out of bed or wanders around at night).

__ It is inconvenient (e.g. because helping takes so much time or it's a long drive over to help).

__ It is a physical strain (e.g. because of lifting in and out of a chair; effort or concentration is required).

__ It is confining (e.g. helping restricts free time, or cannot go visiting).

__ There have been family adjustments (e.g. because helping has disrupted routine; there has been no privacy).

__ There have been changes in personal plans (e.g. had to turn down a job; could not go on vacation/holiday).

__ There have been other demands on my time (e.g. from other family members).

__ There have been emotional adjustments (e.g. because of severe argument).

__ Some behaviour is upsetting (e.g. because of incontinence; .... has trouble remembering things; or .... accuses people of taking things).

__ It is upsetting to find ... has changed so much from his/her former self (e.g. he/she is a different person than he/she used to be).

__ There have been work adjustments (e.g. because of having to take time off).

__ It is a financial strain.

__ Feeling completely overwhelmed (e.g. because of worry about ....; concerns about how you will manage).

__ /13 Total

Reference   Robinson (1983)

Comment

This is the only short measure specifically designed to assess strain on the carer. Its validity was well tested in the original paper. It has not been widely used.

Rivermead Behavioural Memory Test

The test has the following components:

1. Remembering a person's first name and surname, tested by associating the names with a face (photograph) and asking for the names when the photograph is shown again later (without warning).

2. Remembering ten common objects (which the subject is required to name and study), and five faces. The initial stimuli (objects, faces) are represented with the same number of additional distracting objects and the subject is required to identify the objects/faces initially seen.

3. Remembering the gist of a short prose passage, tested immediately and again after a 20-min delay.

4. Following a route around a room visiting five specified points, first immediately after being shown and then 20 min later. (A model or drawing can be used for immobile patients.) The patient is also asked to leave a message (envelope) at one point.

5. Remembering to ask for a personal belonging, which is taken from the patient at the beginning, at the end of the test (20–30 min delay).

6. Remembering a particular question (asking about the next appointment), the question being given initially with instructions to ask it when an alarm bell rings 20 min later.

7. Ten questions to test orientation in time, place, person, and one question asking for the date.

Items scored (for screening score)

1. First name of person in photograph
2. Second name (surname) of person in photograph
3. Remembering hidden belonging
4. Remembering to ask about appointment (question after alarm sounds)
5. Picture (object) recognition (selecting 10 from 20 shown)
6a. Prose recall—immediate (21 ideas)
6b. Prose recall—delayed (20 min)
7. Face recognition (recognizing 5 from 10 shown)
8a. Route—immediate (five places)
8b. Route—delayed (about 20 min)
9. Route—message (envelope to be left)
10. Orientation
11. Date (correct)

References   Wilson *et al.* (1985); Wilson *et al.* (1989)

Comment

An easy-to-use measure, not requiring specialist professional training and relatively short. It can be administered repeatedly (there are parallel versions). It is widely used in many different situations, for example in community surveys and is in regular use at the Rivermead Centre. It originally was scored to give a screening score out of 12 but now a screening score of 24 is used (calculated from the same tests). There is some experience in its use in patients with aphasia. A children's version is being developed.

Rivermead Perceptual Assessment Battery

This battery has 16 components, described by Barer *et al.* (1990) thus:

Test title	Description
Picture matching	Tests the ability to match identical pairs of picture cards, while discriminating from other similar pictures. Given first as a simple task to boost confidence.
Object matching	Tests 'form constancy', through the ability to match real objects according to shape. Colour is kept constant.
Colour matching	Assesses the patient's ability to recognize different shades of the same colour as belonging together. Coloured blocks must be placed in columns below correct stimulus colours.
Size recognition	The patient's ability to recognize and match two dimensional objects despite differences in size is tested, again assessing 'form constancy'.
Series	Patient is asked to arrange a series of pictures in size order, testing ability to sequence.
Animal halves	Tests object completion through the ability to put together two separate parts of familiar figures to complete the whole.
Missing article	Tests ability to recognize that a picture is incomplete, and to select the missing part. Another object completion task.
Figure-ground discrimination*	Patient is asked to recognize individual objects presented as part of a complex picture.
Sequencing pictures*	Tests ability to recognize that a set of pictures forms a sequence; involves understanding picture content.
Body image (a)*	Patient asked to assemble a jig-saw of a body. Assesses ability to recognize the whole and to assemble them in correct relationship.

Body image (b)*	As above, only with the face in isolation.
Right/left copying shapes*	Patient asked to copy shapes to right and left of midline. Tests neglects/inattention and spatial awareness.
Right/left copying words*	As above, only copying words.
Three-dimensional copying*	Patient asked to copy a three-dimensional model. Assesses form constancy and spatial awareness.
Cube copying*	Patient asked to copy two-dimensional design using cubes. Tests spatial awareness (and IQ). Like block design of WAIS.
Cancellation*	Patient asked to cancel selected letters from an array containing many letters. Assesses neglect, concentration and visual scanning.
Body image, self-identification	Patient asked to copy the assessor's bodily actions.

References   Whiting *et al.* (1985); Lincoln and Edmans (1989); Barer *et al.* (1990)

Comment
The Rivermead Perceptual Assessment Battery (RPAB) is designed to be used by occupational therapists who wish to assess perception. In practice it takes about two hours to complete; it is difficult to interpret; and each test can be influenced by several impairments. A useful collection of tests, well-tested but not very useful as a whole. The tests should be used selectively as needed. This has been made easier because Lincoln and Edmans (1989) have shown that selected sub-tests provide almost as much information: the sub-tests forming their version 'B' are identified by an asterisk. This reduces the time taken by 32 per cent but other selections can reduce the time by 45 per cent.

Wechsler Adult Intelligence Scales

The most widely used test of intelligence has the following subscales, divided into two domains: verbal intelligence and performance (non-verbal) intelligence.

Verbal	*Performance*
Information (general knowledge)	Digit-symbol
Comprehension	Picture completion
Arithmetic	Block design
Similarities (between objects)	Picture arrangement
Digit span	Object assembly
Vocabulary (meaning of words)	

References   Wechsler (1981); Lezak (1983)

Comment
The standard measure for assessing intelligence. Often results are prorated from a selection of the subtests.

Wechsler Memory Scale

A less widely used test which may now be superseded, for example by the Rivermead Behavioural Memory Test. It has seven components which may form three factors (Skilbeck and Woods 1980).

Orientation factor
  Personal information
  Orientation

Attention/concentration factor
  Mental control (e.g. count backwards from 20 to 1)
  Digit span

Memory/learning factor
  Logical memory (paragraph recall)
  Visual reproduction (recall of drawings)
  Paired associates (learning word pairs)

References   Wechsler (1945); Skilbeck and Woods (1980); Lezak (1983)

Comment
This test is limited and testing of specific aspects of memory requires specific tests (see Lezak 1983). The paragraph recall relates best to everyday performance (Sunderland *et al.* 1983).

Behavioural Inattention Test

Six conventional tests
- Line crossing (Albert's test)
- Letter cancellation
- Star cancellation
- Figure and shape copying
- Line bisection
- Representational drawing

Nine behavioural tests
- Picture scanning
- Telephone dialling
- Menu reading
- Article reading
- Telling and setting the time (digital clock)
- Coin sorting
- Address and sentence copying
- Map navigation
- Card sorting

References   Wilson *et al.* (1987*a*, *b*); Halligan *et al.* (1989)

Comment

A standard battery for detecting and measuring severity of visuospatial neglect. The Star Cancellation Test is the most sensitive at detecting neglect (Halligan *et al.* 1989). The line cancellation is Albert's Test (Albert 1973; Fullerton *et al.* 1986). Testing for tactile inattention may be the most economic method of detecting significant (i.e. prognostically important) neglect after stroke (Barer 1990).

References

Adams, D.L. (1969). Analysis of a life satisfaction index. *Journal of Gerontology*, **24**, 470–4.

Adams, R.J., Meador, K.J., Sethi, K.D., Grotta, J.C., and Thompson, D.S. (1987). Graded neurologic scale for use in acute hemispheric stroke treatment protocols. *Stroke*, **18**, 665–9.

Affleck, J.W., Aitken, R.C.B., Hunter, J.A.A., McGuire, R.J., and Roy, C.W. (1988). Rehabilitation status: a measure of medicosocial dysfunction. *Lancet*, **1**, 230–3.

Aggrell, B. and Dehlin, O. (1989). Comparison of six geriatric rating scales in geriatric stroke patients. *Stroke*, **20**, 1190–4.

Agre, J.C., Magness, J.L., Hull, S.Z. *et al.* (1987). Strength testing with a portable dynamometer: reliability for upper and lower extremities. *Archives of Physical Medicine and Rehabilitation*, **68**, 454–8.

Ahlsio, B., Britton, M., Murray, V., and Theorell, T. (1984). Disablement and quality of life after stroke. *Stroke*, **15**, 886–90.

Alba, A., Trainor, F.S., Ritter, W., and Dacso, M.M. (1968). A clinical rating scale for Parkinson patients. *Journal of Chronic Disease*, **21**, 507–22.

Albert, M.L. (1973). A simple test of visual neglect. *Neurology*, **23**, 658–64.

Allen, C.M.C. (1983). Clinical diagnosis of the acute stroke syndrome. *Quarterly Journal of Medicine*, **52**, 515–23.

Allen, C.M.C. (1984). Predicting the outcome of acute stroke: a prognostic score. *Journal of Neurology, Neurosurgery and Psychiatry*, **47**, 457–80.

Andres, P.L., Hedlund, W., Finison, L., Conlon, T., Felmus, M., and Munsat, T.L. (1986). Quantitative motor assessment in amyotrophic lateral sclerosis. *Neurology*, **36**, 937–41.

Andrews, K. and Stewart, J. (1979). Stroke recovery: he can but does he? *Rheumatology and Rehabilitation*, **18**, 43–8.

Annett, M. and Kilshaw, D. (1983). Right and left hand skill. *British Journal of Psychology*, **74**, 269–83.

Applegate, W.B., Blass, J.P., and Williams, T.F. (1990). Instruments for the functional assessment of older patients. *New England Journal of Medicine*, **322**, 1207–14.

Artiola i Fortuny, L., Briggs, M., Newcombe, F., Ratcliffe, G., and Thomas, C. (1980). Measuring the duration of post-traumatic amnesia. *Journal of Neurology, Neurosurgery and Psychiatry*, **43**, 377–9.

Ashburn, A. (1982). Assessment of motor function in stroke patients. *Physiotherapy*, **68**, 109–13.

Bamford, J.M. (1988). The classification and natural history of acute cerebrovascular disease. Unpublished. M.D. thesis. University of Manchester.

Bard, G. and Hirschberg, G.G. (1965). Recovery of voluntary motion in upper extremity following hemiplegia. *Archives of Physical Medicine and Rehabilitation*, **46**, 567–72.

Barer, D.H. (1989a). Continence after stroke: useful predictor or goal of therapy? *Age and Ageing*, **18**, 183–91.

Barer, D.H. (1989b). The natural history and functional consequences of dysphagia after hemisphere stroke. *Journal of Neurology, Neurosurgery and Psychiatry*, **52**, 236–41.

Barer, D.H. (1990). The influence of visual and tactile inattention on predictions for recovery from acute stroke. *Quarterly Journal of Medicine*, **273**, 21–32.

Barer, D. and Nouri, F. (1990). Measurement of activities of daily living. *Clinical Rehabilitation*, **3**, 179–87.

Barer, D.H., Edmans, J.A., and Lincoln, N.B. (1990). Screening for perceptual problems in acute stroke patients. *Clinical Rehabilitation*, **4**, 1–11.

Barlow, D.H. and Hersen, M. (1984) *Single case experimental designs. Strategies for studying behaviour change.* Pergamon Press, New York.

Beatty, W.W. and Goodkin, D.E. (1990). Screening for cognitive impairment in multiple sclerosis. An evaluation of the Mini-Mental State Examination. *Archives of Neurology*, **47**, 297–301.

Bebbington, A.C. (1977). Scaling indices of disablement. *British Journal of Preventive and Social Medicine*, **31**, 122–6.

Beck, A.T., Ward, C.H., Mendelson, M., Mock, J.E., and Erbaugh, J.K. (1961). An inventory for measuring depression. *Archives of General Psychiatry*, **4**, 561–71.

Bendall, M.J., Bassey, E.J., and Pearson, M.B. (1989). Factors affecting walking speed of elderly people. *Age and Ageing*, **18**, 327–32.

Benjamin, J. (1976). The Northwick Park ADL index. *British Journal of Occupational Therapy*, **39**, 301–6.

Berglund, K. and Fugl-Meyer, A.R. (1986). Upper extremity function in hemiplegia: a cross-validation study of two assessment methods. *Scandinavian Journal of Rehabilitation Medicine*, **18**, 155–7.

Bergner, M., Bobbitt, R.A., Carter, W.B., and Gibson, B.S. (1981). The Sickness Impact Profile: development and final revision of a health status measure. *Medical Care*, **19**, 789–805.

Bland, J.M. and Altman, D.G. (1986). Statistical methods for assessing agreement between two methods of clinical measurement. *Lancet*, **1**, 307–10.

Bleecker, M.M.L., Bolla-Wilson, K., Kawas, C., and Agnew, J. (1988). Age-specific norms for the minimental state exam. *Neurology*, **38**, 1565–8.

Blessed, G., Tomlinson, B.E., and Roth, M. (1968). The association between quantitative measures of dementia and of senile change in the cerebral grey matter of elderly subjects. *British Journal of Psychiatry*, **114**, 797–811.

Bohannon, R.W. (1989a). Is the measurement of muscle strength appropriate in patients with brain lesions? *Physical Therapy*, **69**, 225–30.

Bohannon, R.W. (1989b). Correlation of lower limb strengths and other variables with standing performance in stroke patients. *Physiotherapy Canada*, **41**, 198–202.

Bohannon, R.W. (1989c). Selected determinants of ambulatory capacity in patients with hemiplegia. *Clinical Rehabilitation*, **3**, 47–53.

Bohannon, R.W. and Andrews, A.W. (1987a). Interrater reliability of hand-held dynamometry. *Physical Therapy*, **67**, 931–3.

Bohannon, R.W. and Andrews, A.W. (1987*b*). Relative strength of seven upper extremity muscle groups in hemiparetic stroke patients. *Journal of Neurological Rehabilitation*, **1**, 161–5.

Bohannon, R.W. and Andrews, A.W. (1990). Correlation of knee extensor muscle torque and spasticity with gait speed in patients with stroke. *Archives of Physical Medicine and Rehabilitation*, **71**, 330–3.

Bohannon, R.W. and Smith, M.B. (1987). Interrater reliability of a modified Ashworth scale of muscle spasticity. *Physical Therapy*, 1987, **67**, 206–7.

Bracken, M.B., Webb, S.B., and Wagner, F.C. (1977–8). Classification of the severity of acute spinal cord injury: implications for management. *Paraplegia*, **15**, 319–26.

Bradstater, M.E., de Bruin, H., Gowland, C., and Clarke, B.M. (1983). Hemiplegic gait: analysis of temporal variables. *Archives of Physical Medicine and Rehabilitation*, **64**, 583–7.

Broadbent, D.E., Cooper, P.F., FitzGerald, P., and Parkes, K.R. (1982). The Cognitive Failures Questionnaire (CFQ) and its correlates. *British Journal of Clinical Psychology*, **21**, 1–16.

Brott, T., Adams, H.P., Olinger, C.P. *et al.* (1989). Measurements of acute cerebral infarction: a clinical examination scale. *Stroke*, **20**, 864–70.

Brown, R.G., MacCarthey, B., Gotham, A.M., Der, G.J., and Marsden, C.D. (1988). Depression and disability in Parkinson's Disease: a follow-up of 132 cases. *Psychological Medicine*, **18**, 49–55.

Brown, R.G., MacCarthey, B., Jahanshahi, M., and Marsden, D. (1989). Accuracy of self-reported disability in patients with parkinsonism. *Archives of Neurology*, **46**, 955–9.

Burke, R.E., Fahn, S., Marsden, D., Bressman, S.B., Moskowitz, C., and Friedman, J. (1985). Validity and reliability of a rating scale for the primary torsion dystonias. *Neurology*, **35**, 73–7.

Butland, R.J.A., Pang, J., Gross, E.R., Woodcock, A.A., and Geddes, D.M. (1982). Two, six, and twelve minute walking tests in respiratory disease. *British Medical Journal*, **284**, 1604–8.

Canter, G.J., De la Torre, R., and Mier, M. (1961). A method for evaluating disability in patients with Parkinson's Disease. *Journal of Nervous and Mental Diseases*, **133**, 143–7.

Capildeo, R. and Clifford Rose, F. (1979). The assessment of neurological disability. In *Progress in stroke research* (ed. R.M. Greenhalgh and F. Clifford Rose), pp. 106–16. Pitman Medical, London.

Carnwath, T.C.M. and Johnson, D.A.W. (1987). Psychiatric morbidity among spouses of patients with stroke. *British Medical Journal*, **294**, 409–11.

Carr, J.H., Shepherd, R.B., Nordholm, L. and Lynne, D. (1985). Investigation of a new motor assessment scale for stroke patients. *Physical Therapy*, **65**, 175–80.

Carroll, D. (1965). A quantitative test of upper extremity function. *Journal of Chronic Diseases*, **18**, 479–91.

Carroll, R.A., Borstein, S.S., and Hoffman, S.G. (1984). Rehabilitation networking: a solution for the future. In *Functional assessment in rehabilitation medicine* (ed. C.V. Granger and G.E. Gresham), pp. 364–77. Williams & Wilkins, Baltimore.

Charlton, J.R.H. (1989). Measuring disability in a longitudinal survey. In *Disablement in the community* (ed. D.L. Patrick and H. Peach), pp. 62–80. Oxford University Press.

Chien, C-P, Jung, K., and Ross-Townsend, A. (1980). Methodologic approach to measurement of tardive dyskinesia: piezoelectric recording and concurrent validity test on five clinical scales. In *Tardive dyskinesia; research and treatment* (ed. W.E. Fann, R.C. Smith, J.M. Davis, and E.F. Domino), pp. 233–66. Spectrum Publications, New York.

Chiou, I.L. and Burnett, C.N. (1985). Values of activities of daily living: a survey of stroke patients and their home therapists. *Archives of Physical Medicine and Rehabilitation*, **65**, 901–6.

Collen, F.M., Wade, D.T., and Bradshaw, C.M. (1990). Mobility after stroke: reliability of measures of impairment and disability. *International Disability Studies*, **12**, 6–9.

Collen, F.M., Wade, D.T., Robb, G.F., and Bradshaw, C.M. (1991). The Rivermead Mobility Index: a further development of the Rivermead Motor Assessment. *International Disability Studies*, **13**, in press.

Collin, C., Wade, D.T., Davis, S., and Horne, V. (1988). The Barthel ADL index: a reliability study. *International Disability Studies*, **10**, 61–3.

Collin, C. and Wade, D. (1990). Assessing motor impairment after stroke: a pilot reliability study. *Journal of Neurology, Neurosurgery and Psychiatry*, **53**, 576–9.

Cooper, P., Osborn, M., Gath, D., and Feggetter, G. (1982). Evaluation of a modified self-report measure of social adjustment. *British Journal of Psychiatry*, **141**, 68–75.

Corcoran, P.J., Jebson, R.H., Brengelman, G.L., and Simons, B.C. (1970). Effects of plastic and metal leg braces on speed and energy cost of hemiparetic ambulation. *Archives of Physical Medicine and Rehabilitation*, **51**, 69–77.

Corrigan, J.D. (1989). Development of a scale for assessment of agitation following traumatic brain injury. *Journal of Clinical and Experimental Neuropsychology*, **11**, 261–77.

Cote, R., Battista, R.N., Wolfson, C.M., and Hachinski, V. (1988). Stroke assessment scales: guidelines for development, validation, and reliability assessment. *Canadian Journal of Neurological Sciences*, **15**, 261–5.

Cote, R., Battista, R.N., Wolfson, C., Boucher, J., Adam, J., and Hachinski, V. (1989). The Canadian Neurological Scale: validation and reliability assessment. *Neurology*, **39**, 638–43.

Cramer, J.A., Smith, D.B., Mattson, R.H. *et al.* (1983). A method of quantification for the evaluation of antiepileptic drug therapy. *Neurology 33 Suppl*, **1**, 26–37.

Creed, P.J., Black, D., Anthony, P., Osborn, M., Thomas, P., and Tomenson, B. (1990). Randomised controlled trial of day patient versus inpatient psychiatric treatment. *British Medical Journal*, **300**, 1033–7.

Crow, J.L., Lincoln, N.N.B., Nouri, F.M., and De Weerdt, W. (1989). The effectiveness of EMG biofeedback in the treatment of arm function after stroke. *International Disability Studies*, **11**, 155–60.

Cunningham, D.A., Rechnitzer, P.A., Pearce, M.E., and Donner, A.P. (1982). Determinants of self-selected walking pace across ages 19 to 66. *Journal of Gerontology*, **37**, 560–4.

Demeurisse, G., Demol, O., and Robaye, E. (1980). Motor evaluation in vascular hemiplegia. *European Neurology*, **19**, 382–9.

DePaulo, J.R., Folstein, M.F., and Gordon, B. (1980). Psychiatric screening on a neurological ward. *Psychological Medicine*, **10**, 125–32.

DeSouza, L.H., Langton Hewer, R., and Miller, S. (1980). Assessment of recovery of arm control in hemiplegic stroke patients. Arm function test. *International Rehabilitation Medicine*, **2**, 3–9.

DeWeerdt, W.J.G. and Harrison, M.A. (1985). Measuring recovery of arm-hand function in stroke patients: a comparison of the Brunnstrom–Fugl-Meyer test and the Action Research Arm test. *Physiotherapy Canada*, **37**, 65–70.

Deyo, R.A. (1984). Measuring functional outcomes in therapeutic trials for chronic disease. *Controlled Clinical Trials*, **5**, 223–40.

Diamond, S.G. and Markham, C.H. (1983). Evaluating the evaluations: or how to weigh the scales of parkinsonian disability. *Neurology*, **33**, 1098–9.

Dick, J.P.R., Guiloff, R.J., Stewart, A., Blackstock, ., Bielawska, C., Paul, E.A., and Marsden, C.D. (1984). Mini-mental state examination in neurological patients. *Journal of Neurology, Neurosurgery and Psychiatry*, **47**, 496–9.

Donald, C.A., Ware, J.E., Brook, R.H., and Davies-Avery, A. (1978). *Conceptualisation and measurement of health for adults in the health insurance study*: Vol. IV. *Social Health*. Rand Pub No. R-1987/4-HEW, Santa Monica.

Donaldson, S.W., Wagner, C.C., and Gresham, G.E. (1973). A unified ADL evaluation form. *Archives of Physical Medicine and Rehabilitation*, **54**, 175–9.

Drummond, M.F. (1987). Resource allocation decisions in health care: a role for quality of life assessments? *Journal of Chronic Disease*, **40**, 605–16.

Duckworth, D. (1984). The need for a standard terminology and classification of disablement. In *Functional assessment in rehabilitation medicine* (ed. C.V. Granger and G.E. Gresham), pp. 1–13. Williams & Wilkins, Baltimore.

Duncan, P.W., Propst, M., and Nelson, S.G. (1983). Reliability of the Fugl-Meyer assessment of sensorimotor recovery following cerebrovascular accident. *Physical Therapy*, **63**, 1606–10.

Dyck, P.J. and O'Brien, P.C. (1989). Approaches to quantitative cutaneous sensory assessment. In *Quantification of neurologic deficit* (ed. T.L. Munsat), Chapter 15, pp. 187–95. Butterworths, Stoneham, MA 02180.

Eakin, P. (1989). Assessments of Activities of Daily Living: a critical review. *British Journal of Occupational Therapy*, **52**, 11–15.

Ebrahim, S., Nouri, F., and Barer, D. (1985). Measuring disability after stroke. *Journal of Epidemiology and Community Health*, **39**, 86–9.

Ebrahim, S., Barer, D., and Nouri, F. (1986). Use of the Nottingham Health Profile with patients after stroke. *Journal of Epidemiology and Community Health*, **40**, 166–9.

Enderby, P.M., Wood, V.A., Wade, D.T., and Langton Hewer, R. (1986). The Frenchay Aphasia Screening Test: a short, simple test for aphasia appropriate for non-specialists. *International Rehabilitation Medicine*, **8**, 166–70.

Epstein, A.M., Stern, R.S., Tognetti, J. *et al.* (1988). The association of patients' socioeconomic characteristics with the length of hospital stay and hospital charges within diagnosis-related groups. *New England Journal of Medicine*, **318**, 1579–85.

Fahn, S. (1989). Assessment of the primary dystonias. In *Quantification of neuro-logic deficit* (ed. T.L. Munsat), Chapter 19, pp. 241–70. Butterworths, Stoneham, MA 02180.

Fazio, A.F. (1977). *A concurrent validational study of the NCHS General Well-Being Schedule*. US Department of Health, Education and Welfare, National Centre for Health Statistics. (Vital and Health Statistics Series 2, No. 73. DHEW Publication No (HRA) 78-1347).

Feinstein, A.R., Josephy, B.R., and Wells, C.K. (1986). Scientific and clinical problems in indexes of functional disability. *Annals of Internal Medicine*, **105**, 413–20.

Fleiss, J.L. (1971). Measuring nominal scale agreement among many raters. *Psychological Bulletin*, **76**, 378–82.

Folstein, M.F. and Luria, R. (1973). Reliability, validity and clinical application of the visual analogue mood scale. *Psychological Medicine*, **3**, 479–86.

Folstein, S.E., Jensen, B., Leigh, J., and Folstein, M.F. (1983). The measurement of abnormal movement: methods developed for Huntington's disease. *Neuro-behavioural Toxicology and Teratology*, **5**, 605–9.

Frankel, H.L., Hancock, D.O., Hyslop, G. *et al.* (1969). The value of postural reduction in the initial management of closed injuries of the spine with paraplegia and tetraplegia. *Paraplegia*, **7**, 179–92.

Froberg, D.G. and Kane, R.L. (1989). Methodology for measuring health-state preferences: I: Measurement strategies; II: Scaling methods; III: Population and context effects; IV: Progress and a research agenda. *Journal of Clinical Epidemiology*, **42**, 345–54; 459–71; 585–92; 675–85.

Fugl-Meyer, A.R., Jaasko, L., Leyman, I., Olsson, S., and Steglind, S. (1975). The post-stroke hemiplegic patient. 1. A method for evaluation of physical performance. *Scandinavian Journal of Rehabilitation Medicine*, **7**, 13–31.

Fullerton, K.J., McSherry, D., and Stout, R.W. (1986). Albert's Test: a neglected test of perceptual neglect. *Lancet*, **1**, 430–2.

Galasko, D., Klauber, M.R., Hofstetter, R., Salmon, D.P., Lasker, B., and Thal, L.J. (1990). The Mini-Mental State Examination in the early diagnosis of Alzheimer's disease. *Archives of Neurology*, **47**, 49–52.

Garraway, W.M., Akhtar, A.J., Gore, S.M., Prescott, R.J., and Smith, R.G. (1976). Observer variation in the clinical assessment of stroke. *Age and Ageing*, **5**, 233–9.

Gilleard, C.J. and Pattie, A.H. (1977). The Stockton Geriatric Rating scale: a shortened version with British normative data. *British Journal of Psychiatry*, **131**, 90–4.

Goetz, C.G., Tanner, C.M., Wilson, R.S., and Shannon, K.M. (1987). A rating scale for Gilles de la Tourette's syndrome: description, reliability and validity data. *Neurology*, **37**, 1542–4.

Goldberg, D.P. (1972). *The detection of psychiatric illness by questionnaire*. Maudsley Monograph No. 21. Oxford University Press, Oxford.

Goldberg, D.P. and Hillier, V.F. (1979). A scaled version of the General Health Questionnaire. *Psychological Medicine*, **9**, 139–45.

Goldfarb, B.J. and Simon, S.R. (1984). Gait patterns in patients with amyotrophic lateral sclerosis. *Archives of Physical Medicine and Rehabilitation*, **65**, 61–5.

Goldstein, L.B., Bertels, C., and Davis, J.N. (1989). Interrater reliability of the NIH stroke scale. *Archives of Neurology*, **46**, 660–2.

Goodkin, R. and Diller, L. (1973). Reliability among physical therapists in diagnosis and treatment of gait deviations in hemiplegics. *Perceptual and Motor Skills*, **37**, 727–34.

Goodkin, D.E., Hertsgaard, D., and Seminary, J. (1988). Upper extremity function in multiple sclerosis: improving assessment sensitivity with box-and-block and nine-hole peg tests. *Archives of Physical Medicine and Rehabilitation*, **69**, 850–4.

Gordon, C., Langton Hewer, R., and Wade, D.T. (1987). Dysphagia in acute stroke. *British Medical Journal*, **295**, 411–14.

Gouvier, W.D., Blanton, P.D., LaPorte, K.K., and Nepomuceno, C. (1987). Reliability and validity of the Disability Rating Scale and the Levels of Cognitive Functioning Scale in monitoring recovery from severe head injury. *Archives of Physical Medicine and Rehabilitation*, **68**, 94–7.

Granger, C.V. (1984). A conceptual model for functional assessment. In *Functional assessment in rehabilitation medicine* (ed. C.V. Granger and G.E. Gresham), pp. 14–25. Williams & Wilkins, Baltimore.

Granger, C.V. and McNamara, M.A. (1984). Functional assessment utilisation: the Long-Range Evaluation System (LRES). In *Functional assessment in rehabilitation medicine* (ed. C.V. Granger and G.E. Gresham), pp. 99–121. Williams & Wilkins, Baltimore.

Granger, C.V., Albrecht, G.L., and Hamilton, B.B. (1979). Outcome of comprehensive medical rehabilitation: measurement by PULSES profile and the Barthel index. *Archives of Physical Medicine and Rehabilitation*, **60**, 145–54.

Granger, C.V., Hamilton, B.B., and Sherwin, F.S. (1986). *Guide for the use of the uniform data set for medical rehabilitation*. Uniform Data System for Medical Rehabilitation Project Office, Buffalo General Hospital, New York 14203, USA.

Gresham, G.E. and Labi, M.L.C. (1984). Functional assessment instruments currently available for documenting outcomes in rehabilitation medicine. In *Functional assessment in rehabilitation medicine* (ed. C.V. Granger and G.E. Gresham), pp. 65–85. Williams & Wilkins.

Gresham, G.E., Philips, T.F., and Labi, M.L.C. (1980). ADL status in stroke: relative merits of three standard indexes. *Archives of Physical Medicine and Rehabilitation*, **61**, 355–8.

Gronwall, D.M.A. (1977). Paced Auditory Serial Addition Task: a measure of recovery from concussion. *Perceptual and Motor Skills*, **44**, 367–73.

Gronwall, D. and Wrightson, P. (1974). Delayed recovery of intellectual function after minor head injury. *Lancet*, **2**, 605–9.

Gronwall, D. and Wrightson, P. (1975). Cumulative effect of concussion. *Lancet*, **2**, 995–7.

Gronwall, D. and Wrightson, P. (1980). Duration of Post-traumatic Amnesia after mild head injury. *Journal of Clinical Neuropsychology*, **2**, 51–60.

Gross, C.R., Shinar, D., Mohr, J.P. *et al.* (1986). Interobserver agreement in the diagnosis of stroke type. *Archives of Neurology*, **43**, 893–8.

Grynderup, V. (1969). A comparison of some rating scales in multiple sclerosis. *Acta Neurologica Scandinavica*, **45**, 611–22.

Guyatt, G.H., Pugsley, S.O., Sullivan, M.J. *et al.* (1984). Effect of encouragement on walking test performance. *Thorax*, **39**, 818–22.

Guyatt, G., Walter, S., and Norman, G. (1987). Measuring change over time: assessing the usefulness of evaluative instruments. *Journal of Chronic Disease*, **40**, 171–8.

Hachinski, V.C., Iliff, L.D., Zilhka, E. *et al.* (1975). Cerebral blood flow in dementia. *Archives of Neurology*, **32**, 632–7.

Hall, K., Cope, N., and Rappaport, M. (1985). Glasgow Outcome Scale and Disability rating scale: comparative usefulness in following recovery in traumatic head injury. *Archives of Physical Medicine and Rehabilitation*, **66**, 35–7.

Halligan, P.W., Marshall, J.C., and Wade, D.T. (1989). Visuospatial neglect: underlying factors and test sensitivity. *Lancet*, **2**, 908–10.

Hamilton, M. (1967). Development of a rating scale for primary depressive illness. *British Journal of Social and Clinical Psychology*, **6**, 278–96.

Hanley, J. and McAndrew, L. (1987). A survey of the younger chronic sick and disabled in the community in Lothian Region. *International Disability Studies*, **8**, 74–7.

Harcherik, D.F., Leckman, J.F., Detlor, J., and Cohen, D.J. (1984). A new instrument for clinical studies of Tourette's syndrome. *Journal of American Academy Child Psychiatry*, **23**, 153–60.

Hauser, S.L., Dawson, D.M., Lehrich, J.R. *et al.* (1983). Intensive immuno-suppression in progressive multiple sclerosis: a randomised, three-arm study of high-dose intravenous cyclophosphamide, plasma exchange, and ACTH. *New England Journal of Medicine*, **308**, 173–80.

Heller, A., Wade, D.T., Wood, V.A., Sunderland, A., Langton Hewer, R., and Ward, E. (1987). Arm function after stroke: measurement and recovery over the first three months. *Journal of Neurology, Neurosurgery and Psychiatry*, **50**, 714–19.

Hodkinson, H.M. (1972). Evaluation of a mental test score for assessment of mental impairment in the elderly. *Age and Ageing*, **1**, 233–8.

Hoehn, M.M. and Yahr, M.D. (1967). Parkinsonism: onset, progression and mortality. *Neurology*, **17**, 427–42.

Hogarty, G.E. and Katz, M.M. (1971). Norms of adjustment and social behaviour. *Archives of General Psychiatry*, **25**, 470–80.

Holbrook, M. and Skilbeck, C.E. (1983). An activities index for use with stroke patients. *Age and Ageing*, **12**, 166–70.

Holden, M.K., Gill, K.M., Magliozzi, M.R., Nathan, J., Piehl-Baker, L. (1984). Clinical gait assessment in the neurologically impaired: reliability and meaningfulness. *Physical Therapy*, **64**, 35–40.

Holden, M.K., Gill, K.M., and Magliozzi, M.R. (1986). Gait assessment for neurologically impaired patients. Standards for outcome assessment. *Physical Therapy*, **66**, 1530–9.

House, A. (1987). Mood disorders after stroke: a review of the evidence. *International Journal of Geriatric Psychiatry*, **2**, 211–21.

House, A., Dennis, M., Molyneux, A., Warlow, C., and Hawton, K. (1989*a*). Emotionalism after stroke. *British Medical Journal*, **298**, 991–4.

House, A., Dennis, M., Hawton, K., and Warlow, C. (1989*b*). Methods of identifying mood disorders in stroke patients: experience in the Oxfordshire Community Stroke Project. *Age and Ageing*, **18**, 371–9.

Hoyt, D.R. and Creech, J.C. (1983). The life satisfaction index: a methodological and theoretical critique. *Journal of Gerontology*, **38**, 111–16.

Hunt, S.M., McKenna, S.P., McEwan, J. *et al.* (1980). A quantitative approach to perceived health status: a validation study. *Journal of Epidemiology and Community Health*, **34**, 281–6.

Hunt, S.M., McKenna, S.P., and Williams, J. (1981). Reliability of a population survey tool for measuring perceived health problems: a study of patients with osteo-arthritis. *Journal of Epidemiology and Community Health*, **35**, 297–300.

Hunter, J. (1986). What does 'virtually unable to walk' mean? *British Medical Journal*, **292**, 172–3.

Hutchinson, T.A., Body, N.F., Feinstein, A.R. *et al.* (1979). Scientific problems in clinical scales, as demonstrated by the Karnofsky Index of performance status. *Journal of Chronic Disease*, **32**, 661–6.

Iwasaki, Y., Kinoshita, M., Ikeda, K., Takamiya, K., and Shiojima, T. (1990). Cognitive impairment in amyotrophic lateral sclerosis and its relation to motor disabilities. *Acta Neurologica Scandinavica*, **81**, 141–3.

Jackson, H.F., Hopewell, A.C., Glass, C.A., Ghadliali, E., and Warburg, R. (   ). The Katz adjustment scale: modification for use with victims of traumatic brain and spinal injury. *Brain Injury*—submitted for publication.

Jagger, J., Jane, J.A., and Rimel, R. (1983). The Glasgow Coma Scale: to sum or not to sum? *Lancet*, **2**, 97.

Jebsen, R.H., Taylor, N., Trieschmann, B.B., Trotter, M.J., and Howard, L.A. (1969). An objective and standardised test of hand function. *Archives of Physical Medicine and Rehabilitation*, **50**, 311–19.

Jennett, B. and Bond, M. (1975). Assessment of outcome after severe brain damage. A practical scale. *Lancet*, **1**, 480–4.

Jennett, B., Snoek, J., Bond, M.R. *et al.* (1981). Disability after severe head injury; observations on the use of the Glasgow Outcome Scale. *Journal of Neurology, Neurosurgery and Psychiatry*, **44**, 285–93.

Jette, A.M. and Clearly, P.D. (1987). Functional Disability Assessment. *Physical Therapy*, **67**, 1854–9.

Kaplan, R.M. and Bush, J.W. (1982). Health-related quality of life measurement for evaluation research and policy analysis. *Health Psychology*, **1**, 61–80.

Kaplan, R.M., Bush, J.W., and Berry, C.C. (1978). The reliability, stability and generalisability of a health status index. *American Statistical Association Proceedings of the Social Statistics Section*, pp. 704–9.

Karnofsky, D.A., Burchenal, J.H., Armistead, G.C. *et al.* (1951). Triethylene melamine in the treatment of neoplastic disease. *Archives of Internal Medicine*, 1951, **87**, 477–516.

Kase, C.S., Wolf, P.A.A., Chodosh, E.H. *et al.* (1989). Prevalence of silent stroke in patients presenting with initial stroke: the Framingham study. *Stroke*, **20**, 850–2.

Katz, M.M. and Lyerly, S.B. (1963). Methods for measuring adjustment and social behaviour in the community: 1. Rational, description, discriminative validity and scale development. *Psychological Reports*, **13**, 503–35.

Katz, S., Ford, A.B., Moskowitz, R.W., Jackson, B.A., and Jaffe, M.W. (1963). Studies of illness in the aged. The index of ADL: a standardised measure of biological and psychosocial function. *Journal of the American Medical Association*, **185**, 914–19.

Katzman, R., Brown, T., Fuld, P., Peck, A., Schechter, R., and Schimmel, H. (1983). Validation of a short Orientation–Memory–Concentration test of cognitive impairment. *American Journal of Psychiatry*, 1983, **140**, 734–9.

Kellor, M., Frost, J., Silberberg, N., Iversen, I., and Cummings, R. (1971). Hand strength and dexterity. *American Journal of Occupational Therapy*, **25**, 77–83.

Kennedy, P., Fisher, K., and Pearson, E. (1988). Ecological evaluation of a rehabilitative environment for spinal cord injured people: behavioural mapping and feedback. *British Journal of Clinical Psychology*, **27**, 239–46.

King, P. and Barrowclough, C. (1989). Rating the motivation of elderly patients on a rehabilitation ward. *Clinical Rehabilitation*, **3**, 289–91.

Klockgether, T., Schroth, G., Diener, H.C., and Dichgans, J. (1990). Idiopathic cerebellar ataxia of late onset: natural history and MRI morphology. *Journal of Neurology, Neurosurgery and Psychiatry*, **53**, 297–305.

Knaus, W.A., Draper, E.A., Wagner, D.P. *et al.* (1985). APACHE II: a severity of disease classification system. *Critical Care Medicine*, **13**, 818–29.

Kruse, J.A., Thill-Baharozian, M.C., and Carlson, R.W. (1988). Comparison of clinical assessment with APACHE II for predicting mortality risk in patients admitted to a medical intensive care unit. *Journal of the American Medical Association*, **260**, 1739–42.

Kurtzke, J.F. (1955). A new scale for evaluating disability in multiple sclerosis. *Neurology*, **5**, 580–3.

Kurtzke, J.F. (1965). Further notes on disability evaluation in multiple sclerosis, with scale modifications. *Neurology*, **15**, 654–61.

Kurtzke, J.F. (1983). Rating neurologic impairment in multiple sclerosis: an expanded disability status scale (EDSS). *Neurology*, **33**, 1444–52.

Kurtzke, J.F. (1981). A proposal for a uniform minimal record of disability in multiple sclerosis. *Acta Neurologica Scandinavica*, **64** Suppl 87, 110–29.

Kurtzke, J.F. (1989). The Disability Status Scale for multiple sclerosis: apologia pro DSS sua. *Neurology*, **39**, 291–302.

Kuzma, J.W., Namerow, N.S., Tourtellotte, W.W. *et al.* (1969). An assessment of the reliability of three methods used in evaluating the status of multiple sclerosis patients. *Journal of Chronic Disease*, **21**, 803–14.

Landis, J.R. and Koch, G.G. (1977). The measurement of observer agreement for categorical data. *Biometrics*, **33**, 159–74.

Lang, A.E.T. and Fahn, S. (1989). Assessment of Parkinson's Disease. In *Quantification of neurologic deficit* (ed. T.L. Munsat), Chapter 21, pp. 285–309. Butterworths, Stoneham, MA 02180.

LaRocca, N.G. (1989). Statistical and methodologic considerations in scale construction. In *Quantification of neurologic deficit* (ed. T.L. Munsat), Chapter 21, pp. 49–67. Butterworths, Stoneham, MA 02180.

Law, M. and Letts, L. (1989). A critical review of scales of Activities of Daily Living. *American Journal of Occupational Therapy*, **43**, 522–8.

Levin, H.S. and Grossman, R.G. (1978). Behavioural sequelae of closed head injury. *Archives of Neurology*, **35**, 720–7.

Levin, H.S., O'Donnell, V.M., and Grossman, R.G. (1979). The Galveston Orientation and Amnesia Test. A practical scale to assess cognition after head injury. *Journal of Nervous and Mental Disease*, **167**, 675–84.

Levin, H.S., High, W.M., Goethe, K.E. *et al.* (1987). The neurobehavioural rating scale: assessment of the behavioural sequelae of head injury by the clinician. *Journal of Neurology, Neurosurgery and Psychiatry*, **50**, 183–93.

Levy, D.E., Bates, D., Caronna, J.J. *et al.* (1981). Prognosis in non-traumatic coma. *Annals of Internal Medicine*, **94**, 293–301.

Lezak, M.D. (1983). *Neuropsychological assessment* (2nd edn). New York, Oxford University Press.

Li, C., Houlden, D.A., and Rowed, D.W. (1990). Somatosensory evoked potentials and neurologic grades as predictors of outcome in acute spinal cord injury. *Journal of Neurosurgery*, **72**, 600–9.

Lieberman, A.N. (1974). Parkinson's disease: a clinical review. *American Journal of Medical Science*, **267**, 66–80.

Lincoln, N.B. (1981). Discrepancies between capabilities and performance of activities of daily living in multiple sclerosis patients. *International Rehabilitation Medicine*, **3**, 84–8.

Lincoln, N.B. (1982). The Speech Questionnaire: an assessment of functional language ability. *International Rehabilitation Medicine*, **4**, 114–17.

Lincoln, N.B. and Edmans, J.A. (1989). A shortened version of the Rivermead Perceptual Assessment Battery? *Clinical Rehabilitation*, **3**, 199–204.

Lincoln, N.B. and Edmans, J.A. (1990). A re-validation of the Rivermead ADL scale for elderly patients with stroke. *Age and Ageing*, **19**, 9–24.

Lincoln, N. and Leadbitter, D. (1979). Assessment of motor function in stroke patients. *Physiotherapy*, **65**, 48–51.

Lincoln, N.B. and Tinson, D.J. (1989). The relation between subjective and objective memory impairment after stroke. *British Journal of Clinical Psychology*, **28**, 61–5.

Lincoln, N.B., Gamlen, R., and Thomason, H. (1989). Behavioural mapping of patients on a stroke unit. *International Disability Studies*, **11**, 149–54.

Lindblom, U. and Tegner, R. (1989). Quantification of sensibility in mononeuropathy, polyneuropathy, and central lesions. In *Quantification of neurologic deficit* (ed. T.L. Munsat), Chapter 14, pp. 171–85. Butterworths, Stoneham, MA 02180.

Lipkin, D.P., Scriven, A.J., Crake, T., and Poole-Wilson, P.A. (1986). Six minute walking test for assessing exercise capacity in chronic heart failure. *British Medical Journal*, **292**, 653–5.

Livingstone, M.G. and Livingstone, H.M. (1985). The Glasgow Assessment Schedule: clinical and research assessment of head injury outcome. *International Rehabilitation Medicine*, **7**, 145–9.

Loewen, S.C. and Anderson, B.A. (1988). Reliability of the Modified Motor Assessment Scale and the Barthel index. *Physical Therapy*, **68**, 1077–81.

Lucas, J.T. and Ducker, T.B. (1979). Motor classification of spinal cord injuries with mobility, morbidity and recovery indices. *American Surgeon*, **45**, 151–8.

Luker, K.A. (1979). Measuring life satisfaction in an elderly female population. *Journal of Advanced Nursing*, **4**, 503–11.

Lyle, R.C. (1981). A performance test for assessment of upper limb function in physical rehabilitation treatment and research. *International Journal of Rehabilitation Research*, **4**, 483–92.

Maas, A.I.R., Braakman, R., Schouten, H.J.A., Minderhoud, J.M., and Van Zomeren, A.H. (1983). Agreement between physicians on assessment of outcome following severe head injury. *Journal of Neurosurgery*, **58**, 321–5.

McDowell, I. and Newell, C. (1987). *Measuring Health: a Guide to Rating Scales and Questionnaires.* Oxford University Press, Oxford.

McDowell, F., Lee, J.E., Swift, T., Sweet, R.D., Ogsbury, J.S., and Kessler, J.T. (1970). Treatment of Parkinson's syndrome with L Dihydroxyphenylalanine (Levodopa). *Annals of Internal Medicine*, **72**, 29–35.

McGinnis, G.E., Seward, M.L., DeJong, G., and Osberg, J.S. (1986). Program evaluation of physical medicine and rehabilitation departments using self-report Barthel. *Archives of Physical Medicine and Rehabilitation*, **67**, 123–5.

McLenahan, R., Johnston, M., and Denshan, Y. (1990). Misperceptions of comprehension difficulties of stroke patients by doctors, nurses and relatives. *Journal of Neurology, Neurosurgery and Psychiatry*, **53**, 700–1.

McKenna, S., Hunt, S., and McEwan, J. (1981). Weighting the seriousness of perceived health problems using Thurstones method of paired comparisons. *International Journal of Epidemiology*, **10**, 93–7.

MacKenzie, C.R. and Charlson, M.E. (1986). Standards for the use of ordinal scales in clinical trials. *British Medical Journal*, **292**, 40–3.

McLellan, D.L. (1977). Co-contraction and stretch reflexes in spasticity during treatment with baclofen. *Journal of Neurology, Neurosurgery and Psychiatry*, **40**, 30–8.

Marsden, C.D. and Schachter, M. (1981). Assessment of extra-pyramidal disorders. *British Journal of Clinical Pharmacology*, **11**, 129–51.

Martin, J., Meltzer, H., and Elliot, D. (1988). *The prevalence of disability among adults.* Office of Population Censuses and Surveys, HMSO, London.

Mathew, N.T., Meyer, J.S., Rivera, V.M., Charney, J.Z., and Hartmann, A. (1972). Double-blind evaluation of glycerol therapy in acute cerebral infarction. *Lancet*, **2**, 1327–9.

Mathiowetz, V., Kashman, N., Volland, G., Weber, K., Dowe, M., and Rogers, S. (1975). Grip and pinch strength: normative data for adults. *Archives of Physical Medicine and Rehabilitation*, **66**, 69–72.

Mathiowetz, V., Volland, G., Kashman, N., and Weber, K. (1985). Adult norms for the box and block test of manual dexterity. *American Journal of Occupational Therapy*, **39**, 386–91.

Mathiowetz, V., Weber, K., Kashman, N., and Volland, G. (1985). Adult norms for the nine-hole peg test of finger dexterity. *Occupational Therapy Journal of Research*, **5**, 24–37.

May, D., Nayan, U.S.L., and Isaacs, B. (1985). The life-space diary: a measure of mobility in old people at home. *International Rehabilitation Medicine*, **7**, 182–7.

Mayeux, R., Stern, Y., Rosenstein, R., Marder, K., Hauser, A., Cote, L., and Fahn, S. (1988). An estimate of the prevalence of dementia in idiopathic Parkinson's disease. *Archives of Neurology*, **45**, 260–2.

Mickey, M.R., Ellison, G.W., and Myers, L.W. (1984). An illness severity score for multiple sclerosis. *Neurology*, **34**, 1343–7.

Miller, N. (1986). Dyspraxia and its management. Croom Helm, London and Sydney.

Milligan, N.M., Newcombe, R., and Compston, D.A.S. (1987). A double-blind controlled trial of high dose methylprednisolone in patients with multiple sclerosis: 1. Clinical effects. *Journal of Neurology, Neurosurgery and Psychiatry*, **50**, 511–16.

Minden, S.L. and Schiffer, R.B. (1990). Affective disorders in multiple sclerosis. Review and recommendations for clinical research. *Archives of Neurology*, **47**, 98–104.

Minderhoud, J.M., Dassel, H., and Prange, A.J.A. (1984). Proposal for summing the incapacity status or environmental status scores. *Acta Neurologica Scandinavica*, **70 Suppl 101**, 87–91.

Molsa, P.K., Paljarvi, L., Rinne, J.O., Rinne, U.K., and Sako, E. (1985). Validity of clinical diagnosis in dementia: a prospective clinico-pathological study. *Journal of Neurology, Neurosurgery and Psychiatry*, **48**, 1085–90.

Mor, V. and Guadagnoli, E. (1988). Quality of life measurement: a psychometric tower of Babel. *Journal of Clinical Epidemiology*, **41**, 1055–8.

Munsat, T.L. (ed.) (1989). *Quantification of neurologic deficit*. Butterworths, Boston.

Nelson, H.E. and O'Connell, A. (1978). Dementia: the estimation of premorbid intelligence levels using the New Adult Reading Test. *Cortex*, **14**, 234–44.

Neugarten, B.L., Havighurst, R.J., and Tobin, S.S. (1961). The measurement of life satisfaction. *Journal of Gerontology*, **16**, 134–43.

Newton, T., Butler, N.M., and Dawson, I. (1989). Engagement levels on a unit for people with a physical disability. *Clinical Rehabilitation*, **3**, 299–304.

Niemi, M.L., Laaksonen, R., Kotila, M., and Waltimo, O. (1988). Quality of life four years after stroke. *Stroke*, **19**, 1101–7.

Norstrom, T. and Thorslund, M. (1991). The structure of IADL and ADL measures. *Age and Aging*, **20**, 23–8.

Noseworthy, J.H., Vandrvoort, M.K., Wong, C.J., Ebers, G.C., and the Canadian Cooperative MS Study Group. (1990). Interrater variability with the Expanded Disability Status Scale (EDSS) and Functional Systems (FS) in a multiple sclerosis clinical trial. *Neurology*, **40**, 971–5.

Nouri, F.M. and Lincoln, N.B. (1987). An extended activities of daily living scale for stroke patients. *Clinical Rehabilitation*, **1**, 301–5.

O'Neill, P.A., Cheadle, B., Wyatt, R., McGuffog, J., and Fullerton, K.J. (1990). The value of the Frenchay Aphasia Screening Test for dysphasia: better than the clinician? *Clinical Rehabilitation*, **4**, 123–8.

Orgogozo, J.M. (1989). Evaluation of treatments in ischaemic-stroke patients. In *Clinical trial methodology in stroke* (ed. W.K. Amery, M.G. Bousser, and F.C. Rose), Chapter 3, pp. 35–53. Ballière Tindall, London.

Parker, V.M., Wade, D.T., and Langton Hewer, R. (1986). Loss of arm function after stroke: measurement, frequency and recovery. *International Rehabilitation Medicine*, **8**, 69–73.

Partridge, C. and Johnston, M. (1989). Perceived control of recovery from physical disability: measurement and prediction. *British Journal of Clinical Psychology*, **28**, 53–9.

Patrick, D.L. and Peach, H. (eds) (1989). *Disablement in the community*, Appendix 1 and 2. Oxford University Press, Oxford.

Patrick, D.L., Bush, J.W., and Chen, M.M. (1973). Methods for measuring levels of well being for a Health Status Index. *Health Services Research*, **10**, 181–98.

Pattie, A.H. and Gilleard, C.J. (1975). A brief psychogeriatric assessment schedule. Validation against psychiatric diagnosis and discharge from hospital. *British Journal of Psychiatry*, **127**, 489–93.

Pattie, A.H. and Gilleard, C.J. (1978). The two-year predictive validity of the Clifton Assessment Schedule and the shortened Geriatric Rating Scale. *British Journal of Psychiatry*, **133**, 457–60.

Peyser, J.M., Rao, S.M., LaRocca, N.G., and Kaplan, E. (1990). Guidelines for neuropsychological research in multiple sclerosis. *Archives of Neurology*, **47**, 94–7.

Philips, P. (1986). Grip strength, mental performance and nutritional status as indicators of mortality risk among female geriatric patients. *Age and Ageing*, **15**, 53–6.

Piepmeier, J.M. and Jenkins, N.R. (1988). Late neurological changes following traumatic spinal cord injury. *Journal of Neurosurgery*, **69**, 399–402.

Poole, J.L. and Whitney, S.L. (1988). Motor Assessment Scale for stroke patients: concurrent validity and interrater reliability. *Archives of Physical Medicine and Rehabilitation*, **69**, 195–7.

Poser, C.M., Paty, D.W., Scheinberg, L. *et al.* (1983). New diagnostic criteria for multiple sclerosis: guidelines for research protocols. *Annals of Neurology*, **13**, 227–31.

Prescott, R.J., Garraway, W.M., and Akhtar, A.L. (1982). Predicting functional outcome following acute stroke using a standard clinical examination. *Stroke*, **13**, 641–7.

Qureshi, K.N. and Hodkinson, H.M. (1974). Evaluation of a ten-question mental test in the institutional elderly. *Age and Ageing*, **3**, 152–7.

Rai, G.S., Stewart, K., and Scott, L.C. (1990). Assessment of anomalous sentences repetition test. *Journal of Neurology, Neurosurgery and Psychiatry*, **53**, 611–12.

Raimondi, A.J. and Hirschauer, J. (1984). Head injury in the infant and toddler; coma scoring and outcome scale. *Child's Brain*, **11**, 12–35.

Rankin, J. (1957). Cerebral vascular accidents in patients over the age of 60. 2. Prognosis. *Scottish Medical Journal*, **2**, 200–15.

Rappaport, M., Hall, K.M., Hopkins, K., Belleza, T., and Cope, D.N. (1982). Disability rating scale for severe head trauma: coma to community. *Archives of Physical Medicine and Rehabilitation*, **63**, 118–23.

Raven, J.C. (1960). *Guide to the standard progressive matrices*. H.K. Lewis, London.

Raven, J.C. (1965). *Guide to using the coloured progressive matrices*. H.K. Lewis, London.

Read, J.L., Quinn, R.J., and Hoefer, M.A. (1987). Measuring overall health: an evaluation of three important approaches. *Journal of Chronic Disease*, **40** Suppl 1, 7S–21S.

Roberts, R.C., Shorvon, S.D., Cox, T.C.S., and Gilliatt, R.W. (1988). Clinically unsuspected cerebral infarction revealed by computed tomography scanning in late onset epilepsy. *Epilepsia*, **29**, 190–4.

Robinson, B.C. (1983). Validation of a caregiver strain index. *Journal of Gerontology*, **38**, 344–8.

Robinson, J.L. and Smidt, G.L. (1981). Quantitative gait evaluation in the clinic. *Physical Therapy*, **61**, 351–3.

Rosser, R.M. and Watts, V.C. (1972). The measurement of hospital output. *International Journal of Epidemiology*, **1**, 361–8.

Rosser, R.M. and Kind, P. (1978). A scale of valuations of states of illness—is there a social consensus? *International Journal of Epidemiology*, **7**, 347–58.

Roy, C.W., Tognneri, J., Hay, E., and Pentland, B. (1988). An inter-rater reliability study of the Barthel index. *International Journal of Rehabilitation Research*, **11**, 67–70.

Sackett, D.L. and Torrance, G.W. (1978). The utility of different health states as perceived by the general public. *Journal of Chronic Disease*, **31**, 697–704.

Salkind, M.R. (1969). Beck depression inventory in general practice. *Journal of Royal College General Practitioners*, **18**, 267–71.

Sandercock, P.A.G., Allen, C.M.C., Corston, R.N., Harrison, M.J.G., and Warlow, C.P. (1985). Clinical diagnosis of intracranial haemorrhage using Guy's Hospital score. *British Medical Journal*, **291**, 1675–7.

Sandford, J.R.A. (1975). Tolerance of debility in elderly dependents by supporters at home: its significance for hospital practice. *British Medical Journal*, **3**, 471–3.

Schindler, J.S., Brown, R., Welburn, P., and Parkes, J.D. (1987). Measuring the quality of life of patients with Parkinson's Disease. In *Quality of life: assessment and application* (ed. S.R. Walker and R.M. Rosser), pp. 223–34. MTP Press.

Schoening, H.A. and Iversen, I.A. (1968). Numerical scoring of self-care status: a study of the Kenny self care evaluation. *Archives of Physical Medicine and Rehabilitation*, **49**, 221–9.

Schoening, H.A., Anderegg, L., Bergstrom, D., Fonda, M., Steinke, N., and Ulrich, P. (1965). Numerical scoring of self-care status of patients. *Archives of Physical Medicine and Rehabilitation*, **46**, 689–97.

Schwab, R.S. and England, A.C. (1969). Projection technique for evaluating surgery in Parkinson's Disease. In *Third symposium on Parkinson's Disease* (ed. F.J. Gillingham and M.C. Donaldson), pp. 152–7. Livingstone, Edinburgh.

Shah, S., Vanclay, F., and Cooper, B. (1989). Improving the sensitivity of the Barthel index for stroke rehabilitation. *Journal of Clinical Epidemiology*, **42**, 703–9.

Shapiro, A., Susak, Z., Malkin, C., and Mizrahi, J. (1990). Preoperative and post-operative gait evaluation in cerebral palsy. *Archives of Physical Medicine and Rehabilitation*, **71**, 236–40.

Sheikh, K. (1986). Disability scales: assessment of reliability. *Archives of Physical Medicine and Rehabilitation*, **67**, 245–9.

Sheikh, K., Smith, D.S., Meade, T.W., Goldenberg, E., Brennan, P.J., and Kinsella, G. (1979). Repeatability and validity of a modified activities of daily living (ADL) index in studies of chronic disability. *International Rehabilitation Medicine*, **1**, 51–8.

Shinar, D., Gross, C.R., Mohr, J.P. *et al.* (1985). Interobserver variability in the assessment of neurologic history and examination in the stroke data bank. *Archives of Neurology*, **42**, 557–65.

Shoulson, I. and Fahn, S. (1979). Huntington's disease: clinical care and evaluation. *Neurology*, **29**, 1–3.

Shrout, P.E. and Fleiss, J.L. (1979). Intraclass correlations: uses in assessing rater reliability. *Psychological Bulletin*, **86**, 420–8.

Siegel, S. and Castellan, N.J. (1988). *Non-parametric statistics for the behavioural sciences* (2nd edn). McGraw-Hill, New York.

Sipe, J.C., Knobler, R.L., Braheny, S.L., Rice, G.P.A., Panitch, H.S., and Oldstone, M.B.A. (1984). A neurologic rating scale (NRS) for use in multiple sclerosis. *Neurology*, **34**, 1368–72.

Sisk, C., Zeigler, D.K., and Zileli, T. (1970). Discrepancies in recorded results from duplicate neurological history and examination in patients studied for prognosis in cerebrovascular disease. *Stroke*, **1**, 14–18.

Skilbeck, C.E. and Woods, R.T. (1980). The factorial structure of the Wechsler Memory Scale: samples of neurological and psychogeriatric patients. *Journal of Clinical Neuropsychology*, **2**, 293–300.

Slevin, M.L., Plant, H., Lynch, D., Drinkwater, J., and Gregory, W.M. (1988). Who should measure quality of life, the doctor or the patient? *British Journal of Cancer*, **57**, 109–12.

Smaje, J.C. and McLellan, D.L. (1981). Depth sense aesthesiometry: an advance in the clinical assessment of sensation in the hands. *Journal of Neurology, Neurosurgery and Psychiatry*, **44**, 950–6.

Smith, A. (1987). Qualms about QALYs. *Lancet*, **1**, 1134–6.

Smith, D.L., Akhtar, A.J., and Garraway, W.M. (1983). Proprioception and spatial neglect after stroke. *Age and Ageing*, **12**, 63–9.

Smith, D.S., Goldenberg, E., Ashburn, A. *et al.* (1981). Remedial therapy after stroke: a randomised, controlled trial. *British Medical Journal*, **282**, 517–20.

Snaith, R.P., Ahmed, S.N., Mehta, S., and Hamilton, M. (1971). Assessment of severity of primary depressive illness: Wakefield self assessment depression inventory. *Psychological Medicine*, **1**, 143–9.

Snaith, R.P., Constantopoulos, A.A., Jardine, M.Y., and McGuffin, P. (1978). A clinical scale for the self-assessment of irritability. *British Journal of Psychiatry*, **132**, 164–71.

Snaith, R.P., Baugh, S.J., Clayden, A.D., Husain, A., and Sipple, M.A. (1982). The clinical anxiety scale: an instrument derived from the Hamilton Anxiety Scale. *British Journal of Psychiatry*, **141**, 518–23.

Spaulding, S.J., McPherson, J.J., Strachota, E., Kuphal, M., and Ramponi, M. (1988). Jebsen hand function test: performance of the uninvolved hand in hemiplegia and of right-handed, right and left hemiplegic persons. *Archives of Physical Medicine and Rehabilitation*, **69**, 419–22.

Stanczak, D.E., White, J.G., Gouview, W.D. *et al.* (1984). Assessment of level of consciousness following severe neurological insult. A comparison of the psychometric qualities of the Glasgow Coma Scale and the Comprehensive Level of Consciousness Scale. *Journal of Neurosurgery*, **60**, 955–60.

Starr, L.B., Robinson, R.G., and Price, T.R. (1983). Reliability, validity and clinical utility of the Social Functioning Exam in the assessment of stroke patients. *Experimental Aging Research*, **9**, 101–6.

Steer, R.A., Beck, A.T., and Garrison, B. (1986). Applications of the Beck depression inventory. In *Assessment of depression* (ed. N. Santorius and T. Ban). Springer-Verlag, Heidelberg.

Stein, R.E.K., Gortmaker, S.L., Perrin, E.C., Perrin, J.M., Pless, I.B., Walker, D.K., and Weitzman, M. (1987). Severity of illness: concepts and measurements. *Lancet*, **2**, 1506–9.

Stern, Y., Hesdorffer, D., Sano, M., and Mayeux, R. (1990). Measurement and prediction of functional capacity in Alzheimer's disease. *Neurology*, **40**, 8–14.

Stewart, A., Ware, J.E., Brook, R.H., and Davies-Avery, A. (1978). *Conceptualisation and Measurement of Health for Adults in the Health Insurance Study*: Vol. 2. *Physical Health in terms of Functioning*. Rand Pub No. 1987/2-HEW, Santa Monica.

Stonier, P.D. (1974). Score changes following repeated administration of mental status questionnaires. *Age and Ageing*, **3**, 91–6.

Sugiura, K., Muraoka, K., Chishiki, T., and Baba, M. (1983). The Edinburgh-2 Coma Scale: a new scale for assessing impaired consciousness. *Neurosurgery*, **12**, 411–15.

Sunderland, A. (1990). Single-case experimental design in neurological rehabilitation. *Clinical Rehabilitation*, **4**, 181–92.

Sunderland, A., Harris, J.E., and Baddeley, A.D. (1983). Do laboratory tests predict everyday memory? A neuropsychological study. *Journal of Verbal Learning and Verbal Behaviour*, **22**, 341–57.

Sunderland, A., Harris, J.E., and Gleave, J. (1984). Memory failures in everyday life following severe head injury. *Journal of Clinical Neuropsychology*, **6**, 127–42.

Sunderland, A., Watts, K., Baddeley, A.D., and Harris, J.E. (1986). Subjective memory assessment and test performance in elderly adults. *Journal of Gerontology*, **41**, 376–84.

Sunderland, A., Tinson, D., Bradley, L., and Langton Hewer, R. (1989). Arm function after stroke. An evaluation of grip strength as a measure of recovery and a prognostic indicator. *Journal of Neurology, Neurosurgery and Psychiatry*, **52**, 1267–72.

Sunderland, A., Tinson, D.J., Bradley, E.L., Fletcher, D., Langton Hewer, R., and Wade, D.T. (1991). Enhanced physical therapy improves recovery of arm function after stroke. A randomised controlled trial. *Journal of Neurology, Neurosurgery and Psychiatry*. (In press.)

Teasdale, G. and Jennett, B. (1974). Assessment of coma and impaired consciousness. A practical scale. *Lancet*, **2**, 81–3.

Teasdale, G., Knill-Jones, R., and Van der Sande, J. (1978). Observer variability in assessing impaired consciousness and coma. *Journal of Neurology, Neurosurgery and Psychiatry*, **41**, 603–10.

Teasdale, G., Murray, G., Parker, L., and Jennett, B. (1979). Adding up the Glasgow Coma Scale. *Acta Neurochirurgica*, **Suppl 28**, 13–16.

Thompson, C. (ed.) (1989). *The instruments of psychiatric research*. John Wiley, Chichester.

Thompson, A.J., Kermode, A.G., MacManus, D.G. *et al.* (1990). Patterns of disease activity in multiple sclerosis: clinical and magnetic resonance imaging study. *British Medical Journal*, **300**, 631–4.

Tinson, D.J. (1989). How stroke patients spend their days. *International Disability Studies*, **11**, 45–9.

Tinson, D.J. and Lincoln, N.B. (1987). Subjective memory impairment after stroke. *International Disability Studies*, **9**, 6–9.

Tomasello, F., Mariani, F., Fieschi, C. *et al.* (1982). Assessment of interobserver differences in the Italian multicenter study on reversible cerebral ischaemia. *Stroke*, **13**, 32–4.

Torrance, G.W. (1987). Utility approach to measuring health-related quality of life. *Journal of Chronic Disease*, **40**, 593–600.

Trobe, J.D., Acosta, P.C., Krischer, J.P., and Trick, G.L. (1981). Confrontation visual field techniques in the detection of anterior visual pathway lesions. *Annals of Neurology*, **10**, 28–34.

Turton, A.J. and Fraser, C.M. (1986). A test battery to measure the recovery of voluntary movement control following stroke. *International Rehabilitation Medicine*, **8**, 74–8.

Van den Berg, J.P. and Lankhorst, G.J. (1990). Inter-rater and intra-rater reliability of disability ratings based on the modified D code of the ICIDH. *International Disability Studies*, **12**, 20–1.

Van der Ploeg, R.J.O., Oosterhuis, H.J.G.H., and Reuvekamp, J. (1984). Measuring muscle strength. *Journal of Neurology*, **231**, 200–3.

Van Knippenberg, F.C.E. and De Haes, J.C.J.M. (1988). Measuring the quality of life of cancer patients: psychometric properties of instruments. *Journal of Clinical Epidemiology*, **41**, 1043–53.

Van Swieten, J.C., Koudstaal, P.J., Visser, M.C., Schouten, H.J.A., and Van Gijn, J. (1988). Interobserver agreement for the assessment of handicap in stroke patients. *Stroke*, **19**, 604–7.

Van Zomeren, A.H. and Brouver, W.H. (1987). Head injury and concepts of attention. In *Neurobehavioural recovery from head injury* (ed. H.S. Levin, J. Grafman, and H.M. Eisenberg), pp. 398–415. Oxford University Press.

Viitanen, M., Fugl-Meyer, K.S., Bernspang, B., and Fugl-Meyer, A.R. (1988). Life satisfaction in long-term survivors after stroke. *Scandinavian Journal of Rehabilitation Medicine*, **20**, 17–24.

Wade, D.T. (1988). Measurement in rehabilitation. *Age and Ageing*, **17**, 289–92.

Wade, D.T. (1989). Measuring arm impairment and disability after stroke. *International Disability Studies*, **11**, 89–92.

Wade, D.T. and Collin, C. (1988). The Barthel ADL index: a standard measure of physical disability? *International Disability Studies*, **10**, 64–6722.

Wade, D.T. and Langton Hewer, R. (1985a). Hospital admission for acute stroke: who, for how long, and to what effect? *Journal of Epidemiology and Community Health*, **39**, 347–52.

Wade, D.T. and Langton Hewer, R. (1985b). Outcome after an acute stroke: urinary incontinence and loss of consciousness compared in 532 patients. *Quarterly Journal of Medicine*, **221**, 347–52.

Wade, D.T. and Langton Hewer, R. (1987a). Functional abilities after stroke: measurement, natural history and prognosis. *Journal of Neurology, Neurosurgery and Psychiatry*, **50**, 177–82.

Wade, D.T. and Langton Hewer, R. (1987b). Motor loss and swallowing difficulty after stroke: frequency, recovery and prognosis. *Acta Neurologica Scandinavica*, **76**, 50–4.

Wade, D.T., Langton Hewer, R., Wood, V.A., Skilbeck, C.E., and Ismail, I.M. (1983). The hemiplegic arm after stroke: measurement and recovery. *Journal of Neurology, Neurosurgery and Psychiatry*, **46**, 521–4.

Wade, D.T., Skilbeck, C.E., Langton Hewer, R., and Wood, V.A. (1984). Therapy after stroke: amounts, determinants and effects. *International Rehabilitation Medicine*, **6**, 105–10.

Wade, D.T., Legh-Smith, J., and Langton Hewer, R. (1985). Social activities after stroke: measurement and natural history using the Frenchay Activities Index. *International Rehabilitation Medicine*, **7**, 176–81.

Wade, D.T., Parker, V., and Langton Hewer, R. (1986a). Memory disturbance after stroke: frequency and associated losses. *International Rehabilitation Medicine*, **8**, 60–4.

Wade, D.T., Legh-Smith, J., and Langton Hewer, R. (1986b). Effects of living with and looking after survivors of a stroke. *British Medical Journal*, **293**, 418–20.

Wade, D.T., Wood, V.A., Heller, A., Maggs, J., and Langton Hewer, R. (1987a). Walking after stroke: measurement and recovery over the first three months. *Scandinavian Journal of Rehabilitation Medicine*, **19**, 25–30.

Wade, D.T., Legh-Smith, J., and Hewer, R.L. (1987b). Depressed mood after stroke. A community study of its frequency. *British Journal of Psychiatry*, **151**, 200–5.

Wade, D.T., Skilbeck, C.E., and Langton Hewer, R. (1989). Selected cognitive losses after stroke. Frequency, recovery and prognostic importance. *International Disability Studies*, **11**, 34–9.

Webster, D.D. (1968). Critical analysis of the disability in Parkinson's disease. *Modern Treatment*, **5**, 257–82.

Wechsler, D. (1945). A standardised memory scale for clinical use. *Journal of Psychology*, **19**, 87–95.

Wechsler, D. (1981). *WAIS-R Manual*. Psychological Corporation, New York.

Weeks, D.J. (1988). The Anomalous Sentences Repetition Test. NFER Nelson, Windsor.

Weissman, M.M. and Bothwell, S. (1976). Assessment of social adjustment by patient self-report. *Archives of General Psychiatry*, **33**, 1111–15.

Whiting, S. and Lincoln, N. (1980). An ADL assessment for stroke patients. *British Journal of Occupational Therapy*, **43**, 44–6.

Whiting, S.E., Lincoln, N.B., Bhavnani, G., and Cockburn, J. (1985). The Rivermead Perceptual Assessment Battery. NFER-Nelson, Windsor.

Wiles, C.M. and Karni, Y. (1983). The measurement of strength in patients with peripheral neuromuscular disorders. *Journal of Neurology, Neurosurgery and Psychiatry*, **46**, 1006–113.

Williams, R.G.A. (1979). Theories and measurement in disability. *Epidemiology and Community Health*, **33**, 32–47.

Willoughby, E.W. and Paty, D.W. (1988). Scales for rating impairment in multiple sclerosis: a critique. *Neurology*, **38**, 1793–8.

Wilson, B.A., Cockburn, J., and Baddeley, A.D. (1985). The Rivermead Behavioural Memory Test. Thames Valley Test Company, Titchfield, Hants.

Wilson, B.A., Cockburn, J., and Halligan, P. (1987). Behavioural Inattention Test. Thames Valley Test Company, Titchfield, Hants.

Wilson, B.A., Cockburn, J., and Halligan, P. (1987). Development of a behavioural test of visuospatial neglect. *Archives of Physical Medicine and Rehabilitation*, **68**, 98–102.

Wilson, B.A., Cockburn, J., Baddeley, A.D., and Hierns, R.W. (1989). The development and validation of a test battery for detecting and monitoring everyday memory problems. *Journal of Clinical Experimental Neuropsychology*, **11**, 855–70.

Wolfson, L., Whipple, R., Amerman, P., and Tobin, J.N. (1990). Gait assessment in the elderly: a gait abnormality rating scale and its relation to falls. *Journal of Gerontology*, **45**, M12–19.

Wood, V., Wylie, M.L., and Sheafor, B. (1969). An analysis of a short self-report measure of life satisfaction: correlation with rater judgements. *Journal of Gerontology*, **24**, 465–9.

Wood-Dauphinee, S.L., Opzoomer, A., Williams, J.I., Marchand, B., and Spitzer, W.O. (1988). Assessment of global function: the Reintegration to Normal Living index. *Archives of Physical Medicine and Rehabilitation*, **69**, 583–90.

Wood-Dauphinee, S.L., Williams, J.I., and Shapiro, S.H. (1990). Examining outcome measures in a clinical study of stroke. *Stroke*, **21**, 731–9.

World Health Organisation. (1980). *The International Classification of Impairments, Disabilities, and Handicaps*. World Health Organisation, Geneva.

Wykes, T. and Sturt, E. (1986). The measurement of social behaviour in psychiatric patients: an assessment of the reliability and validity of the SBS schedule. *British Journal of Psychiatry*, **148**, 1–11.

Yahr, M.D., Duvoisin, R.C., Schear, M.J. *et al.* (1969). Treatment of Parkinsonism with levodopa. *Archives of Neurology*, **21**, 343–54.

Yen, J.K., Bourke, R.S., Nelson, L.R., and Popp, A.J. (1978). Numerical grading of clinical neurological status after serious head injury. *Journal of Neurology, Neurosurgery and Psychiatry*, **41**, 1125–30.

Zigmond, A.S. and Snaith, R.P. (1983). The Hospital Anxiety and Depression scale. *Acta Psychiatrica Scandinavica*, **1983**, **67**, 361–70.

Zillmer, E.A., Fowler, P.C., Gutnick, H.N., and Becker, E. (1990). Comparison of two cognitive bedside screening instruments in nursing home residents: a factor analytic study. *Journal of Gerontology*, **45**, P69–74 (psychological sciences).

Zung, W.W.K. (1965). A self-rating depression scale. *Archives of General Psychiatry*, **12**, 63–70.

Appendix   Sources of measures mentioned in the text

- Anomalous Sentences Repetition Test
- Frenchay Aphasia Screening Test (FAST)
- Rivermead Perceptual Assessment (RPA)
- General Health Questionnaire (GHQ)

   All from: NFER-Nelson, Darville House, 2 Oxford Road East, Berkshire SL4 1DF, UK.

- Rivermead Behavioural Memory Test (RBMT)
- Behavioural Inattention Test (BIT)

   From: Thames Valley Test Company, 7–9 The Green, Flempton, Bury St. Edmunds, Suffolk IP28 6EL, UK.

- Some of the measures in this book are available with up-to-date information as top copies (for copying), both in a single use and repeated use format. The Nine-hole Peg Test is also available. For details and cost please write with request to: Dr D.T. Wade, Rivermead Rehabilitation Centre, Abingdon Road, Oxford OX1 4XD, UK.

Index

This index includes entries which will lead the reader to component parts of large indices where the author has felt that the component is unusual or useful. **Bold type** = major entry; *Italics* = scale shown.